Practical Management of Meningomyelocele

Practical Management of Meningomyelocele

Edited by

John Mark Freeman, M.D.
Associate Professor of Pediatrics and Neurology
Johns Hopkins Hospital
Baltimore, Maryland

Director, National Foundation-March of Dimes
Birth Defects Treatment Center
Johns Hopkins Hospital
Baltimore, Maryland

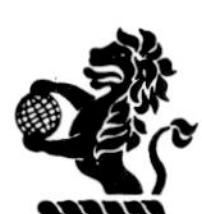

UNIVERSITY PARK PRESS
Baltimore • London • Tokyo

University Park Press
International Publishers in Science and Medicine
Chamber of Commerce Building
Baltimore, Maryland 21202

Printed in the United States of America by The Maple Press Company

Library of Congress Cataloging in Publication Data

Freeman, John Mark.
Practical management of meningomyelocele.

1. Myelomeningocele. I. Title. [DNLM: 1. Spina bifida—In infancy and childhood. 2. Spina bifida—Therapy. WE 730 F855p 1973]
RJ255.F73 617'.375 72-12706
ISBN 0-8391-0639-4

We would like to dedicate this book to the children of the Birth Defects Treatment Center at the Johns Hopkins Hospital, and to their families. Both have taught us what little we know about the problems associated with spina bifida. We also dedicate this book to the National Foundation-March of Dimes, whose support of treatment centers at Hopkins and elsewhere has provided these children with their best chances for life, mobility, and the pursuit of happiness.

Contents

List of Contributors

Johanna R. Bengel, E.T.
Enterostomal Therapy Center
Baltimore City Hospitals

Charlotte L. Blackmon, E.T.
Enterostomal Therapy Center
Baltimore City Hospitals

Rainer M. E. Engel, M.D.
Associate Professor of Urology
The James Buchanan Brady Urological Institute
Johns Hopkins School of Medicine, and
Urologist, Birth Defects Treatment Center
Johns Hopkins Hospital

John M. Freeman, M.D.
Associate Professor of Pediatrics and Neurology
Johns Hopkins School of Medicine
Director,
Birth Defects Treatment Center
Johns Hopkins Hospital

Verna Klein
Coordinator-Councillor
Birth Defects Treatment Center
Johns Hopkins Hospital

Steven F. Kopits, M.D.
Assistant Professor of Orthopedic Surgery
Johns Hopkins School of Medicine,
Orthopedic Surgeon in Charge
Children's Orthopedic Surgery Service, and
Pediatric Orthopedic Surgeon
Birth Defects Treatment Center
Johns Hopkins Hospital

Edward R. Laws, Jr., M.D.
Assistant Professor of Neurosurgery
Johns Hopkins School of Medicine
Neurosurgeon,
Birth Defects Treatment Center
Johns Hopkins Hospital
Present Address:
Department of Neurological Surgery
Mayo Clinic

Marvin M. Schuster, M.D.
Associate Professor of Medicine
Assistant Professor of Psychiatry
Johns Hopkins School of Medicine
Director,
Enterostomal Therapy Center
Baltimore City Hospitals

Issam J. Shaker, M.D.
Fellow in Pediatric Surgery
Johns Hopkins Hospital

George B. Udvarhelyi, M.D.
Professor of Neurosurgery
Associate Professor of Radiology
Johns Hopkins School of Medicine
Neurosurgeon,
Birth Defects Treatment Center
Johns Hopkins Hospital

John J. White, M.D., C.M.
Associate Professor of Surgery, and
Garrett Scholar in Pediatric Surgery
Johns Hopkins School of Medicine
Pediatric Surgeon,
Birth Defects Treatment Center
Johns Hopkins Hospital

Introduction

John M. Freeman, M.D.

The problem of dealing with children with meningomyeloceles is only 10 to 15 years old. This may seem an odd statement to make about the most common major structural birth defect. Prior to the late 1950's, however, when early closure of the spinal defect and intensive therapy of all facets of the defect came into vogue, the majority of children with meningomyeloceles were left to die. Indeed, even today, when one speaks to physicians from many less affluent countries about "the problem of children with meningomyeloceles," they respond, "What problem?"

Children with meningomyeloceles are a problem, or rather they present a series of problems. In these children the back, hydrocephalus, paralysis and dislocations, bladder, and bowels are all medical problems. The reaction and adjustment of the family to the defect and, later, the child's reactions are psychological problems. Intellectual limitations, the needs for special schooling and repeated hospitalization, and enormous medical expenses are sociological problems.

Medical specialization poses the important administrative problem of coordination among the many physicians and agencies involved in the care of an individual child with a meningomyelocele. Few physicians are cognizant of *all* the problems that these children face and of the need for *total* care of these children. The orthopedist may give superb care to the legs and hips, and yet not be aware that the child is receiving inadequate urological care. The child will thus have straight legs and well-fitting braces, but may die of renal decompensation in the teen-age period. The urologist may perform a urinary diversion for hydronephrosis and treat the urinary infections, but never realize that the child's subtle intellectual deterioration may be caused by slowly progressive hydrocephalus. The conscientious pediatrician may ensure that the child has a good neurosurgeon, orthopedist, and urologist, only to find that the family is soon $20,000 in debt for the good care.

It is to provide *coordinated* care that Birth Defects Treatment Centers, such as the one funded at the Johns Hopkins Hospital by the National Foundation-March of Dimes, were started. Providing coordinated care by many specialists is an often frustrating, frequently irritating, but always crucial aspect of the care of children with interdisciplinary problems. However, the benefits of such care are multiple. The child is assured of being seen by each of the crucial specialists—pediatrician, neurosurgeon, urologist, orthopedist, and bowel specialist—as well as by the social worker and psychiatrist. The family can obtain this care in one place instead of going from one physician's office to another for frequent follow-up. Hospitalizations can be coordinated and minimized by integration of procedures. Costs are also minimized.

Coordinated care also benefits the specialists. Not only does each physician acquire a wider experience with the problems of children with meningomyeloceles, but he and his co-workers are better able to evaluate the results of their work and to challenge each specialty's preconceptions. They learn that the child is greater than the sum of his organs. Interdisciplinary discussion leads to an awareness of the differences between what can be done technically and what should be done for the overall benefit of the child. For example, is the child to be a sitter or a walker? A child who will be sitting, with little back support, may require different placement of the loop stoma than the child who will be ambulatory. The child with advanced renal disease and a developing scoliosis could have her back fused, but the months spent in bed and in a cast may not be the best use of her limited future. The research opportunities that result from treating these children in one location are obvious.

This book grew out of our experiences in the Birth Defects Treatment Center at the Johns Hopkins Hospital. It is written for the *nonspecialist*. Its purpose is to provide each physician dealing with children who have meningomyeloceles with a basic knowledge of the dilemmas and approaches of his colleagues. It is not written to teach the neurosurgeon the latest neurosurgical approaches or to teach the orthopedist problems of ileo-psoas transfers. Rather, its purpose is to enable each to learn the multiple problems of the child with a meningomyelocele and the imperatives of multidisciplinary care. If we have achieved that end, we have been successful.

Acknowledgments

We would like to express our appreciation to the many people who have made this book possible: James Donovan and the Baltimore Chapter of the National Foundation-March of Dimes for their diligent efforts in support of the Birth Defects Treatment Center; to Dr. Judson Force and Eva Morton of the Maryland Crippled Children's Service for their help in providing financial and other assistance to our children; and Verna Klein, who has faithfully administered this clinic for many years and eased the burden of the staff physicians. I would especially like to thank my wife, who has assumed much of the editorial burden, and Deborah Sando, who has typed the manuscript more times than I would care to remember.

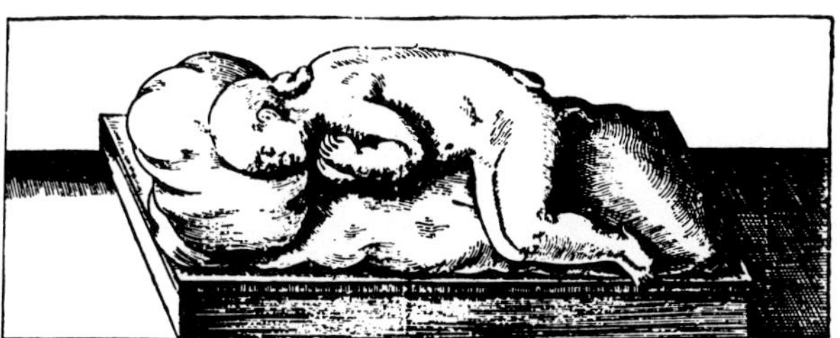

Medieval copperplate engraving of an infant with a meningomyelocele, from a pamphlet describing a sympus; Cologne, 1597. From R. Herrlinger. 1961. History of Medical Illustration from Antiquity to 1600. British Book Center, Elmsford, New York.

1

Terminology

John M. Freeman, M.D.

The terminology of defects of closure of the spinal canal has been confused by the plethora of names used by authors. The same terminology has been used and misused for conditions which vary anatomically and clinically. Terms such as myeloschisis, myelorachischisis, myelocele, and lipomeningocele, as well as the more familiar terms meningomyelocele and meningocele, have been used interchangeably. Here are our definitions of the terms.

Spinal dysraphism is a generic term which might be applied to all defects of closure of the spinal cord. Since all these defects are associated with nonfusion of the lamina of the spinal arches, the term spina bifida may also be applied to the group. Essentially there are two clinical forms of spina bifida: spina bifida occulta (no external manifestations) and spina bifida manifesta (a demonstrable abnormality).

Spina bifida occulta is nonfusion of the spinal arches without external manifestations. This common abnormality is of no clinical significance in itself, but may be associated with intraspinal lipomas, dermoids, tethering of the cord, and diastematomyelia.

Spina bifida manifesta is nonfusion of the spinal arches associated with neurological or ectodermal manifestations. Some, but not all, of these abnormalities have been termed spina bifida cystica. The major forms of spina bifida cystica are as follows:

1. *Spina bifida occulta with skin manifestations.* No single term adequately describes this group of children. The term minimal spinal dysraphism might be useful. The association of spina bifida occulta with a hairy patch on the back, a hemangioma, lipoma, a bony spicule, a scar, or a dermal sinus may alert the physician to the possibility of intraspinal processes. These processes may include tethering of the cord, lipomas, diastemato-

myelia and diplomyelia, or pilonidal sinuses. The intraspinal processes may produce neurological impairment. This separate, but important, group is discussed further in Chapter 8.

2. *Meningocele.* This is a spina bifida with a cystic protrusion of the meninges through the defect to the surface without myelodysplasia (abnormalities of the spinal cord). Functional nerve roots may extend into the sac. Since pathological examination of the spinal cord to determine myelodysplasia is not possible, one can only differentiate meningoceles from meningomyeloceles by the neurological deficit accompanying the latter. We therefore use the term meningocele in an operational sense to define that group of symptoms involving a cystic lesion on the back but no motor or sensory deficit of the limbs, bowel, or bladder. A child whose defect falls into this group has an excellent prognosis.

3. *Meningomyelocele* is a spina bifida associated with the cystic distension of the meninges and varying degrees of myelodysplasia (abnormalities of the spinal cord). Myelomeningocele is an identical and interchangeable term. Some degree of neurological impairment is invariably present. Within this group may be included the children with myeloschis (spina bifida aperta) who have myelodysplasia without the cystic dilatation of the meninges, and who have little clinical, therapeutic, or prognostic difference from those with cystic dilatation of the meninges. The clinical picture of both, and their prognosis, will depend on the location of the lesion and the degree of myelodysplasia.

A list of some of the many terms applied to the spina bifida is given in Table 1-1. While the more precise terminology may be of importance to embryologists, the clinical and prognostic features are sufficiently covered by the terms used above.

Table 1-1 Glossary of Terms

1. Diastematomyelia	Splitting of spinal cord, often associated with bony or cartilaginous spur tethering cord
2. Diplomyelia	Reduplication of part of the spinal cord, often associated with diastematomyelia
3. Dysraphism	Incomplete closure of neural tube; may be of variable severity from spina bifida occulta to myeloschisis
4. Lipomeningocele	Overgrowth of fatty tissue which involves the meninges and/or spinal cord and may be associated with tethering of cord
5. Meningocele	Spina bifida cystica without neural elements in the cyst; operationally used for such defects without demonstrable neurological deficit
6. Meningomyelocele	Spina bifida cystica with neural elements in the cystic cavity; operationally any cystic lesion of the spinal coverings with evidence of neurological dysfunction
7. Myelocele	Same as myelocystocele
8. Myelocystocele	Cavitated spinal cord lying in abnormal meningeal sac, often used synonymously with spina bifida aperta or myeloschisis
9. Myelodysplasia	Abnormalities of the spinal cord or roots of varying type, including diplomyelia, myeloschisis, hydromyelia, syringomyelia, and diastematomyelia
10. Myelomeningocele	Synonymous with meningomyelocele
11. Myeloschisis	Split cord, exposed to the surface without cystic coverings, identical to spina bifida aperta
12. Rachischisis	Splitting of the spinal column; should mean same as spina bifida, but is often used to mean nonfusion of neural folds in myeloschisis
13. Spina bifida	Nonfusion of the dorsal arches of the spine of variable degree; the skin, subcutaneous tissue, spinal cord, and contents of spinal canal may or may not be abnormal
14. Spina bifida aperta	Spina bifida with open cord on surface, possibly covered with thin membranes, no cystic covering; identical to myeloschisis and myelocele
15. Spina bifida cystica	Spina bifida associated with a cystic lesion on the back; the cystic lesion consists of dura, meninges, and normal or abnormal skin and may or may not include neural elements; this term includes meningoceles and meningomyeloceles
16. Spina bifida manifesta	Spina bifida associated with external manifestation; abnormalities ranging from hemangioma and skin lesions to an open or covered cord are included

2

Neural Tube Defects: Risks of Occurrence And Recurrence

John M. Freeman, M.D.

The etiology or etiologies of meningomyeloceles and neural tube defects are unknown. A higher occurrence rate in some families, races, and ethnic groups suggests genetic or polygenetic factors. There is evidence that maternal age, social and economic factors, and even seasonal factors may play a role. To provide adequate genetic counseling, one must know the incidence and risk as well as the recurrence rates in individual populations.

INCIDENCE

The incidence of neural tube defects varies markedly between geographic areas. This variability is partially related to case-finding techniques, but is influenced to an even larger extent by the racial and ethnic makeup of the population. The results of some incidence surveys are shown in Table 2-1. The reason for the marked regional differences is postulated to be in part a polygenetic form of inheritance (Carter, 1969). Concordance studies with twins also suggest the possibility of a polygenetic form of inheritance.

Evidence that meningomyeloceles are not purely genetic, however, comes from a study of the incidence in Boston, Mass. (Naggan and MacMahon, 1967). In this study marked ethnic differences in incidence were found between the Irish (4.9 per thousand) and the Jews (0.77 per thousand). But the authors noted that while the incidence in Ireland was 8.7 per thousand, the risk decreased to 4.9 per thousand in children whose mothers had been born in Ireland. The risk decreased still further to 3.1 per thousand in children whose parents were second- or third-generation Irish.

This study suggests the possibility that environmental factors play an additional role in the pathogenesis.

Social class and, presumably, socioeconomic factors also play a role. The incidence within each ethnic group was two to three times higher in the lowest socioeconomic class than in the highest class. An interesting seasonal incidence has been noted in some surveys and experimentally (Kalter and Warkany, 1961).

RECURRENCE RISKS

The risk of having a single infant with anencephaly or a meningomyelocele ranges from less than 1 in 1000 in the Jewish population to as high as 1 in 140 in Wales. However, the risk of recurrence in a family which has had one affected child is 7 to 40 times as high (Laurence, 1969). In Laurence's series, if parents had one child with spina bifida, the risk of having a second child with spina bifida was 3.7%, or 1 in 33. In addition, for these parents the risk of having a child with anencephaly was 2.3%, or 1 in 44. Thus the risk of having a second child with a neural tube defect was 6.1%, or 1 in 17. If the first child had anencephaly, then the risk of having another anencephalic child was greater than the risk of having a child with spina bifida, but the overall risk of a neural tube defect was 4.1%, or 1 in 24.

A number of other studies also show that the overall risk of having a second child with anencephaly or spina bifida manifesta is about 4 to 5%, or 1 in 20 to 25 (Smithells, D'Arcy, and McAllister, 1967; Stevenson et al., 1966; Timson, 1970). Populations with a lower incidence had a higher recurrence rate, thus making the overall recurrence risk similar among various populations.

If two affected children occur in one family, the risk of having a third is about 10%. There is also a two-fold increase in neural tube defects among cousins of the affected child.

It is thus important to provide the family that has a child with meningomyelocele with adequate genetic counseling. When prenatal detection of

Table 2-1 Incidence of Anencephaly and Spina Bifida

		Incidence per 1000 total births	
Location	Reference	Anencephaly	Spina bifida
Dublin, Ireland	Coffey and Jessop, 1957	5.5	4.2
Birmingham, England	McKeown and Record, 1950	2.0	3.0
South Wales	Laurence, 1969	3.5	4.1
Boston, Mass.	Naggan and MacMahon, 1967	1.0	1.3
Israel	Halevi, 1967	0.6	0.7
Atlanta, Ga.	USPHS, 1971	1.1	1.2

a meningomyelocele becomes available, parents who have had an affected child represent a sufficiently high-risk population to warrant prenatal study.

Renwick (1972) has recently provided data suggesting a relationship between blighted potatoes and anencephaly-meningomyelocele. It is postulated that either the fungus causing the blight, or antibiotics produced by the potatoes in response to the blight may be teratogenic. Dr. Renwick feels that 95% of these defects could be prevented if potatoes were avoided during the first month of pregnancy, or if extreme potato epicurism was practiced. Feeding of blighted potatoes to pregnant marmosets (but not rats) produced skull defects in offspring, but not spina bifida or myelomeningoceles (Poswillo et al., 1972). These reports have met considerable challenge (Emanuel, 1972, editorials a and b). This interesting and provocative hypothesis is now the subject of intensive study, but, even if proven, would not account for the incidence in areas such as Taiwan, Egypt, or Nigeria where few potatoes, blighted or otherwise, are ingested.

REFERENCES

Carter, C. O. 1969. Spina bifida and anencephaly. A problem in genetic-environmental interaction. J. Biosoc. Sci. 1:71.

Coffey, V. P., and W. J. Jessop. 1957. Study of 137 cases of anencephaly. Brit. J. Prev. Soc. Med. 11:174.

Emanuel, I. 1972. Non-tuberous. Neural-tube defects. Lancet ii:879; Editorial, 1972. Neural tubers. Lancet ii:222; Editorial, 1972. Can. Med. Ass. J. 107:1160.

Halevi, H. S. 1967. Congenital malformation in Israel. Brit. J. Prev. Soc. Med. 21:66.

Kalter, H., and J. Warkany. 1961. Experimental production of congenital malformation in strains of inbred mice by maternal treatment with hyper-vitaminosis A. Am. J. Path. 38:1.

Laurence, K. M. 1969. Recurrence risk in spina bifida cystica and anencephaly. Develop. Med. Child Neurol. Supp. 20:23.

McKeown, T., and R. G. Record. 1950. Congenital malformations of central nervous system. III. Risk of malformation in sibs of malformed individuals. Brit. J. Prev. Soc. Med. 4:217.

Naggan, L., and B. MacMahon. 1967. Ethnic differences in prevalence of anencephaly in Boston, Mass. New Eng. J. Med. 277:1119.

Poswillo, D. E., D. Sapher, and S. Mitchell. 1972; Experimental induction of Malformation with "Blighted" Potatoes: A Preliminary Report. Nature 239:462.

Renwick, J. H. 1972. Hypothesis. Anencephaly and spina bifida are usually preventable by avoidance of a specific but unidentified substance present in certain potato tubers. Brit. J. Prev. Soc. Med. 26:68.

Renwick, J. H. 1972b. Spina bifida and the potato. New Sci. November:277.

Smithells, R. W., E. E. D'Arcy, and E. F. McAllister. 1967. The outcome of pregnancies before and after the birth of infants with nervous system malformations. Develop. Med. Child Neurol. Supp. 15:16.

Stevenson, A. C., et al. 1966. Congenital malformation: report of study of series of consecutive births in 24 centers. Bull. World Health Org. Supp. 34:127.

Timson, J. 1970. Social factors in the incidence of spina bifida and anencephaly. J. Biosoc. Sci. 2:81.

USPHS Report. June 1971. Congenital malformations surveillance report: Center for Disease Control, Atlanta, Ga.

3

Embryology and Pathogenesis

John M. Freeman, M.D.

Although the classic presentation of a child with a meningomyelocele is familiar to most (Fig. 3-1), the embryogenesis of the nervous system is incompletely understood, and the pathogenesis of the spinal dysraphism remains a matter of debate.

However, some concept of spinal cord development is necessary to an understanding of spinal dysraphism. The normal embryology of the spinal cord is shown in Fig. 3-2 (top). The neural plate is a longitudinal thickening of specialized ectoderm which appears dorsal to the notochord during the middle of the third week of gestation. This neuroectoderm proliferates and becomes a groove which closes to form a tube. The closure proceeds from the mid-dorsal area cephalad to the rostral neuropore and caudad to the caudal neuropore, and is complete by the end of the fourth week.

As the neural tube closes, it is separated from the skin ectoderm by the ingrowth of mesodermal tissue, which later becomes the muscle and vertebral column. This closure is complete by the fourth week. At this time the brain is forming its flexures, and the choroid plexus is formed and is relatively large. There is marked dilatation of the telencephalic vesicles, which will later become the lateral ventricles. The roof of the fourth ventricle has not yet perforated to form the foramena of Luschka and Magendi, and cerebrospinal fluid (CSF) fills the central canal of the neurotube, a relative hydromyelia. At the end of the sixth week, the fourth ventricle openings normally appear, and the hydrocephalus and hydromyelia gradually disappear. This disappearance may be the result of the opening of the fourth ventricle, or may be unrelated and due to proliferation of adjacent neural tissue.

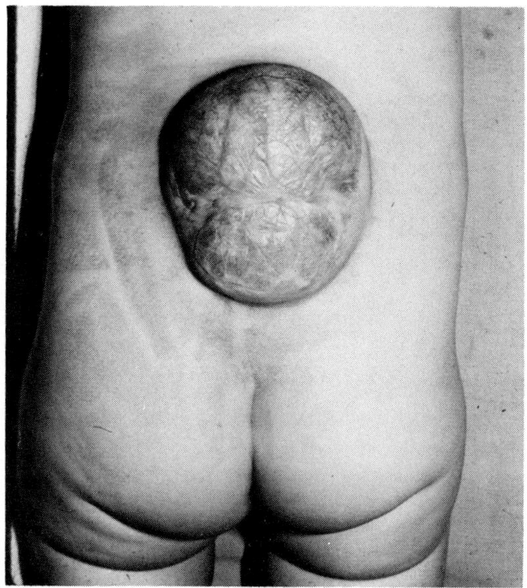

Fig. 3-1 A child with a meningomyelocele.

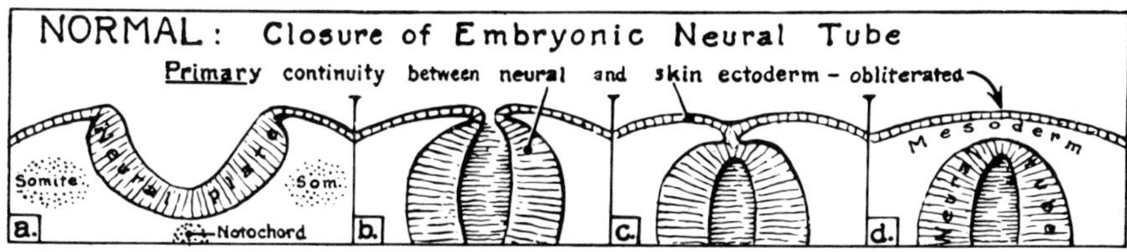

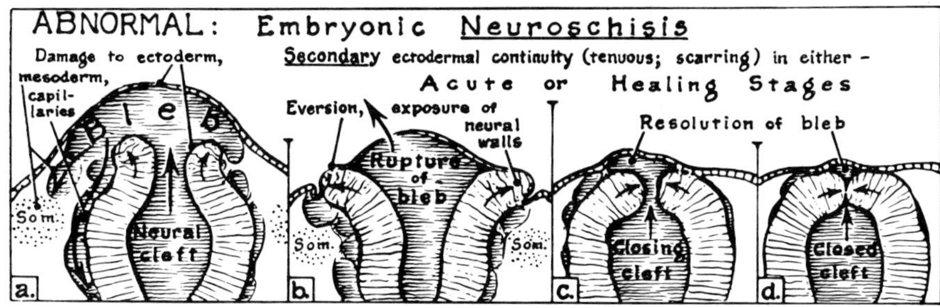

Fig. 3-2 (top) Schematic representation of the normal embryologic development of the spine and spinal cord. From Padget (1968) with permission.

Fig. 3-3 (bottom) Abnormal development of spine and spinal cord in the formation of spina bifidas. The closed neural tube ruptures, causing a neuroschistic bleb, which in turn damages overlying mesoderm and ectoderm. The degree of damage and the success of healing determine the degree of spinal dysraphism. From Padget (1968) with permission.

ABNORMAL DEVELOPMENT

Two major theories of the pathogenesis of spina bifida have been advanced and recently reviewed (Brocklehurst, 1971; Marin-Padilla, 1970):

1. The failure of closure of the neural tube (Patten, von Recklinghausen, as cited in Brocklehurst).

2. Rupture of the neural tube with damage to the overlying mesoderm and ectoderm (Morgagni, as cited in Brocklehurst; Gardner, 1968; Padget, 1968).

It is the second of these theories, advanced by Padget (1968) and Gardner (1968), which appears best to fit all the abnormalities associated with spinal dysraphism. Padget (1968, 1970) has postulated that in spinal dysraphism there is normal formation and closure of the neural tube. The closed tube then splits open (neuroschisis), allowing the escape of fluid. This fluid causes the formation of "neuroschistic blebs" (Fig. 3-3, bottom) and damage to mesodermal capillaries. The different forms of dysraphism are explained as follows:

1. If the bleb ruptures and the neural cleft edges remain everted, the infant is left with myeloschisis or spina bifida aperta, an open spinal canal without cystic coverings (Fig. 3-4a).

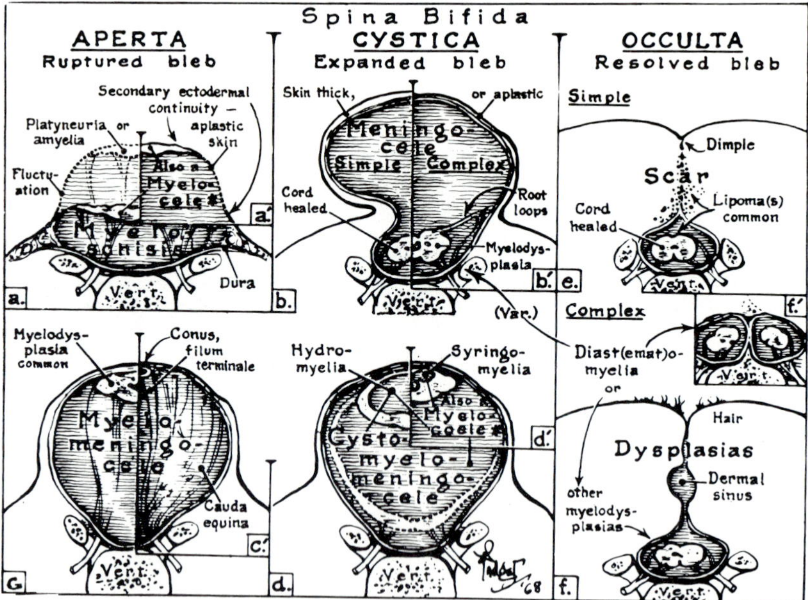

Fig. 3-4 The various forms of spina bifida resulting from the embryonic rupture. a, myeloschisis; b, meningocele; c and d, variations of meningomyelocele; e and f, spina bifida occulta with dermal sinus, diastematomyelia, or lipomata.

2. Persistence of the bleb results in spina bifida cystica. The degree of damage to the neural tube determines whether this spina bifida cystica is a meningocele or a meningomyelocele (Fig. 3-4b, c, d).

3. Spontaneous closure of the neural cleft with variable degrees of scarring results in spina bifida with lipomata, dermoids, diastematomyelia, and cord tethering (Fig. 3-4e, f).

In each case, damage to ectoderm and mesodermal tissues results in the overlying skin manifestations. The neuroschisis may occasionally be asymmetrical, producing hemimyelia and meningomyelocele or anterior meningomyeloceles.

Padget's theory, while not universally accepted, seems to explain the many varieties of spinal dysraphism and their associated abnormalities. It is not necessary, however, to postulate one mechanism for all spinal dysraphism. The widely open spinal defects seen in animals after the administration of a variety of teratogens could be due to nonfusion of the neural groove and overgrowth of the neural tube (Marin-Padilla, 1970). The similarity of these experimental animals to the infant with complete myelorachisis suggests that nonfusion rather than myeloschisis may occasionally play a role in some infants (Warkany, Wilson, and Geiger, 1958; Brocklehurst, 1971). Rupture may occur in other locations in the developing neuroaxis, resulting in encephaloceles or, in severe cases, anencephaly (Padget, 1972).

One must still ask the etiology of the neural tube rupture (neuroschisis) and the reason for the almost constant association of these defects with Arnold-Chiari malformation. One appealing theory is proposed by Gardner (1965) and Williams (1971). From the fourth to the seventh fetal week, before the foramina of Luschka and Magendi are open, there exists marked dilatation of the telencephalic vesicles (lateral ventricles) and of the central canal of the spinal cord, a relative hydrocephalus, and hydromyelia. It is postulated that increased pressure, perhaps due to late opening of the foramena, initiates the rupture (neuroschisis) and escape of fluid. The forcing of fluid down the central canal may result in syringomyelia and hydromyelia (Gardner, 1965) and explain the hydromyelia and syringomyelia found in 60% of spinal cords above the level of meningocele (MacKenzie and Emery, 1971).

The Arnold-Chiari malformation, once erroneously thought to be due to traction on the brainstem, is postulated (Williams, 1971) to result from a pressure differential between the intracranial space and the spinal space, resulting in a pushing down of the cerebellar (MacKenzie and Emery, 1971). Rupture of the neural tube could result in such a pressure differential. Recently, Padget (1972) has shown that premature approximation or fusion of cerebellar primordia within a fourth ventricle and posterior fossa already reduced in size could result in the Arnold-Chiari malformation. Rupture with release of CSF could result in embryonic microcephaly and crowding of the posterior fossa.

SUMMARY

Fetal hydrocephalus could result in hydromyelia and rupture of the neural tube, causing meningomyelocele. The rupture and the release of fluid could explain the crowding of the posterior fossa and the Arnold-Chiari malformation. Lesser degrees of damage to the neural tube and ectoderm may result in other forms of spinal dysraphism. When there is no escape of fluid and the rupture heals, as in cord tethering and diastematomyelia, the lack of a pressure differential between intracranial and spinal contents may prevent the formation of the Arnold-Chiari defect. These postulated mechanisms suggest an appealing hypothesis, but it is not universally accepted.

REFERENCES

Brocklehurst, G. 1971. The pathogenesis of spina bifida: a study of the relationship between observation, hypothesis, and surgical incentive. Devel. Med. Child Neurol. 13:147.

Gardner, W. J. 1965. Hydrodynamic mechanism of syringomyelia: its relationship to myelocele. J. Neurol. Neurosurg. Psychiat. 28:247.

Gardner, W. J. 1968. Myelocele: rupture of the neural tube. Clin. Neurosurg. 15:57.

MacKenzie, N. G., and J. L. Emery. 1971. Deformities of the cervical cord in children with neurospinal dysraphism. Devel. Med. Child Neurol. Supp. 25:58.

Marin-Padilla, M. 1970. Morphogenesis of anencephaly and related malformation. Current Topics in Path. 51:145.

Padget, D. 1968. Spina bifida and embryonic neuroschisis—a causal relationship. Johns Hopkins Med. Bull. 123:233.

Padget, D. H. 1970. Neuroschisis and human embryonic maldevelopment. J. Neuropath. Exp. Neurol. 29:192.

Padget, D. H. 1972. Development of so-called dysraphism with embryologic evidence of clinical Arnold-Chiari and Dandy-Walker malformation. Johns Hopkins Med. J. 130:127.

Warkany, J., J. G. Wilson, and J. F. Geiger. 1958. Myeloschisis and myelomeningocele produced experimentally on the rat. J. Comp. Neurol. 109:35.

Williams, B. J. 1971. Further thoughts on the valvular action of the Arnold-Chiari malformation. Devel. Med. Child Neurol. Supp. 25:105.

4

To Treat or Not to Treat

John M. Freeman, M.D.

Ethical decisions in medicine have become increasingly difficult as the technical capabilities of medical science have increased. The dilemmas are particularly difficult for the physician confronted with an infant who has a congenital malformation often associated with mental retardation. Before congenital heart disease was operable, the physician did not have to make a decision about the closure of a cardiac lesion in a mongoloid child. He could not withhold treatment; no treatment was available, and thus no ethical decision was involved. Prior to the mid 1950's when new shunt techniques were devised, the operative results of treatment of hydrocephalus were little better than the incidence of spontaneous arrest (Laurence, 1966). Therefore, the surgeon was not withholding treatment from the hydrocephalic infant by making a decision not to operate. Ingraham (Ingraham and Hamlin, 1943), summarizing his experience with spina bifida, recommended delay in treatment until the child was one year to 18 months old, by which time epithelization of the sac was complete, the hydrocephalus stabilized, and the mental endowment assessable. This was the best surgical management at the time.

Advances in anesthesia and surgery of the newborn have now made it technically possible to close the meningomyelocele shortly after birth. Advances in shunt technology and the use of antibiotics have made possible more successful treatment of the hydrocephalus.

Sharrard in 1962 demonstrated that muscular innervation to the lower extremities was better preserved after early operation, and in a controlled trial of early therapy (Sharrard et al., 1963), found decreased mortality, decreased duration of hospitalization, lesser incidence of meningitis, and improvement in motor function in children operated upon during the first 48 hours of life. He concluded that immediate closure of the meningomyelocele was a surgical necessity.

Early closure was thus thought to improve the quality of some of the survivors, but in addition had a dramatic effect in increasing the quantity of survivors and decreasing the number of "stillbirths" (Forrest, 1967). Rickham and Mawdsley (1966) found that prior to early surgery only 16% of infants survived, but that 56% of infants operated upon within 24 hours survived to two years of age. Indeed, in the past three years at Hopkins, not a single child whose defect was closed at birth has died. Thus modern medical care has made it technically feasible to increase the number of surviving children with meningomyeloceles and to improve the intellectual and motor function of many of the survivors. These technical advances have also dramatically increased the social problems for the child, the family, and society.

Since early surgery will improve both the quality and the quantity of survivors, ethical problems now exist which were not present before. Is it moral to encourage the survival of a child who will be paraplegic, incontinent, and will require multiple surgical procedures for hydrocephalus, orthopedic deformity, and bladder dysfunction? If the back is closed, should the hydrocephalus be treated? Are we to treat these two acute problems and allow a child to die slowly of renal decompensation? If we elect *not* to treat a child, what becomes of him? Is he to be fed and watered while the physician waits for him to develop meningitis? Is he to be sedated and fed inadequately so that he dies slowly of starvation without making too much noise? Are we to kill him overtly? Or covertly? Actively rather than passively? Or are we to embark on the long, difficult, and costly total care of such a child? These are major, crucial, immediate issues which face every physician dealing with a newborn infant with a meningomyelocele.

One might begin by asking the question: Who is to decide? Is it to be the physician, the parents, society by fiat, or some special committee? It is my personal bias that the ultimate decision rests with the physician. While parents are obviously involved in the decision and their prejudices should be given considerable weight, it is *not* possible in the short time available to educate parents adequately to the long-term aspects of this disease. Similarly, nonphysicians, and even physicians not working with children with meningomyeloceles, rarely appreciate the chronic problems involved. Therefore, I feel the decision to treat, or not to treat, must ultimately be made by a physician from the team which will be responsible for the long-term care of that child—a physician who is aware of his own prejudices toward the problem. This is not to say that the desires of the parents and the opinions of other associates should not heavily influence the physician's decision. When a parent strongly desires therapy, no ethical decision is involved.

To make such decisions the physician must be intimately familiar with the consequences of the alternative decisions. If he decides to treat, he must know the prognosis for ambulation and the intellectual outlook for that child. He must know the facilities and quality of the future medical care for the infant, and the community's ability to provide physical and educational support for the child. He must know the monetary costs of the disease and the family's ability to cope with these costs, or the community's ability to assume them. He must know the parents' desires and whether they are physically and emotionally capable of handling the physically handicapped child.

The physician must also know the prognosis for the child who is not treated. He must be aware that many untreated children do not die quickly, and some do not die at all. If the infant does not develop meningitis, is the doctor willing to allow the child to develop progressive hydrocephalus without treatment? What about the renal disease?

Each child, and each family, is a unique problem. Blanket rules that every child should be operated upon, or that no child with a certain degree of deficit should be operated upon, are easier for the physician to live with, for they evade the ethical and moral dilemmas and the necessity for decisions.

Lorber (1971) has attempted to develop some guidelines for selection of patients for treatment. These helpful guidelines will be discussed below. But physicians who wish to individualize care for each child and family must carefully assess the consequences when helping the family to decide whether or not to embark on the life-long therapy needed by most children with meningomyeloceles.

THE PROGNOSIS OF UNTREATED MENINGOMYELOCELE

Studies of children with meningomyeloceles who have received no therapy are few. Laurence (1964 and 1966), studying children with encephaloceles and spina bifida cystica born in South Wales between 1956 and 1962, before active surgical treatment was available, found that 16% survived 2½ to 9 years. These children received "elementary hygiene to the spinal lesion and antibiotic cover, or no treatment at all." Knox (1967) followed 132 patients with spina bifida cystica with or without an accompanying encephalocele who had received no systematic therapy, and found that 24% were alive at one year. Of the 27 surviving, 13 had no neurological deficit or hydrocephalus, and presumably represent meningoceles. Fourteen of the survivors had neurological disability; only 4 of these had early closure; 4 had shunts and late operation (6 weeks to 10 months); and 4 received no therapy. Thus, even with no therapy, approximately 20% of children will survive.

The figures from these two series, while the best available, are in a sense misleading. They indicate that there is a significant survival rate, and that the children who survive have a significantly greater mental and neurological handicap than they would have if they had been treated. The data do not tell us enough, however, about the children who died, about the weeks and months of chronic care while waiting for death to come. The series thus give little information about the considerable morbidity involved in not treating.

Indeed, even the figures on survival are fallacious, as is indicated by a look at the incidence of stillbirths. Stillbirths account for 25% of the mortality in Laurence's series and 22% in Knox's series. It is of note that in London the incidence of stillbirths with meningomyelocele dropped precipitously from a high of 40% of the births with this defect in 1958 to zero in 1962. The drop in "stillbirths" was concomitant with increasing optimism and enthusiasm about treatment (Forrest, 1967). In marvelous English understatement, Forrest states that "the percentage of stillbirths is by no means as fixed and unalterable as has generally been supposed." Knox states that only 6 of the 29 stillbirths in his series had additional defects considered incompatible with survival.

In Laurence's and Knox's series, an additional 4% to 9% of the infants died in the first 24 hours; therefore, total mortality under 24 hours of age was 30% in both series. The number of these infants who could have been salvaged cannot be ascertained. However, even if we accept the figures from these studies, at least 70% of infants born with meningomyeloceles are potentially treatable. The true figure is probably considerably higher.

Since we are concerned with the potential for surgery, we could take the infants from the series alive at 24 hours as the potentially treatable group and ask what happens if they are left untreated (Table 4-1). In Laurence's series, of the 297 infants alive at 24 hours, 188 (63%) were alive at one month; 136 (46%) were alive at two months, and 96 (32%) were alive at six months. Sixty-eight (22%) survived more than two years. In Knox's series, 71% survived one month; 52% survived six months; 35% survived one year, and 30% survived five years (Laurence, 1966).

Table 4-1 Survival of Untreated Meningomyelocele Alive at 24 Hours

	Stillborn or die within 24 hr	Alive					
		24 hr	1 mo	2 mo	6 mo	1 yr	2 yr
Laurence (1966)	126	297 (100%)*	188 (63%)	136 (46%)	96 (32%)	—	68 (22%)
Knox (1967)	41	91 (100%)*	65 (71%)	—	48 (52%)	32 (35%)	—
Hide (1972)†	9	90 (100%)*	58 (64%)		21 (23%)	7 (8%)	4 (5%)

*Per cent of infants alive at 24 hr who survive to varying ages.
†Includes only "severely" affected children.

Using a different form of analysis of selected patients between 1947 and 1956, during the antibiotic era but before enthusiastic surgery and shunting procedures became available, Laurence found that a newborn infant had a 35% chance of survival to age 12. A two-month-old infant with a meningomyelocele had a 44% chance of surviving 12 years.

The important facts to be gained from these series are that many children who are left unoperated do *not* die, and that many of those that succumb exist for months. Physicians are reluctant to document their role, active or passive, in the deaths of these children, particularly children who are inoperable or unoperated. Therefore, just as the incidence of stillbirths was found to be alterable, the physician's role in the "natural history" of meningomyeloceles in these series is open to question. The *true* "natural history" may have even more survivors.

Two examples of infants who were untreated pose the problem the physician faces.

One, a baby born with a meningomyelocele at T_{12}, had complete paraplegia with no voluntary movement. Since closure of the sac could not preserve function, no surgery was performed. The infant was sent home to the mother, who was told the baby would contract meningitis and die. At six weeks the infant returned with hydrocephalus. The sac had leaked, but the mother had kept it clean, and it had sealed. Because the infant had not acquired meningitis, because of the nursing problems posed by an infant with a large head, and because of the mother's attachment to the child, a shunt was inserted. Over the next year the shunt was revised once, and kidney infections were treated. Intellect appeared to be normal. An ileal loop was performed at one year because of developing hydronephrosis. The meningomyelocele sac was cleared at 14 months because of ulceration and to enable the child to be braced. Thus, while perhaps nothing was lost by delay in operation, little was gained, and the parents were put through the problems of care of an open, leaking lesion, and the anxieties of waiting for their child to die. Significantly, the child's name is Hope.

A second child with a T_{12} lesion was not operated on at birth because of paraplegia. The child was given no therapy and the parents were told that the child would die. After 5½ months in an acute hospital he was transferred to a state institution for the retarded. By 10 months the hydrocephalus was becoming marked and constituted a nursing problem. Therefore, the child was shunted and the meningomyelocele repaired. The child's dislocated hips were also repaired at that time. He was returned to the institution. At age 5 he was found to have an I.Q. of 75, but to be blind secondary to optic atrophy. Because of hydronephrosis an ileal loop was performed at age 6½. However, because of the marked kyphosis and the lack of abdominal wall when sitting, there was marked difficulty keeping the loop appliance in place.

The child was first seen in our clinic at age 8½. He has marked optic atrophy and blindness, a dislocated hip with bilateral equinus positioning of the feet, and a verbal I.Q. of 75. He is currently in a school for the blind. The scoliosis and kyphosis impair his sitting position as well as care of the urinary drainage. At this point we plan to fuse the kyphosis to allow better sitting position and adequate urinary drainage. The mother has openly rejected this child as might be expected from having spent a number of years waiting for the child to die. We have involved the family in psychotherapy to help them adapt to managing this child.

Early comprehensive care could certainly have prevented the major psychological problems for the child and his family. His blindness, an additional severe handicap in a child with paraplegia, was also probably preventable. Unfortunately, this child did not follow the physician's pronouncement and die either quickly or slowly.

Lorber (1971) states: "The large majority of infants do not live long if untreated." This is true, but the *large* minority do live long, and at best have more neurological deficit than if treated. At worst they represent significant nursing and emotional problems at home or in institutions for professional personnel as well as for parents, because of massive enlargement of the head or an open wound. Since hydrocephalus is the major cause of death from three months of life on, shunting at a "late" stage will only increase the number of these survivors. Therefore, if one, elects not to treat the child with a meningomyelocele, he must be prepared to cope with the child who survives.

PROGNOSIS OF VIGOROUSLY TREATED MENINGOMYELOCELES

Early operation and new techniques for shunting have led many groups to enthusiastic treatment of all children with meningomyeloceles. Sharrard et al. (1963), in a controlled series, found decreased mortality, infection, length of hospital stay, and dysfunction in the lower extremities in those treated early. In another series Sharrard, Zachary, and Lorber (1966) reviewed patients referred to them and operated on at varying times. They found that operation within the first four days decreased the mortality in comparison with those operated on after four days or managed conservatively. Mortality was higher in infants with hydrocephalus than in those without, but the incidence of hydrocephalus was not increased by early operation. Early operation decreased the mortality of those with hydrocephalus. The authors found that infants operated upon on the third or fourth day of life had more paralysis than those operated upon earlier, but less than those with no operation. Of infants surviving three years, 35% of those with early operation had normal or near-normal lower extremities. Only 12% of those with late closure had this degree of function. Only in sacral lesions was there no difference in residual paralysis with early operation. Sharrard, Zachary, and Lorber (1966) concluded that "there was no place for selection of patients for conservative rather than operative treatment on the grounds of paralysis, deformity, or hydrocephalus present at birth." In another series, Mawdsley and Rickham (1969) found that 70% of operated cases survived, and that only 10% required special schooling because of mental impairment. Almost half could walk reasonably well with crutches.

Lorber, in a recent review of the Sheffield patients (1971), was less enthusiastic about treatment for all patients. In reviewing his large series of vigorously treated patients, he found that only 7% of patients vigorously

Table 4-2 Quality of Survivors of Vigorously Treated Patients (From Lorber, 1971)

Physical handicap	Intellect	Admissions, %	Survivors, %
1. Mild–moderate	Normal	7	18
2. Severe	Normal	20	49
3. Severe	Moderately retarded, 61–79	9	21
4. Severe	Severe retardation, 60	5	12
	Dead	59	

treated "have less than grossly crippling disability and may be considered to have a quality of life not inconsistent with self respect, earning capacity, happiness, and even marriage." Eighteen per cent of the survivors are severely handicapped physically and are retarded, and 59% of the patients are dead. These figures are summarized in Table 4-2. In addition, 15% of the survivors have severe hydronephrosis and a limited life expectancy.

Lorber also found that patients with hydrocephalus had more severe sequelae and higher mortality. The prognosis was also related to the site of the lesion, mainly because of the hydrocephalus. Children with cervical, thoracic, or sacral defects had a lower incidence of hydrocephalus, a higher rate of survival, and less intellectual handicap.

In order to "spare children and their families prolonged suffering and to give better attention to those who are more likely to benefit from total care," Lorber has developed criteria for selection of those who should *not* be treated. These criteria are (1) paralysis $L_{2\text{-}3}$ or above, (2) marked hydrocephalus, (3) kyphosis, and (4) other congenital abnormalities or birth injuries. Let us review his data for each of these criteria:

1. The results of treatment according to the degree of paralysis are shown in Table 4-3. Patients who had paralysis from $L_{2\text{-}3}$ or higher with no movement from the legs, or only hip flexion and quadriceps activity, had a 50% survival rate and 20% chance of normal intellect. The 48 survivors had undergone 127 operations. Nineteen had hydronephrosis with or without urinary diversion.

2. Hydrocephalus was the major adverse factor related to the intellectual sequelae. Of the 36 infants whose head circumference at birth exceeded the ninetieth percentile by 2 cm, 61% were dead, 20% were extremely retarded, and only 8% had normal intellect.

3. Extreme kyphosis was treated by spinal osteotomy at birth. Of children with this complication, 55% died and 75% of the survivors are retarded in addition to having a severe physical handicap.

4. Other major abnormalities or birth injuries carried a 90% mortality and 100% risk of severe intellectual disability.

Patients having the adverse criteria 2 through 4 without the severe paralysis had a similar outlook to those with paralysis.

Table 4-3 Survival and Handicap Related to Paralysis (From Lorber, 1971)

Initial examination	No.	Survivors	Motor handicap	Normal intellect	Comment
No movement or hip flexion only*	51	26 (51%)	Severe	9 (34%)	6/17 with no other adverse criteria have normal IQ 9/26 have hydronephrosis
Lesion L_{2-3}*	44	22 (50%)	Severe	11 (50%)	Hydronephrosis 50%
Total*	95	48 (50%)	Severe	20 (41%)	
Lesion L_4 or below	106	77 (72%)	None 3% Moderate 29% Severe 68%	60 (77%)	15/106 had adverse criteria other than paralysis

*Patients who should not be operated on, by Lorber's criteria.

In summary, Lorber finds that of patients having major adverse criteria at birth, including severe paralysis, 50% are dead, but 40% of the survivors have normal IQ. Of the patients who had no adverse criteria at birth, 23% are dead, but 50% have severe sequelae, and 14% are retarded. Dr. Lorber concludes this thoughtful review by stating that "only those should be given active treatment who may look forward to a life without grave handicaps."

If one accepts Lorber's figures as showing the best that medicine can do, then the end result of the enormous time, money, and effort expended on these children is disappointing. However, ethicists still contend that it is better *for the child* to be severely handicapped than to be dead. There is no doubt that we can do nothing to repair the neurological deficit of children with meningomyeloceles. Therefore, approximately 50% of the afflicted children will always have severe degrees of paralysis. This degree of paralysis is largely predictable at birth: early surgery can only preserve function.

The mortality from hydrocephalus, ventriculitis, and renal disease *is*, however, susceptible to considerable improvement, and the intellectual residua should also improve with the care of the hydrocephalus and ventriculitis. There is a possibility that Lorber's bleak figures are not the final word. At Johns Hopkins Hospital, *no* child has died of hydrocephalus or of a blocked shunt in the last three years. None of the newborns has developed ventriculitis, and ventriculitis related to the shunt has been amenable to therapy. With close attention to renal function and hydronephrosis, and the early performance of ileal loops, none of our children is dying of renal decompensation. While we have far fewer patients with meningomyeloceles than Sheffield has, this may be an advantage in providing optimum care for them. Similar results have been reported by Ames and Schut (1972).

In summary, there are three alternatives open to the physician faced with a child with a meningomyelocele:

1. To actively treat—closing the back, shunting the hydrocephalus, and offering continuing orthopedic, urologic, and psychological care.

2. Not to treat—with the attendant high morbidity but high rate of survival until the patient *eventually* succumbs to meningitis, increasing hydrocephalus, or chorinc renal disease.

3. To terminate life, actively or passively.

Active euthanasia might be the most humane course for the *most severely* affected infants, but it is illegal. "Passive euthanasia" is legal, but is hardly humane. Therefore, in an ambivalent fashion we feel that *virtually* every child should be given optimal care.

Our ambivalence toward this conclusion will appear often when we talk about providing optimal therapy. This ambivalence comes from a desire to do what is "best" for the child and the family, and for society as a whole, and the feeling that "best" cannot always be equated with life. It comes from a personal projection into the parents' and child's situation, from the feeling that in *some* instances the optimal medical and psychological care we have to offer will be inadequate, and that the child's survival will be severely detrimental to the siblings and to the family as a whole. It comes from the feeling that the family has rights, just as the affected child has rights, and that with a severely affected child the "best" for everyone concerned may be the death of the child.

Since the editor feels that a slow, natural death over weeks or months is not humane for the child, the family, or the staff forced to care for the infant, he is left in the schizophrenic position of advocating either active euthanasia or vigorous treatment. Until active euthanasia for the most severely affected children becomes acceptable to society, we must opt for vigorous treatment, to make these children and their families as intact as we are able.

ADDENDUM

Since preparation of this manuscript there has been growing literature on untreated cases (Smith and Smith, 1973; Hunt et al., 1973; Lorber, 1973; Shaw, 1973), and a major shift towards taking the easy path of not treating children who will inevitably have major neurological deficit. To a large degree this brings about a self-fulfilling prophesy. Children with little or no paralysis at birth are naturally more ambulatory later and, therefore, become "better results." The smaller number of children treated allows better care of the survivors, therefore fewer die of hydrocephalus and of preventable renal decompensation.

This is not to say that a paraplegic child with or without hydrocephalus cannot have a normal intelligence, cannot have a full and active life (if one does not include ambulation in the definition of full), and cannot be a person, provided he or she is given optimal medical care.

REFERENCES

Ames, M. D., and L. Schut. 1972. Results of treatment of myelomeningoceles. Pediat. 50:466.

Forrest, D. M. 1967. Modern trends in the treatment of spina bifida. Proc. Roy. Soc. Med. 60:763.

Hide, D. W., H. P. Williams, and H. L. Ellis. 1972. The outlook for the child with a myelomeningocele for whom early surgery was considered inadvisable. Develop. Med. Child. Neurol. 14:304.

Hunt, G., W. Levin, J. Gleave, and D. Gardiner. 1973. Predictive factors in open myelomeningocele with special reference to sensory level. Brit. Med. J. 2:197. 1973.

Ingraham, F. D., and H. Hamlin. 1943. Spina bifida and cranium bifida. New Eng. J. Med. 228:559, 631, 745.

Knox, E. G. 1967. Spina bifida in Birmingham. Develop. Med. Child Neurol. Supp. 13:14.

Laurence, K. M. 1964. The natural history of spina bifida cystica. Arch. Dis. Childh. 39:41.

Laurence, K. M. 1966. The survival of untreated spina bifida cystica. Develop. Med. Child Neurol. Supp. 11:10.

Lorber, J. 1973. Early results of selective treatment of spina bifida cystica. Brit. Med. J. 2:201.

Lorber, J. 1971. Results of treatment of myelomeningocele. An analysis of 524 unselected cases with special reference to possible selection for treatment. Develop. Med. Child Neurol. 13:279.

Mawdsley, T., and P. P. Rickham. 1969. Further follow-up of early operation for open myelomeningocele. Develop. Med. Child Neurol. 20:8.

Rickham, P. P., and T. Mawdsley. 1966. The effect of early operation on the survival of spina bifida cystica. Develop. Med. Child Neurol. Supp. 11:20.

Sharrard, W. J. W. 1962. The mechanism of paralytic deformity in spina bifida. Develop. Med. Child Neurol. 4:310.

Sharrard, W. J. W., R. B. Zachary, J. Lorber, and A. M. Bruce. 1963. A controlled trial of immediate and delayed closure of spina bifida cystica. Arch. Dis. Childh. 38:18.

Sharrard, W. J. W., R. B. Zachary, and J. Lorber. 1966. Survival and paralysis in open myelomeningocele with special reference to the time of repair of the spinal lesion. Develop. Med. Child Neurol. Supp. 13:35.

Shaw, A. 1973. Dilemmas of "informed consent" in children. New Eng. J. Med. 289:885.

Smith, G. K., and E. D. Smith. Selection for treatment in spina bifida cystica. Brit. Med. J. 2:189.

5

Neurological Examination

John M. Freeman, M.D.

Every infant with a meningomyelocele deserves a complete assessment immediately after birth. It is on the basis of this assessment that prognosis for life and for the eventual minimal degree of handicap *can* be made and that ethical decisions regarding therapy *will* be made.

The birth of a child with a meningomyelocele is a relatively uncommon event; consequently, few pediatricians, general practitioners, or obstetricians acquire sufficient familiarity with the detailed assessment of the infant or with the long-range aspects of the problem to assist the family in the difficult decisions regarding therapy. Thus, whenever possible, these children should be referred immediately to centers actively involved in the care of meningomyeloceles. There the team approach can permit more accurate neurological assessment and present the family with the alternatives needed to make rational decisions. The team is also equipped to undertake optimal treatment.

CARE AND TRANSPORTATION

Infection and drying of the meningomyelocele sac increase neurological disability. Therefore, immediate attention at birth should be given to the protection and sterility of the defect. The infant should be kept on its stomach. The defect should be handled (if at all) with sterile gloves, should be kept covered with a nonadherent sterile covering such as Xerofoam gauze, and should be protected from rupture with a gauze doughnut held on by a loose gauze dressing.

The infant should not be fed, but should be transported in a warm, portable incubator as soon as possible to the regional center. Since the infant's GI tract is sterile for the first 24 hours, local infection and ventriculitis can often be prevented by early operation, and remaining neurological functions can be preserved. Therefore, time is an important factor in optimal care.

HISTORY

Since most infants are referred to a regional center, the history must be obtained from the father. Communication with the mother at this critical period is, unfortunately, limited. Important aspects of the history include:

1. Details of the pregnancy, such as infections, bleeding, drugs, etc.
2. Details of the labor and delivery and the Apgar score, which may give a clue to additional birth injury.
3. A family history of neonatal problems, which may assist in the prediction of medical problems unrelated to the meningomyelocele.
4. A family history of central nervous system malformations in siblings and other relatives, which will influence genetic counseling.
5. A knowledge of the family: the number of children, the difficulties the mother had in getting pregnant, attitudes toward the child's future degree of disability. These are all important considerations in the decision regarding therapy. Often conversations with the family physician about the family structure may help in the determination of therapy.

PHYSICAL EXAMINATION

A complete pediatric examination should be carried out on every infant. This includes examination of the fundi for chorioretinitis or congenital abnormalities of the optic nerve, which may suggest cerebral anomalies, as well as a search for cardiac defects, pulmonary problems, organomegaly, cleft palate, imperforate anus, and genital abnormalities.

The neurological examination should be carried out on a warm infant. Hypothermia may interfere with the examination by producing a lethargic, unresponsive infant.

EXAMINATION OF THE DEFECT AND SPINE

The size and location of the defect should be noted. The location of the lesion on the back will give an indication of the risk of hydrocephalus (Table 5-1). In general, the higher the lesion, the greater the neurological deficit and the higher the risk of hydrocephalus. Leakage of CSF from the defect is an indication for immediate surgery. A marked kyphosis, scoliosis, or gibbus may require removal of bone for adequate closure and may require the assistance of an orthopedic surgeon at the time of initial surgery (see Chapter 8). The size of the lesion is of interest, but few defects are too large for primary closure. Large lesions may require skin flaps and the assistance of a plastic surgeon (see Chapter 6).

While the defect is of major importance, it is also important to examine the remainder of the back for other areas of spina bifida or scoliosis which might influence therapy.

EXAMINATION OF THE LOWER LIMBS

Lesions of the spinal cord associated with meningomyelocele may take several forms:

Table 5-1 Location of Lesion and Its Relation to Prognosis

Lesion	Motor/sensory level	Risk of hydrocephalus	Prognosis for ambulation	Comment
Cervical and high thoracic	Usually none	None	Good	Usually these are menin-goceles, high chance of scoliosis
Thoraco-lumbar	T_{12}–L_2	96%	Complete paraplegia	Kyphosis important for sitting and pelvic band of braces
Lumbar	L_{3-4}	86%	May ambulate with braces and crutches	High risk of paralytic hip dislocation
Lumbo-sacral	L_5–S_1	60%	Will ambulate with or without short leg braces	Outlook excellent

1. Complete dysfunction of the cord and roots below a given level, producing flaccid paralysis.

2. A transection of the cord with an isolated segment below. The transected area results in flaccid paralysis of the affected muscles, but the isolated segments below result in spasticity and reflex activity.

3. The lesion may be incomplete, causing spasticity but allowing some motor function, or it may be asymmetrical and even spotty.

Complete dysfunction below the level of the lesion is the most common condition. Incomplete lesions and lesions with an isolated segment may give erroneous impressions of the amount of neurological disability unless a careful examination is performed. Visual inspection of the posture of the lower extremities and feet usually demonstrates partial abnormalities which correlate with the neurological disability (Stark, 1971; Lorber, 1968; Stark and Baker, 1967).

MOTOR EXAMINATION

A complete motor examination, including each muscle group, takes approximately five minutes. The child should be warm and vigorous. Stimulation with a pin *above* the level of the muscle being tested may stimulate movement without producing misleading reflex activity. The highest level should be tested first. Segmental innervation of the principal muscles to be tested is shown in Table 5-2.

Some muscle groups, such as glutei and abductors, may be difficult to evaluate in the newborn. Spontaneous voluntary activity can usually be observed. If necessary, voluntary activity may be stimulated by a pin *above*

Table 5-2 Segmental Innervation of the Lower Limbs (Summarized from Sharrard, 1964)

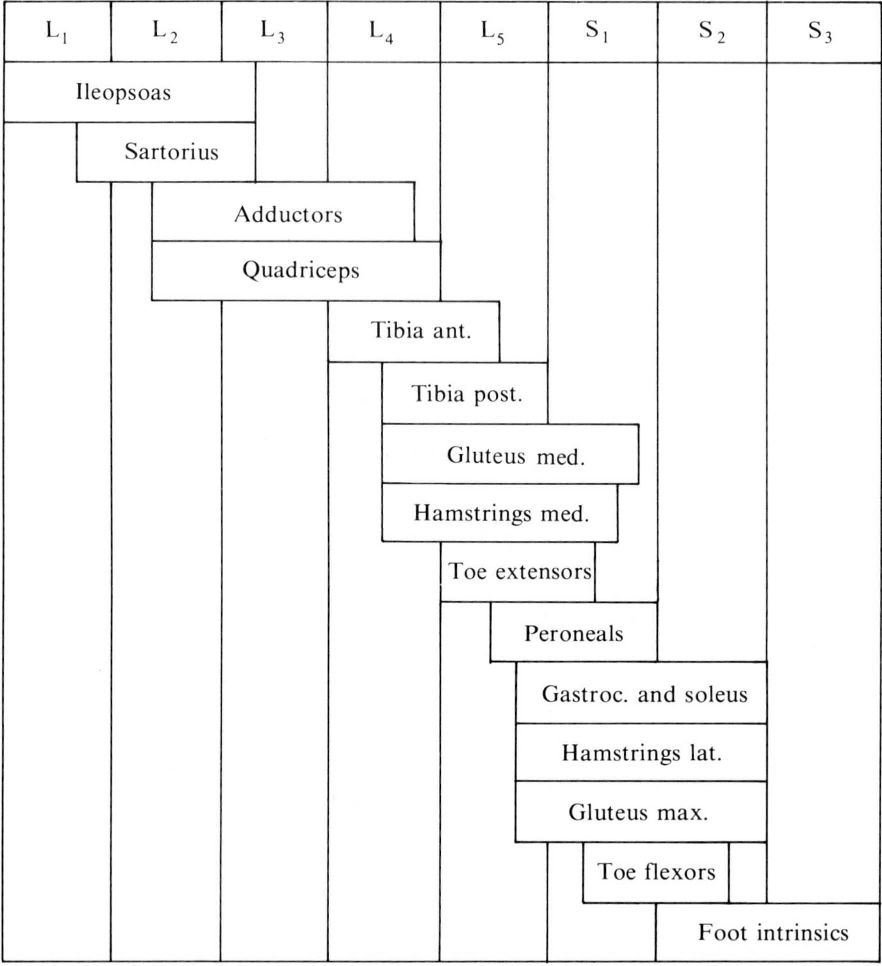

the level of the lesion to avoid reflex activity. The degree of function of each muscle group should be recorded (Table 5-3). Reflex activity of the muscle groups may be assessed by stimulation below the level of the lesion. This activity is an indication of an isolated cord segment with an intact reflex arc and will be of no functional use to the child. It is mentioned only to emphasize that it should *not* be confused with spontaneous activity.

Each leg should be examined separately and the strength of individual muscles graded. Deformities of the feet, legs, or hips are usually secondary to imbalance between antagonistic muscles and can be used to deduce the level of the lesion (Stark, 1971).

Table 5-3 Chart for Testing Infants with Meningomyeloceles

Name ______________ Date and time of examination ______

Date and time of birth ______ Head circ. ______ Percentile ____

Condition of infant ______ Other abnormalities ______

______________ ______________

Motor examination: G—good F—fair P—poor 0—none R—reflex

Joint	Movement	Main muscle	Level of innervation	Right	Left
Hip	Flexion	Psoas	L_1–L_3	______	______
	Extension	Gluteus max.	L_5–S_1	______	______
	Abduction	Gluteus med.	L_4–S_1	______	______
	Adduction	Adductors	L_2–L_4	______	______
Knee	Flexors	Hamstrings med.	L_4–S_1	______	______
		Hamstrings lat.	L_5–S_2	______	______
	Extensors	Quadriceps	L_2–L_4	______	______
Ankle	Plantar flex	Gastroc. and soleus	L_5–S_2	______	______
	Dorsi flex	Tibia ant.	L_4–L_5	______	______
Subtalar	Inversion	Tibia post.	L_4–L_5	______	______
	Eversion	Peroneal	L_5–S_1	______	______
Toes	Flexion	Long flexors	S_1–S_2	______	______
		Short flexors	S_2–S_3	______	______
	Extension	Common extensors	L_5–S_1	______	______
		Short extensors	S_2–S_3	______	______

Motor level ______________

SENSORY EXAMINATION

Nerve conduction in the newborn is slow; therefore, one should wait 3–5 seconds before concluding that the stimulus is not appreciated. Change in facial appearance or crying in response to a pin prick indicates that the stimulus has reached the level of awareness. Withdrawal from such a stimulus may be a local reflex phenomenon and cannot be used to determine the sensory level. The sensory dermatomes are shown in Fig. 5-1. Sensation should be tested proceeding from the sacral areas.

The sensory level may be higher or lower than the motor level and may be asymmetrical.

BOWEL AND BLADDER

Dribbling of urine when the infant cries, or when abdominal pressure is applied, indicates bladder involvement, usually a flaccid bladder. The absence of dribbling does not, however, indicate normal bladder function. The anal wink and anal tone may similarly indicate rectal problems, but the anal wink may be present with isolated cord segments. Further neurological evaluation is deferred until the back is closed.

HYDROCEPHALUS

The head should be measured and plotted on a standard head growth chart (Figs. 5-2 and 5-3). Hydrocephalus of marked degree is unusual at birth,

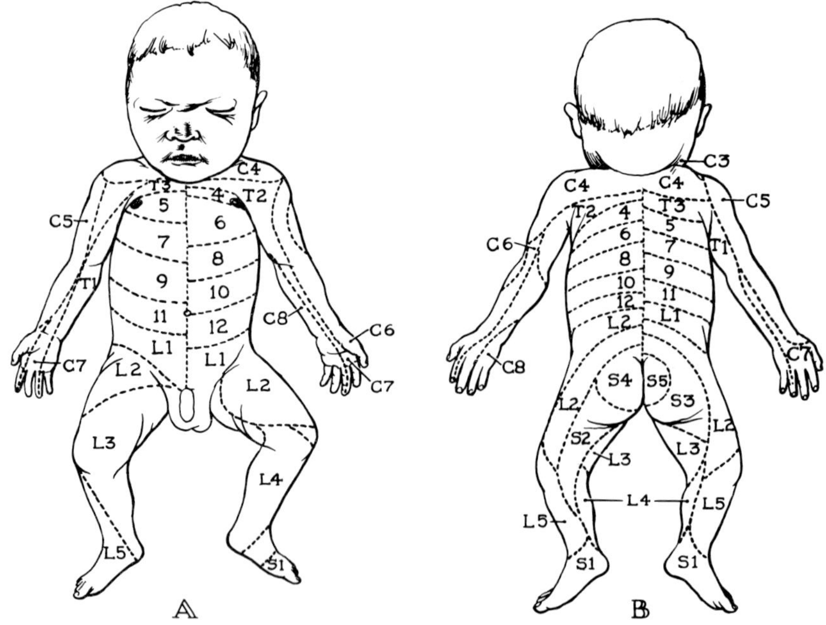

Fig. 5-1 Sensory dermatomes of the infant.

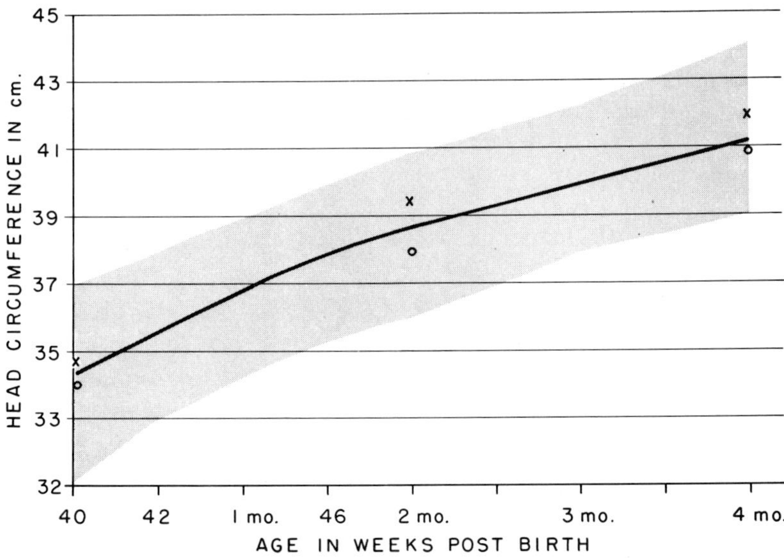

Fig. 5-2 Head growth of full-term infants. Redrawn from O'Neill (1961).

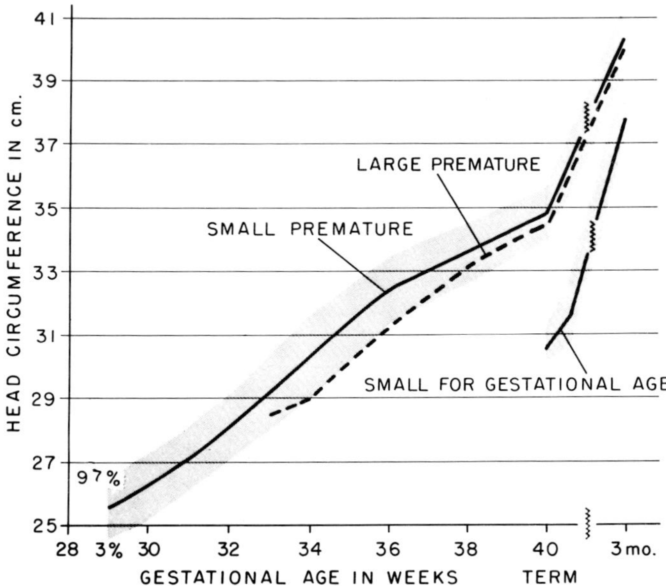

Fig. 5-3 Head growth of low-birth-weight infants both premature and small for gestational age. Redrawn from Babson (1970).

but baseline measurements are important for determining future growth rate. Bulging of the fontanelle, with the infant quiet in an upright position, and separation of the sutures may suggest hydrocephalus. Skull defects may delineate encephaloceles or sinus tracts.

ANCILLARY STUDIES

Electromyographic studies and electrical stimulation and response of individual muscle groups have been utilized by some centers, but do not appear to be of practical importance.

X-rays of the total spine for scoliosis and other spinal abnormalities should be performed prior to surgery, as should x-rays of the chest.

Echoencephalography may be utilized by experienced hands to assess accurately cortical mantle thickness and ventricular size. When used serially, it is a useful technique for the determination of hydrocephalus, particularly after closure of the spinal defect.

SUMMARY

The careful neurological examination in the newborn period can delineate with a high degree of certainty the neurological deficit of the infant. This knowledge should permit reasonably accurate prognostication for ambulation, and the risks of hydrocephalus, bowel and bladder problems, and major orthopedic abnormalities. With this information the physician can rationally determine his future course of management.

REFERENCES

Babson, S. G. 1970. Growth of low-birth-weight infants. J. Pediat. 77, 11.

Lorber, J. 1968. Neurologic assessment of neonates with spina bifida. Clin. Pediat. 7:676.

O'Neill, E. M. 1961. Normal head growth and the prediction of head size in infantile hydrocephalus. Arch. Dis. Childh. 36:241.

Sharrard, W. J. W. 1964. The segmental innervation of the lower limb muscles in man. Ann. Roy. Coll. Surgeons of Eng. 35:106.

Stark, G. D. 1971. Neonatal assessment of the child with myelomeningocele. Arch. Dis. Childh. 46:539.

Stark, G. D., and G. C. W. Baker. 1967. The neurological involvement of the lower limbs in myelomeningocele. Develop. Med. Child Neurol. 9:732.

6

Neurosurgical Management of Meningomyelocele

Edward R. Laws, Jr., M.D.

INITIAL CONSIDERATIONS

As noted in previous chapters, patients with meningomyeloceles come into the world with predictable regularity and need medical attention from the moment of birth through every stage of the remainder of their lives. If one of these patients is to be given the optimal medical care available today, he will need the services of medical specialists in pediatrics, neurosurgery, neurology, urology, orthopedics, rehabilitation medicine, and, frequently, psychiatry. This care will often be elaborate, requiring interrelationships between specialties. It is hoped that this chapter may provide a practical guide for the neurosurgical aspects of care.

There is considerable variation in the anatomy and location of the various forms of spina bifida manifesta. From a practical standpoint, they all include abnormal bony formation of the spine, and all have abnormalities of the membraneous coverings of the spinal cord and nerve roots. The most common form of spina bifida manifesta is the meningomyelocele, where the malformation includes the spinal cord and nerve roots. This involvement of neural elements is the key to the prognosis for the infant and for the timing and nature of the neurosurgical repair.

It is frequently possible to tell, upon inspection of the cystic lesion at birth, whether or not it contains neural elements. A meningocele, a simple sac filled with fluid, without a central neural plaque and adherent nerve roots, carries a very favorable prognosis for neurological function. Unfortunately, these simple meningoceles are far outnumbered by the more devastating meningomyeloceles. In either case, the cystic sac over the opening in the spine is often very thin and filmy, and may transude a yellowish fluid and appear to leak CSF. A considerable number of sacs rupture during delivery, resulting in a frank leak of CSF with collapse of the sac. The presence of a ruptured sac and a CSF leak must obviously influence the speed with which the lesion is closed.

The anatomical level of the lesion is less important than the functional level of neurological deficit in predicting future motor function. The assumption and maintenance of the sitting posture requires that motor function be intact through the L_1 spinal cord level. Infants in whom the lesion interrupts function in the level above L_1 have a limited prognosis.

Occasionally, the bony abnormality underlying the cystic lesion may be more severe than a simple spina bifida or laminar defect. These bony malformations may include sacral dysplasia or agenesis, kyphosis or gibbus formation, severe scoliosis and abnormal fusion of lateral spinal elements, or ventral defects in the spinal column. Some may be corrected by orthopedic procedures, but some may be severe enough to prevent the assumption of the sitting posture and, therefore, limit prognosis for the patient. Foot deformities are common and are of no initial concern.

Hydrocephalus ultimately occurs in more than 90% of patients with meningomyeloceles and occasionally may be manifest at birth. Patients with obvious hydrocephalus at birth carry a poor prognosis for normal mental development. Likewise, neurogenic urinary incontinence with associated urinary reflux, hydro-ureter, and hydronephrosis eventually occurs in more than 95% of patients with meningomyeloceles (Rose and Smith, 1963). These lesions are rarely present at birth, but some infants may be born with structural damage to the upper urinary tracts.

Finally, a small number of infants with meningomyeloceles have major congenital anomalies in other systems, which will influence the course and management of the infant, and may require additional specialty consultations for evaluation and treatment.

To summarize, the initial evaluation of a patient with spina bifida manifesta includes the following points: (1) Is the cyst intact, or is there a leak of CSF? (2) Is the lesion well covered by a cystic sac, or are neural elements exposed? (3) What is the approximate anatomical level of the lesion (cervical, thoracic, thoraco-lumbar, lumbar, or sacral)? (4) Is motor function present in the lower extremities, and, if so, to what extent? (5) Are serious spinal deformities such as kyphosis or scoliosis present? (6) Does the child have other obvious congenital anomalies?

The answers to these questions enable the physician to give the parents a guarded assessment of the patient's condition and prospects. Only rarely should these factors inhibit referral to a team of physicians experienced in the problems of meningomyeloceles.

As soon as possible, the lesion should be covered by a sterile, nonadherent dressing and protected from all forms of irritation. Prompt arrangements should be made for transfer to a neurosurgical center, preferably within the first six hours after birth.

NEUROSURGICAL EVALUATION

Once it has been ascertained that the infant has survived the transfer with normal vital signs and body temperature, a complete physical and neurological examination is performed, and blood is taken for hematological work-up and the cross matching of 250 to 500 cc of blood.

The examination of the infant has been discussed in Chapter 5. The most important facets from the neurosurgical standpoint are the following:

1. *The head:* The head circumference is measured, and the patient is examined for bulging of fontanelles, widening or separation of sutures, and abnormal cranial or sutural defects.

2. *The back:* The lesion on the back is carefully inspected, measured and, if possible, photographed (Figs. 6-1, 6-2, 6-3). The area over the meningomyelocele is cultured whether or not a frank CSF leak is present. These cultures are almost always sterile during the first 12 to 24 hours of life. Using *sterile gloves*, the physician palpates the bony defect above, below, and around the lesion and takes note of the extent of the spinal deformity. Transillumination of the sac may be performed, but is not ordinarily helpful.

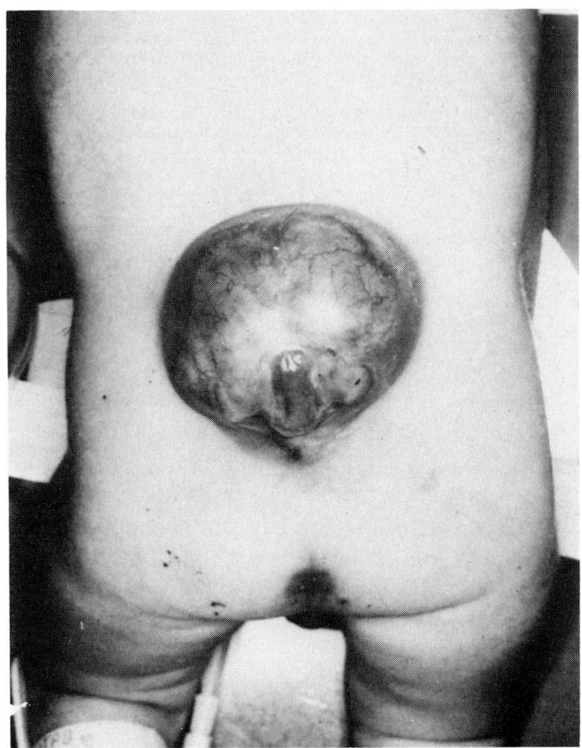

Fig. 6-1 Lumbar meningomyelocele, preoperative, 12 hours of age.

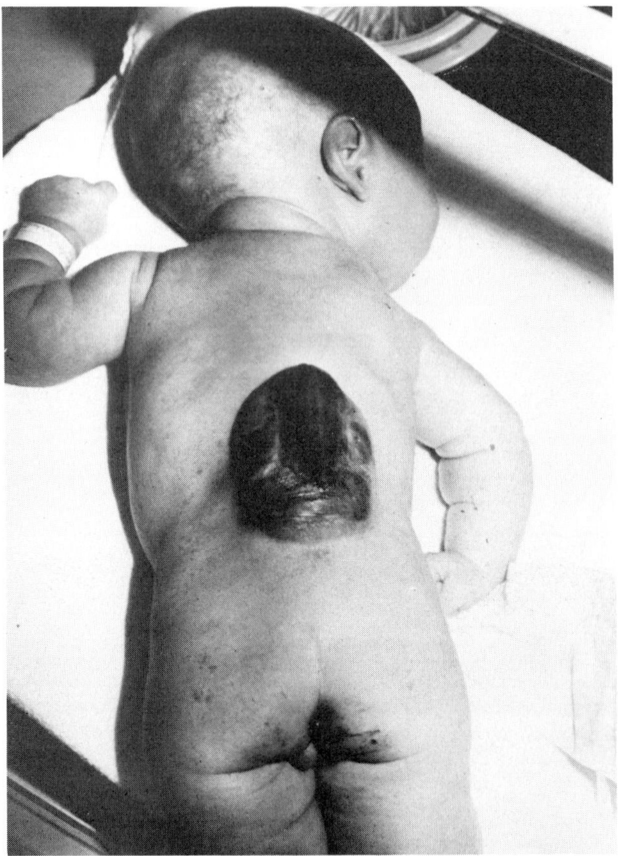

Fig. 6-2 Thoraco-lumbar meningomyelocele. The central neural plaque is visible.

3. *The lower extremities:* Inspection of the lower extremities often reveals foot deformities, most commonly valgus, secondary to abnormal muscle balance resulting from neurological deficits (Fig. 6-4). The extent of spontaneous movements in the lower extremities is noted, and then specific muscle testing in response to noxious stimuli is performed in a systematic manner to determine the lowest level of motor function (see neurological examination). Sensory examination is performed using pin pricks. This is done several times on both sides of the body, and the level of initial response by withdrawal or crying is recorded. Since there is frequently a considerable time delay between stimulus and response, this systematic examination must be done carefully and slowly. The anatomy of the neural plaque within a meningomyelocele is such that the sensory portions of the spinal cord and dorsal sensory nerve roots are more liable to injury and deformation than are the ventral motor roots. Because of this, the level of sensory anesthesia is often significantly higher than the level of motor function. In the examina-

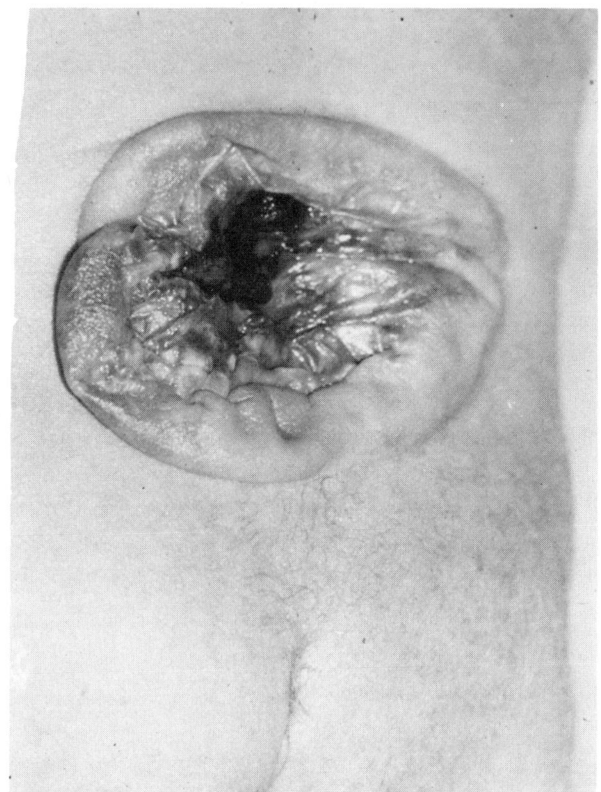

Fig. 6-3 Lumbar meningomyelocele with collapsed ulcerated sac.

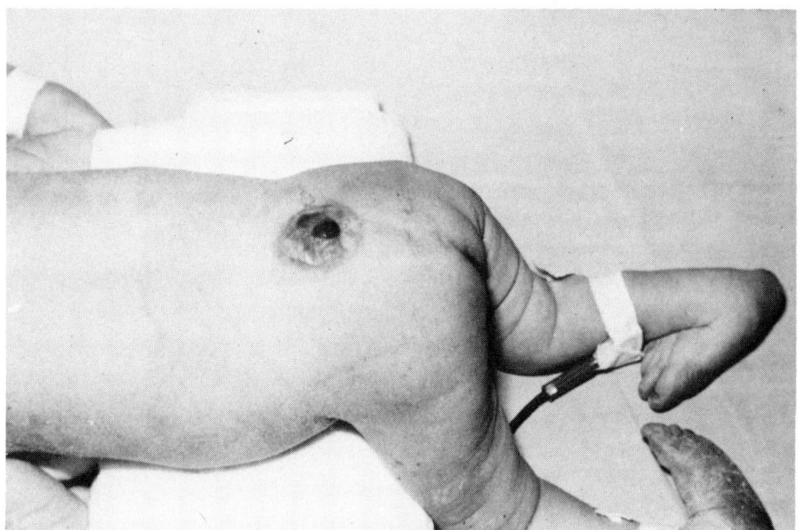

Fig. 6-4 Lumbo-sacral meningomyelocele. Note foot deformities.

tion of motor responses, it is important to distinguish between voluntary withdrawal motor responses and reflex movements which may occur in otherwise functionless motor groups.

4. *The bladder and rectum:* The anus is inspected, and, if denervated, will bulge or tend to prolapse with increases in intra-abdominal pressure, which may also produce dribbling of urine from a denervated bladder. Digital rectal examination is rarely indicated and does not ordinarily provide useful information.

The above examination completed, the lesion is once again covered with a sterile, nonadherent protective dressing, and x-rays of the skull and spine are performed. Skull films frequently show radiolucent areas of membranous bone (Luckenschadel, Fig. 6-5) and may show diastasis of sutures if hydrocephalus is present. Spine films usually show widening of the interpedicular distance in the region of the lesion (Fig. 6-6a and b), along with malformed, incomplete, or absent laminae. They may also demonstrate gibbus formation, scoliosis, and abnormal fusions (Figs. 6-7a and b and 6-8). An orthopedic consultation is always desirable and is frequently necessary for the proper initial evaluation and treatment.

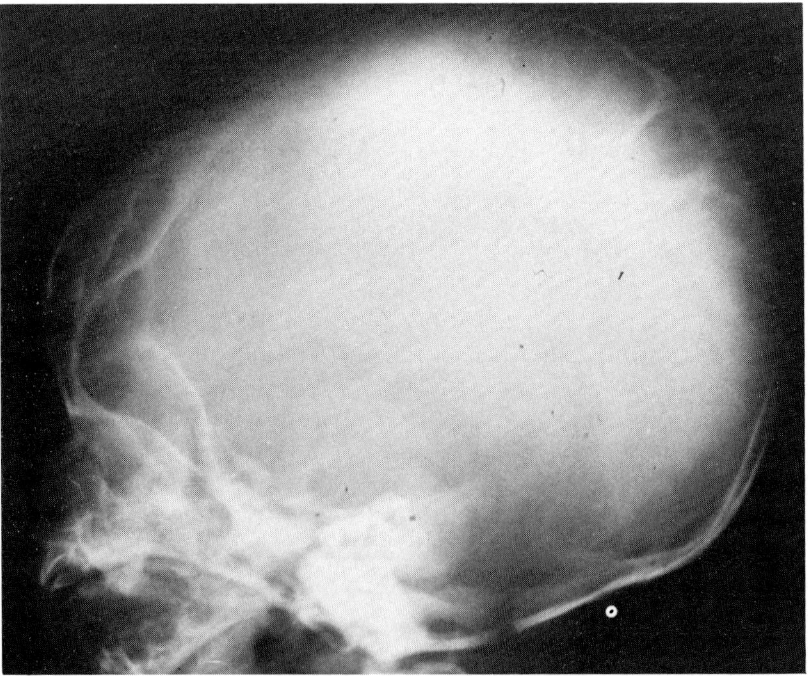

Fig. 6-5 Lateral skull film of newborn with a meningomyelocele. Areas of membranous bone are visible.

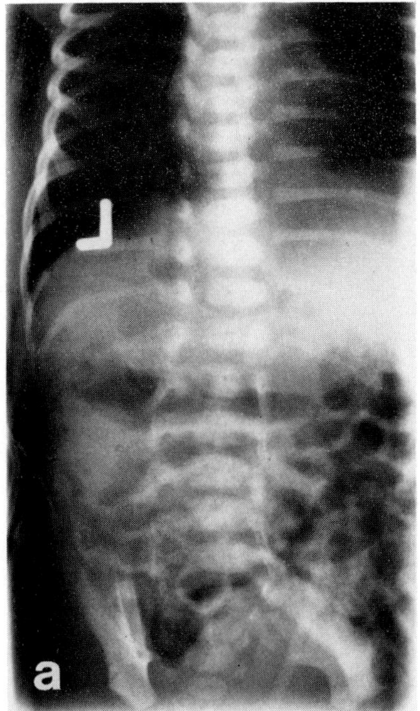

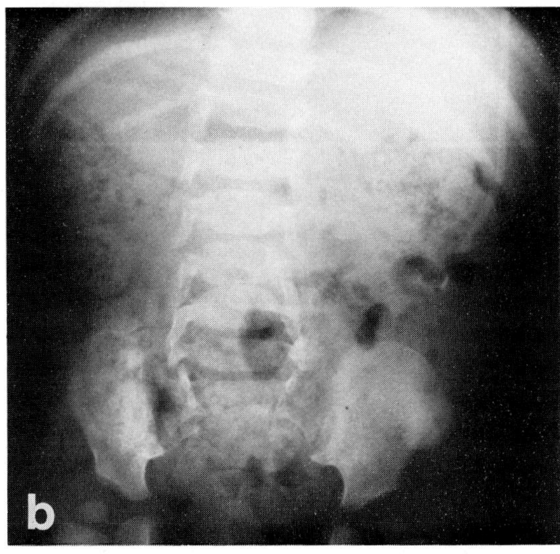

Fig. 6-6 (a) Meningomyelocele patient, AP view of spine at one day of age. Spina bifida is present from T_{11} through the sacrum. (b) Same patient at 10 months of age. Spina bifida and sacral dysplasia are more apparent. Shadows from stool in the large intestine are visible; many of these patients are chronically constipated. The coil-reinforced peritoneal shunt tubing can be seen on the right.

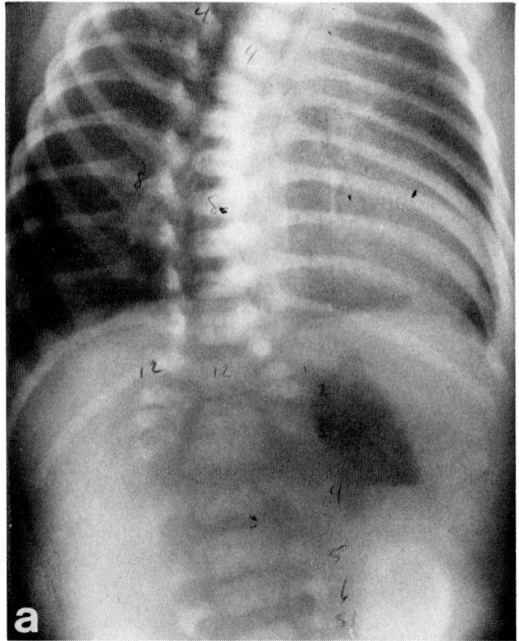

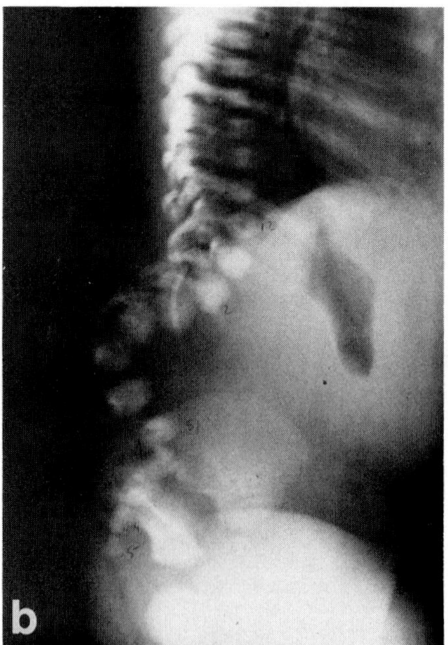

Fig. 6-7 Meningomyelocele patient, (a) AP and (b) lateral views of spine, one day of age. Extensive spina bifida is present from T_{12} through the sacrum. A gibbus with its apex at L_4 is visible in the lateral projection.

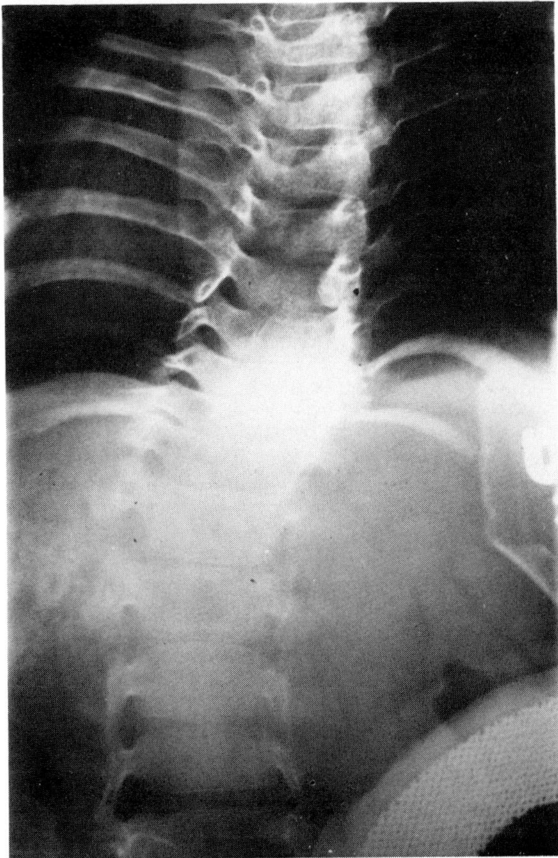

Fig. 6-8 Meningomyelocele patient, AP view of spine, age 5 years. Extensive spina bifida with thoraco-lumbar scoliosis is demonstrated. Shadow of ileal loop appliance is present in lower right corner.

INDICATIONS FOR SURGERY

From the practical standpoint, we feel that the indication for surgery in meningomyelocele cases is the preservation and/or protection of useful neurological function. Any patient with motor function intact through L_1 and motor power and structural spinal elements adequate to support the sitting position later in life, should undergo surgical repair of the lesion for protection and preservation of function.

With the current state of surgical therapy and follow-up, only rarely is a patient actually denied surgical treatment, although it must be kept in mind that once the initial surgical closure of the meningomyelocele defect is performed, one is usually committed to a series of shunt procedures, urinary diversions, and corrective orthopedic procedures.

Those patients with severe hydrocephalus and less than 0.5 cm of cortical mantle in the frontal region have a limited potential for normal mental development, but even in these cases surgical care of the back and hydrocephalus may be indicated. Nursing home placement or custodial care of patients with progressive severe hydrocephalus is extremely difficult if they are untreated.

While ordinarily we do not feel that the aesthetically unpleasing effect of a lesion is itself an adequate indication for cosmetic correction, these lesions are frequently closed to ease the care of the patient during infancy, and to enable the use of braces as supports necessary for proper sitting or standing postures.

TIMING OF SURGERY

There now appears to be no doubt that the ideal time for surgery is within the first 24 hours of life. The most compelling reason, now adequately substantiated with controlled studies (Sharrard et al., 1963; Rickham and Mawdsley, 1966; Guthkelch, 1962; Brocklehurst, Ghave, and Lewin, 1966), is that early operation may forestall worsening of the neurological deficit. If the major goal in surgery is to preserve and protect neurological function, one must advocate early surgery. In addition, the skin and stool of the infant do not ordinarily become colonized with pathogenic microorganisms until after the first 24 hours of life; hence, early operation may also protect the patient against infection.

If proper anesthesia and suitably skilled personnel are available, there is no contraindication to surgery in the newborn. The high hematocrit and the loose skin of the neonate are actually favorable factors in meningomyelocele surgery. We have no hesitation in making the categorical recommendation that the optimal time for surgical repair of a meningomyelocele is within the first 24 hours of life.

It is still not unusual to see patients with meningomyeloceles presented for delayed surgical repair during the first year of life or even later. These patients will rarely regain any function that has been lost, but may be benefited by the release of tethering of the spinal cord and by removal of the protruding meningomyelocele sac. The operative mortality in this group of late repair is somewhat higher than in the neonates, but the overall technical considerations and principles of management are quite similar.

SURGICAL CONSIDERATIONS

In order to preserve neurological function, the neural elements must be covered so that they are protected from exposure and trauma, and the spinal subarachnoid space must be covered and sealed so that CSF leak and meningitis cannot occur. The neural plaque and nerve roots must be carefully dissected to free them from all structures to which they may be fixed or tethered.

The concept of tethering is most important and explains why some of the patients develop a progressive increase in neurological deficit as they grow older. It is well known that with growth before and after birth, a progressive disproportion occurs between the length of the spinal cord and the spinal column. The spinal cord terminates at the L_2-L_4 level at birth, but with growth of the bony elements of the spinal canal, the termination of the spinal cord will, move up to L_1. In a meningomyelocele, the neural plaque and nerve roots are fixed to the skin and subcutaneous tissues with tough fibrous bands, some of which may be intradural. These attachments, if untreated, tether the spinal cord and prevent its normal upward migration, applying traction to and producing progressive dysfunction of the conus medullaris and roots of the cauda equina. Tethering may also be associated with other forms of spina bifida, particularly with subcutaneous lipomas, a hairy patch, or a hemangioma over the back. In these abnormalities similar tethering of the spinal cord may produce progressive neurological impairment (see Chapter 8). Therefore, careful neurological follow-up examination at frequent intervals is indicated for all patients with any form of spina bifida manifesta.

Hydrocephalus occurs in 80% to 90% of infants during the postoperative period. Closure of the sac may appear to precipitate rapidly progressive hydrocephalus, but does not cause hydrocephalus. The mechanisms and treatment of hydrocephalus are discussed in Chapter 7.

OPERATIVE MANAGEMENT

As soon as possible after completion of the preoperative evaluation, the patient is prepared for surgery. Before, during, and after surgery every effort is made to prevent loss of body temperature. Temperature is maintained pre- and postoperatively by the use of a heated isolette. During surgery hypothermia may be prevented by the use of a heating blanket, insulated cotton wrapping for the extremities, and supplementary infrared heat lamps, if necessary. Temperature during surgery is continually monitored by rectal or esophageal probe. The importance of these measures cannot be overemphasized, as loss of temperature can occur precipitously and with disastrous results.

Prior to the induction of anesthesia, a secure intravenous line is started, usually a saphenous cutdown. Blood replacement is rarely necessary in simple meningomyeloceles, but must be anticipated if any bone surgery is planned.

General endotracheal anesthesia is used in all cases. *Special care* is taken not to disturb or contaminate the lesion while the infant is held supine briefly for intubation. Constant monitoring of EKG and heart sounds is employed. The patient is usually placed prone with rolls under the heating blanket to elevate the chest and hips, providing maximum respiratory freedom and maximum laxity of skin around the lesion. The skin is cleansed widely with iodophor, extending laterally as far as possible over the flanks, so that these areas are ready should large flaps or skin grafts be necessary for closure. The back is draped with transparent plastic so that the buttocks and lower extremities may be seen while electrical stimulation of the neural plaque and suspicious nerve roots is performed (Fig. 6-9a and b).

The surgical procedure consists of incision of the skin at the lateral margins of the sac, with careful separation of the splayed-out dura from the underlying lumbo-dorsal fascia and paravertebral musculature. The neural plaque is then separated from the overlying epithelialized sac membrane (Fig. 6-10). It is useful to employ the operating microscope for this part of the procedure; with the magnification and excellent lighting available, the surgeon is better able to preserve nerve roots and remove all epithelial elements.

The dural sac is completely separated from the subcutaneous tissues all around the lesion, and adhesions between nerve roots and connective tissue elements are divided. Occasionally, the nerve roots are fixed or trapped as they traverse the abnormal bony elements, and limited bony removal may be necessary. The objective is to have all the nerve roots and the neural plaque entirely free and untethered, and to remove all epithelioid tissue adherent to the neural plaque. When it is impossible to separate dorsal nerve roots from fibrous attachments to the dura or to subcutaneous lipomatous tissue, electrical stimulation should be utilized. If no motor response or bladder response is present, the roots may be sacrificed without danger to the future development of the patient. However, every effort should be made to preserve *all* neural tissue.

Once all the neural elements are free, a water-tight closure of the dura is performed over which artificial flaps of lumbo-dorsal fascia are placed. A two- or even three-layer closure over the dura is sometimes possible and is attempted in every case.

The surgeon is now faced with a large skin defect. In most cases it is possible to undermine widely the loose subcutaneous tissues of the newborn and to achieve primary wound closure under minimal tension. Very large defects may require rotation of flaps, relaxing incisions, and skin grafts, and the assistance of a plastic surgeon is sought whenever such difficulty is anticipated (Patterson and Till, 1959). In lumbo-sacral and sacral meningomyeloceles of large size, it is sometimes impossible to obtain fascial flaps to cover the dura, since the lumbo-dorsal fascia does not extend down to this region. In these cases, rotational skin flaps can provide good coverage for the meningomyelocele defect. We have found that large flaps may be managed with wound catheters under suction (Fig. 6-11). This helps them adhere rapidly to the underlying tissues and tends to prevent postoperative CSF leak (Fig. 6-12).

The repair of the routine meningomyelocele should take 60 to 90 minutes with a blood loss of 10 to 15 cc. Such a procedure is well tolerated by the

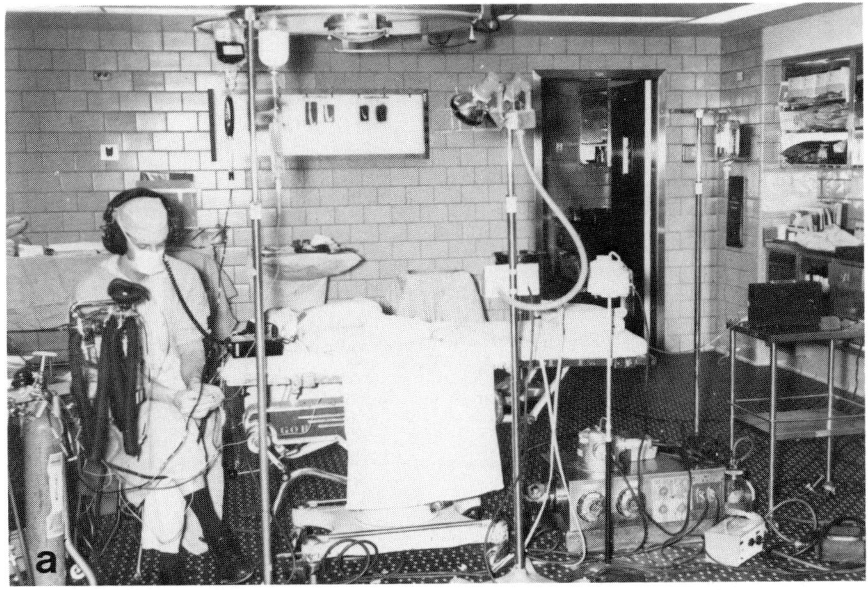

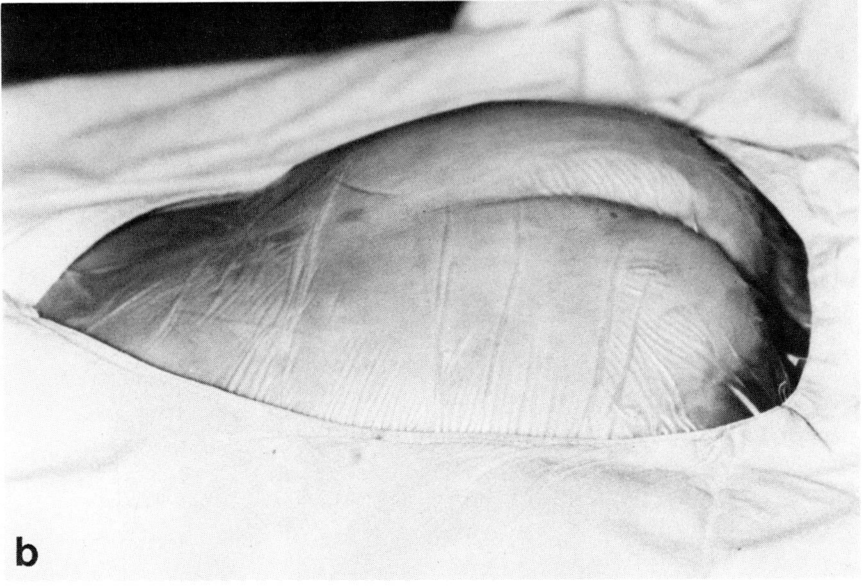

Fig. 6-9 Operating room arrangement for meningomyelocele. (a) Note position with endotracheal tube in place, EKG monitoring, rectal temperature probe, heating blanket beneath patient, infrared external heating lamps, and saphenous vein cutdown for intravenous fluids and blood. (b) Transparent plastic sterile draping in place.

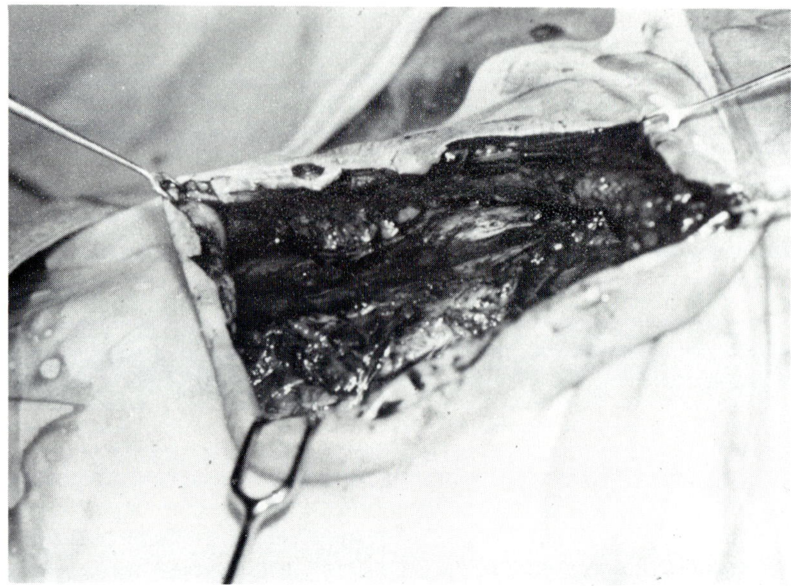

Fig. 6-10 Repair of a meningomyelocele. Intraoperative view of dissection of nerve roots and neural plaque.

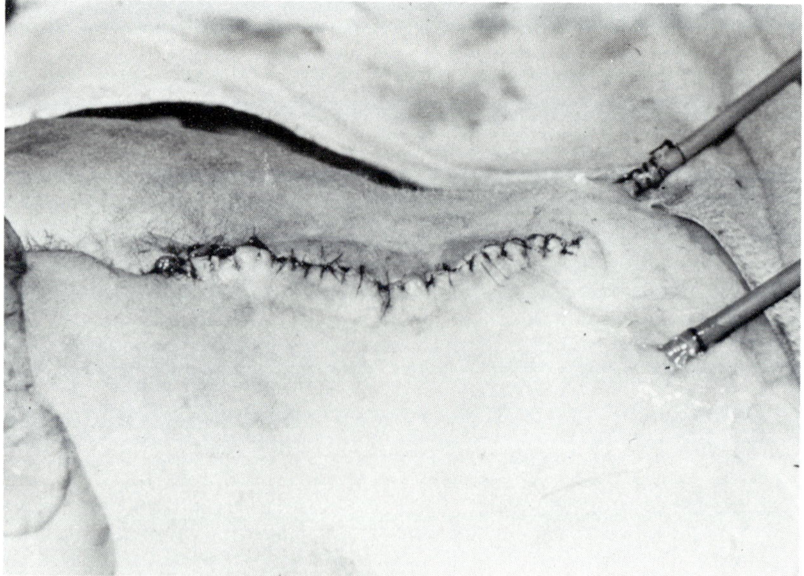

Fig. 6-11 Meningomyelocele repair. Note wound suction catheters.

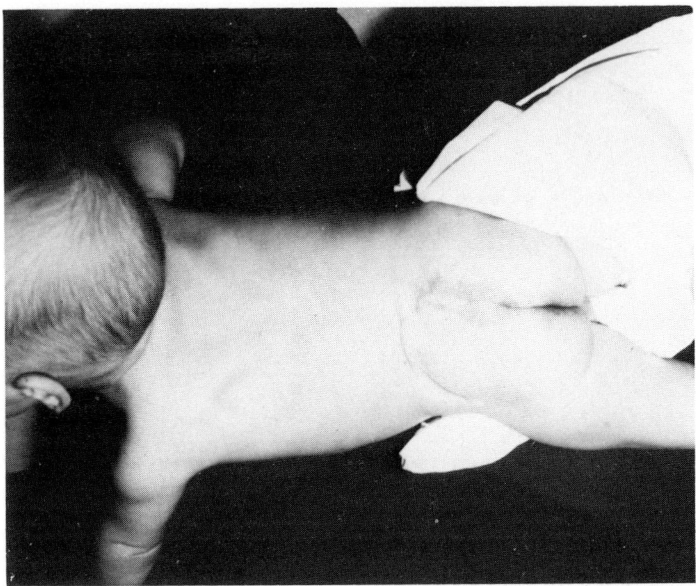

Fig. 6-12 Postoperative result of meningomyelocele closure.

newborn, and we have had no mortality and no morbidity attributable to the surgical procedure during the past six years. Risks are somewhat increased when spinal osteotomy or fusion is performed, but again we have had no operative mortality from these procedures. Postoperatively, the patient is managed in an isolette with a sling, designed to relax tension on the wound, supporting the abdomen (Fig. 6-13). Clear liquid oral feedings may begin as soon as the child is awake.

A head circumference chart should be started immediately. If it appears that the patient has obvious hydrocephalus, with bulging fontanelle and split sutures, continuous ventricular drainage by catheter may be advisable and may be continued safely for a period of 5 to 7 days. Ventricular drainage in this setting prevents further damage to the cortex and may also prevent CSF leakage from the operative site. Continuous drainage is preferable to repeated ventricular taps, since it is more physiological and avoids such complications of tapping as hemorrhage and porencephaly. CSF leakage which does occur in the immediate postoperative period will rarely stop spontaneously unless ventricular drainage or a shunt procedure is done early.

In the postoperative period particular attention should be paid to bladder function, with the Credé maneuver being performed at routine intervals by the nursing staff. Suprapubic taps or catheter drainage may be necessary if urinary retention occurs.

Antibiotics are employed only if the lesion was contaminated preoperatively or if ventricular drainage is used. Unless an organism has been cul-

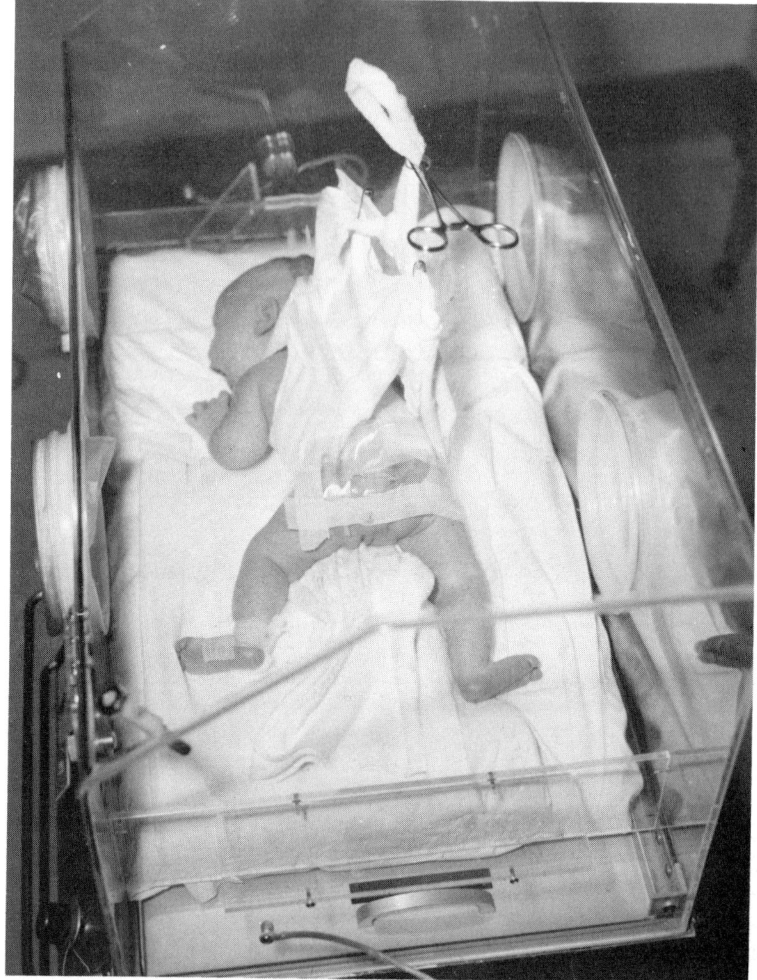

Fig. 6-13 Postoperative nursing arrangement with sling to support abdomen and relieve tension on the wound.

tured, broad-spectrum coverage is utilized, and monitoring of antibiotic levels in CSF and blood may be performed. Ventricular CSF should be cultured prior to the institution of antibiotic therapy, and is recultured at intervals during the period of antibiotic coverage.

Routine daily assessments of head circumference and of motor and sensory function should be made and recorded, and once the patient is stable, the parents should again be counseled. The general comments made to the parents concerning prognosis in the preoperative period should be expanded upon, and the probable need for surgical treatment of hydrocephalus, orthopedic deformities, and urinary incontinence should be reemphasized.

CRANIAL MENINGOCELES AND ENCEPHALOCELES

These lesions are further examples of the dysraphic state, and, while much less common than spina bifida manifesta, the basic principles of management are similar (Fig. 6-14). Ulceration of the sac or frank leakage of CSF are indications for immediate repair except in those patients who have obvious extensive malformations of the brain or other associated congenital defects. If the sac contains no neural tissue, it may be closed simply as an elective procedure. When a sac contains malformed cerebral tissue, adequate closure may necessitate the amputation of small quantities of the brain substance within the sac; this can usually be done without serious compromise of neurological function or potential. Whenever possible, the treatment of cranial encephaloceles should be delayed until the child is able to undergo adequate diagnostic procedures, which may include arteriography and pneumoencephalography, and until enough development has occurred so that one may assess the patient's degree of neurological deficit.

Like meningomyeloceles, cranial meningoceles and encephaloceles may be associated with hydrocephalus. Those lesions which occur at the cranio-cervical junction are frequently accompanied by malformations of structures within the posterior fossa, and hydrocephalus is common.

MANAGEMENT OF POSTOPERATIVE COMPLICATIONS

The most common postoperative complication in children with meningomyeloceles is breakdown of the wound closure. When the defect is closed

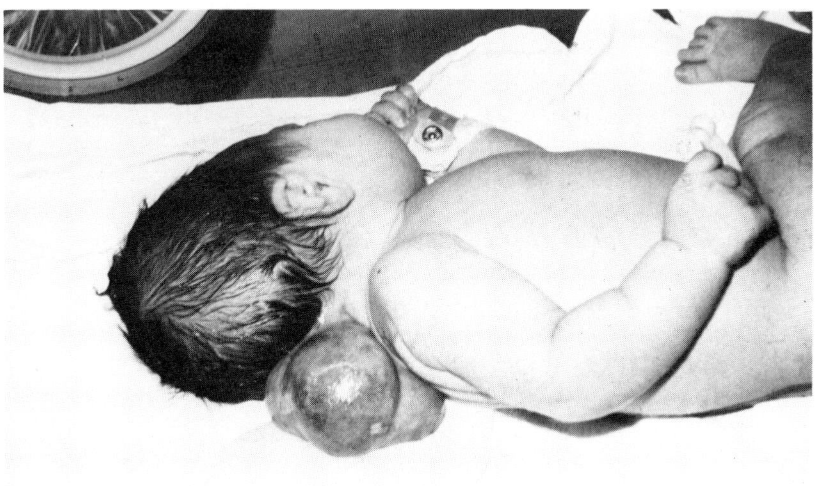

Fig. 6-14 Cranio-cervical meningoencephalocele. This lesion was successfully removed and repaired.

under considerable tension, a small area of dehiscence in the center of the wound, where the tension is the greatest, may occur. Under most circumstances, if adequate coverage of the dural sac has been obtained by means of fascia, and if a good subcutaneous closure has also been achieved, the dehiscence of the external layer of skin is of no consequence. The wound granulates in over a period of 7 to 10 days. In rare cases there is actual necrosis of the edges of the wound where they are closed under tension, and this may produce a wider and more extensive dehiscence, which usually will heal slowly, but may require skin grafting. Wide undermining of the skin flaps prior to the actual closure of the skin at surgery will ordinarily prevent such defects of wound closure. An abdominal sling or support to take tension off the wound edges in the postoperative period is also useful.

Another relatively frequent complication is leakage of CSF from the area of skin breakdown. Once again, the most satisfactory means of preventing this complication is the achievement of a secure, water-tight dural closure with additional flaps of subcutaneous tissue closing the wound in the deeper layers. Occasionally leaks occur even in the presence of a technically adequate repair because of the onset of progressive severe hydrocephalus and increased intracranial pressure transmitted to the lumbar subarachnoid space. When CSF leak does occur, attempts at secondary closure of the wound are usually futile. If the leak persists with the baby in a relatively head-down position, one must resort either to ventricular drainage for a period of 5 to 7 days or to early ventriculography and shunting.

The most disastrous complications following repair of meningomyeloceles are wound infection and the secondary complications of meningitis and ventriculitis. Meticulous sterile technique and vigorous postoperative management of the patient and his wound will help prevent these complications. If the possibility of meningitis or ventriculitis is suspected, no hesitation should be permitted in tapping the ventricle and obtaining samples of CSF for a cell count and culture, and appropriate antibiotic therapy should be instituted immediately.

Nursing care, intelligently designed and diligently executed, is crucial to the prevention of complications. The position of the baby should be explained carefully to the nursing staff, and the necessity for the abdominal sling and its proper fitting, placement, and tension should be demonstrated to all those caring for the patient. They should be instructed in methods of feeding the child, so that tension is not placed on the wound. They must understand that the wound is not to be contaminated in any way. The nursing staff should make every attempt to prevent stool and urine from soiling the area of the wound or the dressings. For this reason, we ordinarily attempt to manage the patients with little or no dressing covering the wound, so that it may be inspected at any time, and so that contamination becomes obvious immediately. The perineal region may be sealed off from the wound by the use of an adhesive plastic drape.

The nursing staff should be taught to pay attention to the patient's urinary output and to perform the Credé maneuver to ensure emptying of the bladder. The physicians caring for the patient must be alert to the possibility of urinary retention. Because of the face-down position in the sling, ulceration of the knees and other pressure points may occur, and this must be guarded against.

Enthusiastic and careful surgery coupled with diligent postoperative care will minimize complications during this initial stage of therapy.

SUMMARY

Neurological and neurosurgical evaluation of the infant with meningomyelocele will permit accurate prognosis of the child's neurological deficit. Early closure of the defect will prevent infection and drying of the neural elements and thus offer the best preservation of existing neurological function. Closure should be done within the first 24 hours. Careful dissection and preservation of the neural elements, removal of lipomatous tissue, and release of the structures tethering the cord will permit optimal neurological function. Meticulous nursing care can help in the prevention of wound breakdown and CSF leaks. The ultimate prognosis of these children is to a large extent related to the diligence and the enthusiasm of the neurosurgeon involved in the child's early care.

BIBLIOGRAPHY

Brocklehurst, G., J. R. W. Ghave, and W. S. Lewin. 1966. Early closure of myelomeningocele with especial reference to leg movement. Develop. Med. Child Neurol. Supp. 13:51.

Cameron, A. H. 1957. The Arnold-Chiari and other neuro-anatomical malformations associated with spina bifida. J. Path. Bact. 73:195.

Campbell, J. B. 1948. Congenital anomalies of the neural axis. Surgical management based on embryologic considerations. Am. J. Surg. 75:231.

Doran, P. A., and A. N. Guthkelch. 1961. Studies in spina bifida cystica. I. General survey and reassessment of the problem. J. Neurol. Neurosurg. Psychiat. 24:331.

Doran, P. A., and A. N. Guthkelch. 1963. Studies in spina bifida. IV. The frequency and extent of paralysis. J. Neurol. Neurosurg. Psychiat. 26:545.

Guthkelch, A. N. 1962. Studies in spina bifida cystica. II. When to repair the spinal defect. J. Neurol. Neurosurg. Psychiat. 25:147.

Ingraham, F. D., H. Swan, H. Hamlin, J. Lowrey, D. Matson, and H. Scott. 1943. Spina bifida and cranium bifidum. Harvard University Press, Boston.

Jackson, I. J., I. M. Thompson, C. A. Hooks, and G. T. Hoffman. 1956. Urinary incontinence in myelomeningoceles due to a tethered spinal cord and its surgical treatment. Surg. Gynec. Obstet. 103:618.

Laurence, K. M. 1960. The natural history of spina bifida cystica. Proc. Roy. Soc. Med. 53:1055.

Laurence, K. M. 1964. The natural history of spina bifida cystica: detailed analysis of 407 cases. Arch. Dis. Childh. 39:41.

Laurence, K. M. 1966. The survival of untreated spina bifida cystica. Develop. Med. Child Neurol. Supp. 11:10.

Lorber, J. 1961. Systematic ventriculographic studies in infants born with meningomyelocele and encephalocele. The incidence and development of hydrocephalus. Arch. Dis. Childh. 36:381.

Lorber, J. 1965. Family history of spina bifida cystica. Pediatrics 35:589.

Lorber, J., and M. Segal. 1962. Bacterial meningitis in spina bifida cystica. A review of 37 cases. Arch. Dis. Childh. 37:300.

Lichtenstein, B. W. 1940. Spinal dysraphism; spina bifida and myelodysplasia. Arch. Neurol. Psychiat. 44:792.

Lichtenstein, B. W. 1942. Distant neuroanatomic complications of spina bifida (spinal dysraphism). Hydrocephalus, Arnold-Chiari deformity, stenosis of the aqueduct of Sylvius, etc., pathogenesis and pathology. Arch. Neurol. Psychiat. 47:195.

Matson, D. D. 1969. Neurosurgery of infancy and childhood. Charles C Thomas, Publisher, Springfield, Ill.

Patterson, T. J. S., and K. Till. 1959. The use of rotation flaps following excision of lumbar myelomeningoceles; an aid to the closure of large defects. Brit. J. Surg. 46:606.

Rickham, P. D., and T. Mawdsley. 1966. The effect of early operation on the survival of spina bifida cystica. Develop. Med. Child Neurol. Supp. 11:20.

Rose, R. S., and J. P. Smith. 1963. Hydronephrosis in infants with meningomyelocele: its early recognition. J. Urol. 90:129.

Russell, D. S., and C. Donald. 1935. The mechanism of internal hydrocephalus in spina bifida. Brain 58:203.

Sharrard, W. J. W., R. B. Zachary, J. Lorber, and A. M. Bruce. 1963. A controlled trial of immediate and delayed closure of spina bifida cystica. Arch. Dis. Childh. 38:18.

Smith, E. D. 1965. Spina bifida and the total care of spinal myelomeningocele. Charles C Thomas, Publisher, Springfield, Ill.

Stark, G. D., and M. Drummond. 1971. The spinal cord lesion in meningomyelocele. Develop. Med. Child Neurol. Supp. 25:1.

7

The Management of Hydrocephalus

Edward R. Laws, Jr., M.D.

Coincident with the embryological defects in neural tube closure resulting in meningomyelocele, congenital defects also occur in midline structures at the upper end of the neuraxis. Thus more than 90% of infants with meningomyeloceles also have abnormalities at the cranio-cervical junction, and/or at the level of the aqueduct of Sylvius, resulting in hydrocephalus (Russell and Donald, 1935; Laurence, 1959; Matson, 1964; Lorber, 1971). Anatomically the most common defect is the Arnold-Chiari malformation (Chiari, 1895; Barry et al., 1957), a downward displacement of the cerebellar tonsils and fourth ventricle, associated with redundancy of the upper cervical spinal cord and lower medulla (McConnell and Parker, 1938) (Fig. 7-1). The Arnold-Chiari defect is frequently accompanied by stenosis, occlusion, or forking of the aqueduct of Sylvius (Lichtenstein, 1959; van Hoytema and van den Berg, 1966). Any of these anomalies has the potential of obstructing the normal pathways of CSF flow and absorption. In most instances hydrocephalus is present at birth (Laurence, 1951) and becomes manifest in the neonatal period. While hydrocephalus may appear to be precipitated by closure of the meningomyelocele defect (Williams, 1971), there is no evidence that closure of the meningomyelocele sac increases the incidence of hydrocephalus.

Once the predisposition of these patients to develop hydrocephalus is recognized, the necessity for a method of clinical evaluation and for the establishment of guidelines for the diagnosis and treatment of the condition is clear.

DIAGNOSIS

Physical findings suggestive of hydrocephalus are searched for at the first examination and monitored daily thereafter. The head circumference is

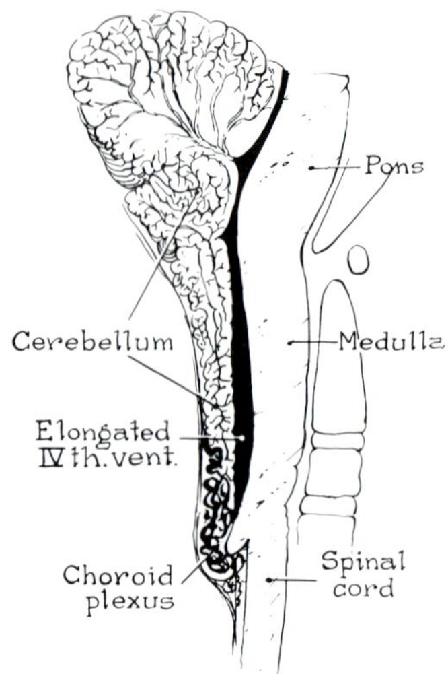

Fig. 7-1 Arnold-Chiari malformation. Note downward displacement of cerebellar tonsils.

carefully measured. The skull is examined for general configuration and proportion, for widening of the sutures, and for conformation and tenseness of the fontanelles. Other signs which may develop as hydrocephalus increases are prominence and distortion of scalp veins and the "setting-sun" appearance of the eyes. These features of the infant are evaluated on a daily basis, and a chart of daily head circumference measurements is kept and compared to norms.

A small percentage of children with meningomyeloceles will have obvious hydrocephalus at birth, and these are detected without difficulty. In the majority, hydrocephalus becomes manifest more or less gradually during the first weeks of life. The most practical and generally available method for following the development of hydrocephalus is measurement of head circumference. The sequential plotting of measurements establishes the rate of increase in head size, which is more important than the absolute measurements in evaluating the progression of hydrocephalus and the necessity for treatment. A rapid rate of growth from the third to the ninety-seventh percentile may be just as significant as growth crossing the ninety-seventh percentile.

Echoencephalography has come to be a reliable tool with which to follow ventricular size in patients with hydrocephalus (Fig. 7-2). In skilled and experienced hands, the echo will demonstrate reproducible reflections of ultrasound from the lateral walls of the lateral ventricles on either side, and frequently the two walls of the third ventricle will give reflections as well. These reflections allow us to follow the thickness of the cortical mantle (the distance from the inner table to the lateral wall of the lateral ventricle)

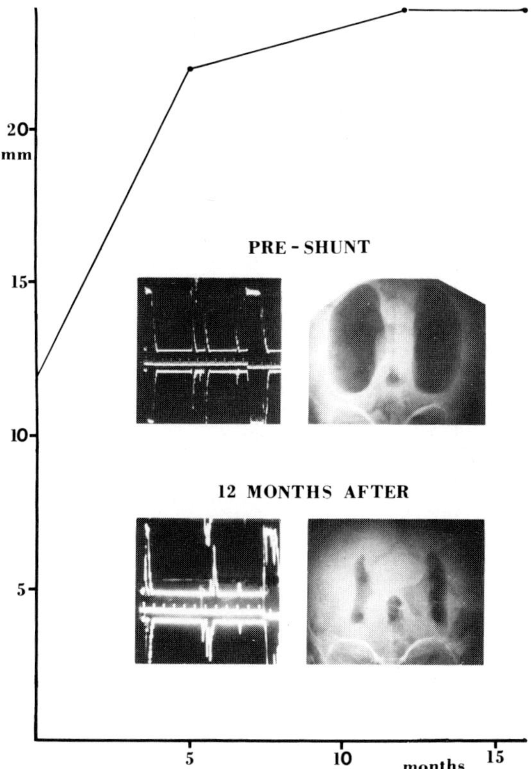

Fig. 7-2 Echoencephalogram in hydrocephalus. Echoes from the lateral ventricles correlate well with ventricular size on pneumoencephalogram and may be followed post-shunting. Graph indicates normal cortical mantle thickness with age. (Courtesy of Dr. Sumio Uematsu.)

and the diameter of the third ventricle as measures of the extent of hydrocephalus. As with head circumference, initial measurements are important, but it is the occurrence of progressive change over time that is crucial for decisions concerning treatment (Fig. 7-3A and B).

DIAGNOSTIC PROCEDURES

The most commonly employed diagnostic procedure for infants with hydrocephalus is air ventriculography. Ordinarily, the right lateral ventricle is punctured through the coronal suture with a 20-gauge needle. CSF pressure is measured and a sample taken for analysis of cell count, protein, glucose, culture, and serology. Then 15 to 50 cc of air are injected, with removal of a nearly equal volume of CSF, and a series of x-rays is taken (Fig. 7-4a, b, and c). These include brow-up, brow-down, and hanging views for demonstration of the aqueduct of Sylvius and the fourth ventricle. Positive contrast ventriculography with pantopaque rarely improves on the results of a care-

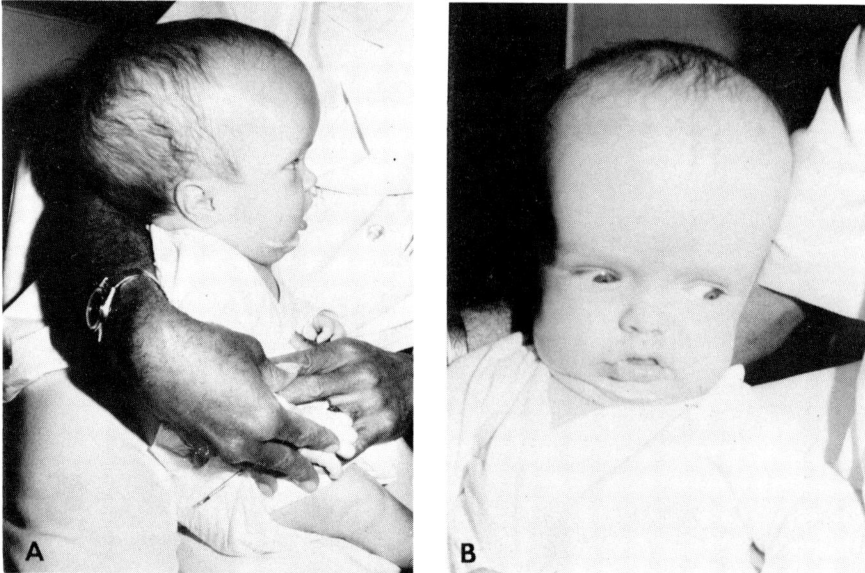

Fig. 7-3 (A and B) Typical appearance of hydrocephalic infant. Note "setting-sun" appearance of eyes and prominent scalp veins.

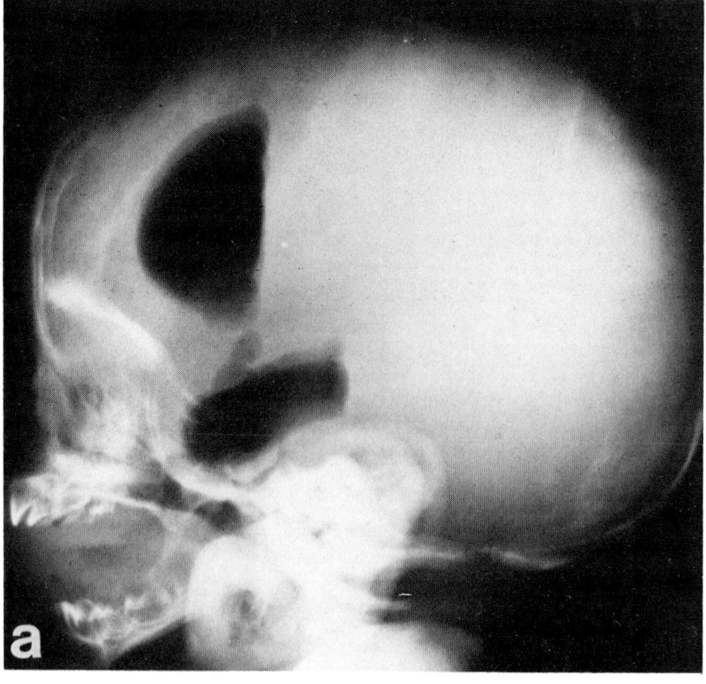

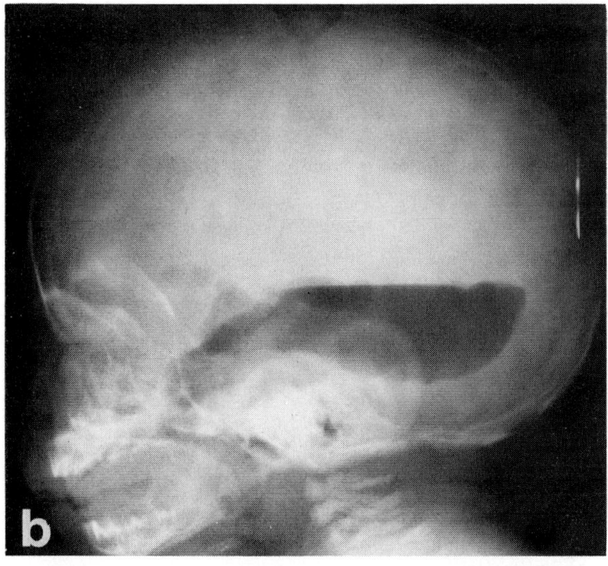

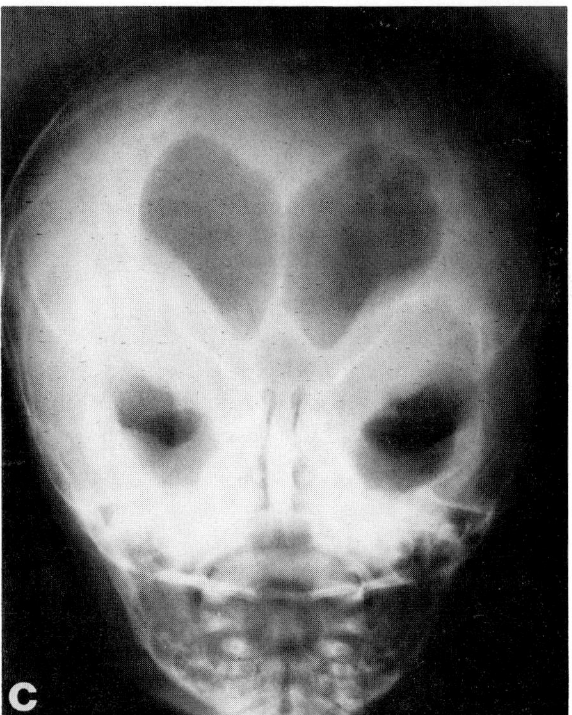

Fig. 7-4 (a, b, and c) Meningomyelocele patient with enlarging head, age 16 days. Trans-coronal ventriculogram demonstrating hydrocephalus secondary to aqueductal stenosis. The posterior fossa is characteristically small and underdeveloped.

ful air study, and is seldom employed. Because of the meningomyelocele in these patients, lumbar air encephalography is hazardous and is, therefore, rarely utilized.

The appropriate time for ventriculography in patients with meningomyeloceles is still a subject of some controversy. Recommendations in the literature range from routine ventriculography shortly after birth to waiting until the head circumference reaches a value 3 cm greater than the ninety-seventh percentile (Laurence, 1959; Lorber, 1971). Our practice is to observe the child closely and to use head circumference and echoencephalography to obtain an estimate of how rapidly the ventricles are enlarging. If the ventricles are growing rapidly, and the head circumference measurements cross percentile lines on the normal growth chart at a rapid rate, reaching the ninety-seventh percentile within the first two weeks of life, then ventriculography is done early, most often between the fifth and twenty-first days of life. If the head circumference grows slowly and shows an indication of leveling off, even if at the ninety-seventh percentile, we prefer to observe the patient if echoencephalography shows a cortical mantle of 15 mm or more.

Ventriculography almost always demonstrates the anatomical cause of the observed hydrocephalus. The majority of our patients with meningomyeloceles who develop hydrocephalus have aqueductal stenosis or occlusion, and no air from the lateral ventricle will enter the aqueduct or fourth ventricle. Most of these patients presumably also have the Arnold-Chiari malformation at the craniocervical junction. In those infants where the aqueduct is patent, one is able to demonstrate downward displacement of the fourth ventricle and herniation of the cerebellar tonsils through the foramen magnum in almost every case (Fig. 7-5). Associated defects which are independent of the hydrocephalus may also be seen by ventriculography. These abnormalities include absence of the septum pellucidum, agenesis of the corpus collosum (cyclops ventricle), midline cysts such as cavum septum pellucidum and cavum vergae, and areas of cerebral agenesis or porencephaly.

Occasionally the timing of ventriculography is affected by exigencies of the meningomyelocele. In a number of patients, the meningomyelocele repair is subjected to great stress or CSF leakage by a rapidly progressive hydrocephalus. These patients are managed by a period of two to seven days of constant ventricular drainage. Either during the period of drainage or just prior to the removal of the catheter, a ventriculogram is performed by injecting air through the drain. Nearly all of these infants require early treatment with a shunt. Some patients with the Arnold-Chiari malformation may develop signs of brainstem decompensation during or following meningomyelocele repair, and these patients may require immediate ventricular drainage and early ventriculography and shunting (Sieben, Hamida, and Shulman, 1971).

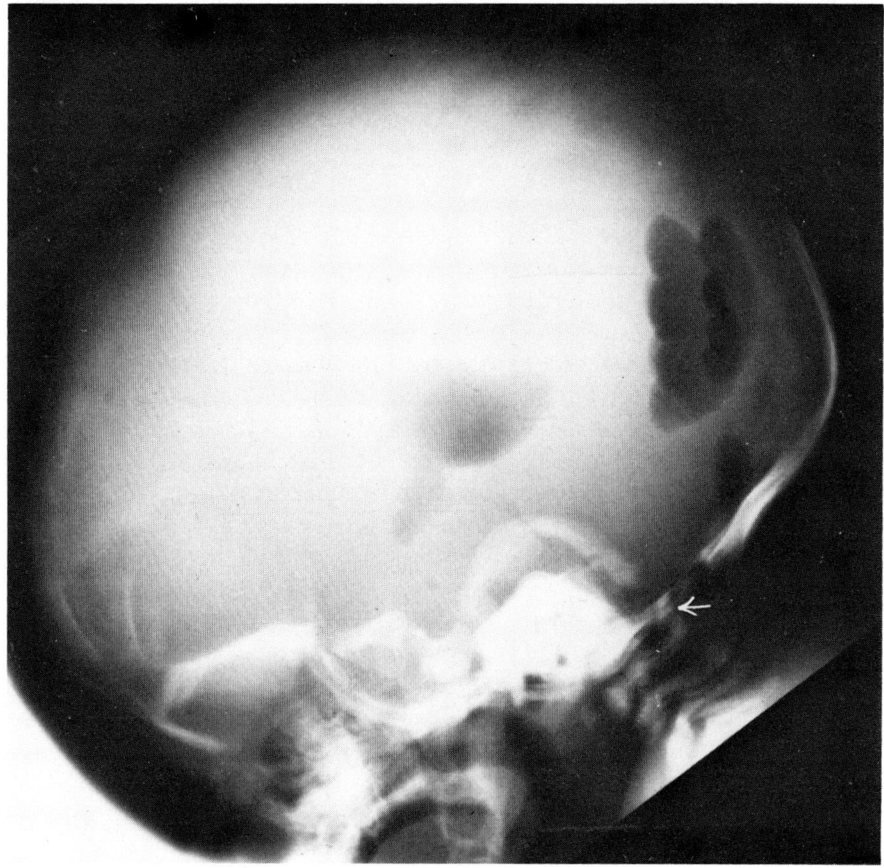

Fig. 7-5 Meningomyelocele patient with enlarging head, age 20 days. Pneumoencephalogram demonstrating abnormally low position of the fourth ventricle (arrow) seen in the Arnold-Chiari malformation.

TREATMENT

At present, the only satisfactory long-term treatment for progressive hydrocephalus is a shunt procedure (Foltz and Shurtleff, 1963; Scarff, 1963; Lorber, 1971). The shunt produces internal diversion of CSF from the ventricular system to a place within the body where it can be absorbed. In an infant with a meningomyelocele and hydrocephalus, the most practical routes for diversion of the 300–600 ml of CSF produced per day are into the venous system or into the peritoneal cavity (Overton and Snodgrass, 1965; Pudenz, 1966; Nulsen and Becker, 1967; Lorber, 1969; Delcour, Grunêwald, and Galebert, 1971). Both ventriculo-jugular (atrial) and ventriculo-peritoneal shunts have been used successfully for some time, and technological aspects of the shunts are constantly improving. Both types of shunt share certain problems, and each has its own peculiar disadvantages.

Shunt devices in current use consist of three parts: a ventricular end, most often positioned in the frontal horn of a lateral ventricle; a flushing device, usually fixed to the skull; and a distal end designed for insertion into either the right atrium of the heart or the peritoneal cavity. At some point in every system there is a pressure-regulated one-way valve, and most components are made of high-grade, low-reactivity silastic.

The surgical procedure for insertion of either type of shunt is relatively simple, and may be performed under local, Ketamine, or general anesthesia. Generally, the operation is well tolerated, even by newborn infants, and takes 30–60 minutes to perform, with minimal anticipated blood loss. The precautions of having a stable intravenous line and cross-matched blood are routinely taken. A curvilinear scalp incision is made, usually in the right parieto-occipital region, and the dura is exposed by a twist-drill or burr hole through the thin skull. A subcutaneous tunnel is then made from the scalp incision to the neck or the abdomen, and the incision made for placement of the distal end of the shunt. The components of the shunt are tested for proper function and opening pressure and then assembled and fixed in place. The skin wounds are carefully closed (Figs. 7-6 and 7-7).

For reasons to be discussed below, we prefer the ventriculo-peritoneal shunt, using a ventricular end designed to prevent occlusion by choroid plexus or ependymal wall, a dome-shaped one-way valve flushing device which may be tapped with a needle for CSF withdrawal or flushing, and a spring-reinforced nonkinking peritoneal end with a calibrated slit valve at its distal end (Raimondi). The incision for the peritoneal end is made in the paraxiphoid region. The peritoneum is opened over the liver, and 20–30 cm of peritoneal catheter are inserted freely into the abdominal cavity and secured with a loose pursestring suture at the peritoneal opening. In most cases, a medium-pressure peritoneal valve opening at a pressure of 40–60 mm of water is employed.

The majority of meningomyelocele patients who have shunt procedures done early in infancy remain dependent on a shunt for the rest of their lives. Even those who do not have aqueductal stenosis when initially shunted run a high risk of developing aqueductal obstruction once a functioning shunt has been in place for a period of time (Foltz and Shurtleff, 1966). A small number of patients with the Arnold-Chiari malformation who need a shunt early in life may eventually outgrow their dependency and reach a state of so-called "arrested" hydrocephalus.

THE MANAGEMENT OF THE PATIENT WITH A SHUNT

The realization of full intellectual potential in a patient with a meningomyelocele and hydrocephalus is dependent in large part on the continued effectiveness of the shunt. Maintaining this effectiveness demands diligent,

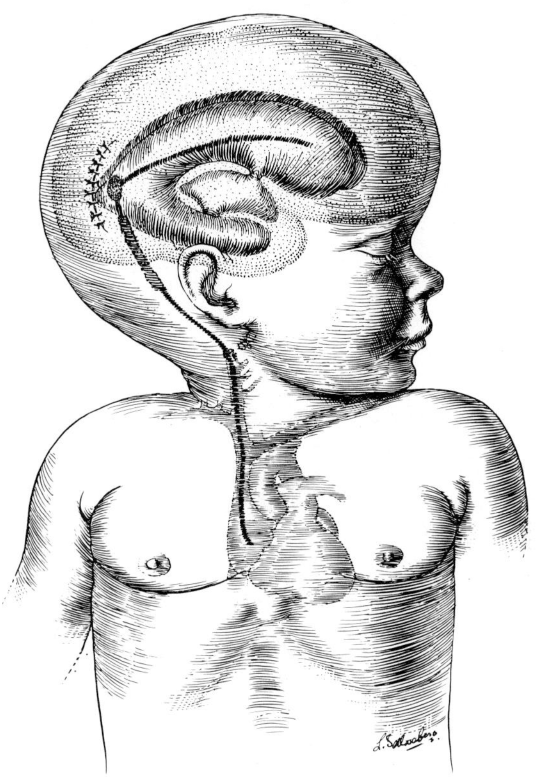

Fig. 7-6 Ventriculo-atrial shunt using Holter valve and Rickham reservoir at cranial end.

careful, and informed follow-up, and prompt, decisive action when shunt malfunction occurs.

The physician following such a patient must know the etiology of the hydrocephalus, since this information may have direct bearing on how shunt-dependent the patient may be. The child with aqueductal stenosis may decompensate much more quickly than the child with communicating hydrocephalus and an Arnold-Chiari malformation. Accurate information on the type of shunt in place is also essential. Pumping devices vary in their characteristics and conformation, and a familiarity with the different types is desirable. It is important, as well, to know whether the patient has an atrial or a peritoneal shunt; the former type tends to block more quickly as growth occurs.

Several techniques may be used in confirming the diagnosis of shunt malfunction or obstruction. The most readily testable feature of the shunt itself is the flushing device attached to the skull. The pump should be easily depressable and should fill out rapidly; if it does not do so, one must suspect that the shunt is *not* functioning properly (Table 7-1). If isotope tracer is

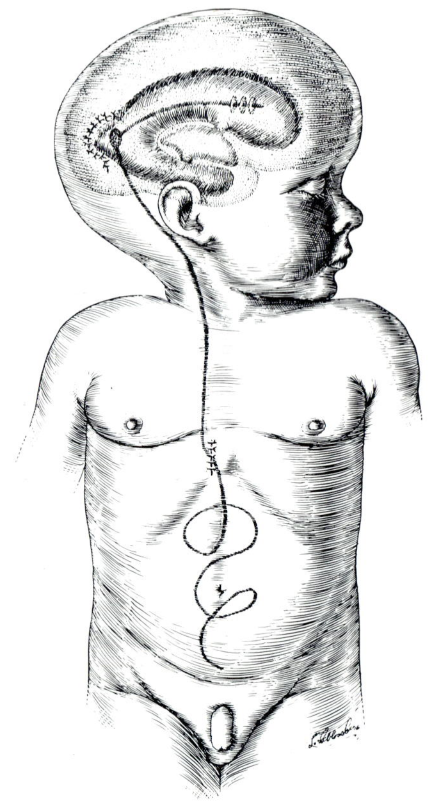

Fig. 7-7 Ventriculo-peritoneal shunt using Pudenz valve at cranial end, multi-perforated flanged ventricular catheter, and Raimondi peritoneal catheter.

injected into the CSF, scanning will demonstrate whether or not isotope in the CSF flows into the right atrium or the peritoneal cavity (depending on the type of shunt present); and this technique may be useful for children with very early and minimal signs of decompensation. It should be emphasized that in the follow-up care of children with hydrocephalus, *any symptoms including changes in the state of consciousness, headache, nausea, or vomiting must be considered as evidence of some malfunction until it is proven otherwise.* It is felt that the diligent application of this principle can markedly decrease the figures for mortality in patients with hydrocephalus and shunts; at the Johns Hopkins Hospital over the past six years, we have had no mortality from shunt obstruction or malfunction.

Infection may occur at any point in the course of treatment. Any child with a shunt who has previously had meningitis, ventriculitis, or septicemia must be considered at risk for repeated infection so long as the foreign material of the shunt is present. It has been our experience that some patients with a history of ventriculitis lose the ability to dilate their lateral ventricles

Table 7-1 "Trouble-Shooting" Chart for Management of Patients with Shunts

Status of patient	Status of shunt	Probable diagnosis	Solution
Normal	Pumps freely Fills freely	Functioning shunt	Routine follow-up
Normal	Pumps freely Fills slowly	Partial obstruction, ventricular end a) plugged with choroid plexus or ependyma b) ventricular collapse around tip of shunt	Close follow-up
Normal	Pumps with difficulty or not at all	Obstruction of distal end, probable compensated hydrocephalus	Close follow-up
Symptomatic	Pumps freely Fills freely	a) Disconnection in shunt system b) Cyst around peritoneal end c) Symptoms not shunt-related, e.g., subdurals, systemic disease	Repair shunt Revise distal end Appropriate diagnostic tests
Symptomatic	Pumps freely Fills slowly or not at all	Obstruction of ventricular end by ependyma, choroid plexus, or fibrin clot	Revise shunt
Symptomatic	Pumps poorly or not at all	Distal obstruction resulting from growth of patient, kinking of tubing, clot, adhesions, etc.	Revise shunt

as compensation for increased intracranial pressure. These patients react as if their ventricular walls had become toughened, and may decompensate rapidly without showing signs of ventricular enlargement. Fortunately, most patients with hydrocephalus react to shunt blockage over a period of time during which symptoms of rapidly increasing intracranial pressure are evident. However, one cannot emphasize too strongly the need for a high index of suspicion and rapid action whenever untoward symptoms develop. We have seen patients have a respiratory arrest within 12 hours of the onset of symptoms due to a blocked shunt.

Shunt malfunction is not the only reason for decompensation in a hydrocephalic patient. One of the most devastating and difficult complications to manage is the occurrence of subdural hematomas as a consequence of the relative lack of intraventricular pressure in the child with a functioning shunt. The development of a hemiparesis or decrease in state of consciousness, particularly following a head injury, may be the result of a subdural hematoma. This complication is relatively rare, but must be kept in mind. Not infrequently the subdural hematomas occur bilaterally, sometimes without lateralizing signs and with no midline shift on echo. Diagnosis is made by subdural tap or arteriography, and treatment consists of drainage. Successful treatment may require temporary interruption of shunt function, but frequently, with careful management, the shunt can be left undisturbed.

ARRESTED HYDROCEPHALUS—OR HOW LONG DOES TREATMENT CONTINUE?

The definition of "arrested hydrocephalus" has classically been that the head has ceased to grow, or grows parallel to the normal rate and within the normal circumference range (Shick and Matson, 1961). Arrest may occur spontaneously even in children with meningomyeloceles (Lorber, 1969), or it may occur after shunting. In the latter case, a child who has been doing well, but whose shunt has clearly ceased to function, is considered "arrested," although the mechanisms by which CSF production and CSF absorption become equilibrated are not entirely clear. It is noteworthy that Matson (1969) states that "many children with spontaneously arrested hydrocephalus do well in development until the age of six to eight years. The discrepancy between their expected and actual level of function in both mental and motor spheres becomes progressively greater." Other children with "arrest" after shunt may also manifest slow intellectual deterioration, or rapid deterioration with minor colds, infections, and head trauma.

The advent of echoencephalography has enabled the assessment of ventricular size without the hazards of anteriography, or the risks of precipitating "active" hydrocephalus by pneumoencephalography. Serial echoencephalography has revealed children with "arrested" hydrocephalus and markedly dilated ventricles who have great improvement in intellectual performance after insertion of a new functioning shunt. This gradual increase of ventricular size may occur without an increase in head circumference.

It is clear that earlier concepts of "arrested hydrocephalus" are not wholly satisfactory and that further work must be done to establish more adequate criteria. For the present it is our policy to follow the condition of every child with hydrocephalus, with or without a shunt, with periodic echoencephalography, performed every three to six months. Periodic psychometric assessment of intellectual performance is also undertaken. Progressive ventricular enlargement and a drop in intellectual performance are utilized as indicators for further evaluation with arteriography or pneumoencephaly.

In children with "arrested" hydrocephalus and a nonfunctioning shunt, the shunt is removed only if it causes physical or psychological distress to the patient.

RESULTS AND COMPLICATIONS OF SHUNT PROCEDURES

Barring immediate technical complications, a shunt procedure may be expected to relieve obstructive hydrocephalus for a period of six months to five or six years, the average being about 1½ years, before revision of the shunt is necessary.

The most frequent cause of shunt malformation is obstruction of the distal catheter. In atrial shunts this occurs with the growth of the child as the distal end is pulled upward out of the right atrium into the superior vena cava where venous occlusion occurs. With peritoneal shunts, distal occlusion also occurs with growth, and the distal end may be pulled up out of the peritoneum. Peritoneal shunts may become occluded by investment of the distal tip with omentum, or by pseudocyst formation, because the reaction of the peritoneal cavity to the continued presence of an in-dwelling foreign body results in a tendency to wall off the peritoneal end of the shunt. Recent changes in materials and design of the peritoneal catheter and the placement of 20–30 cm of tubing within the peritoneal cavity have tended to decrease the frequency of these causes of distal occlusion with peritoneal shunts.

Both basic types of shunts are prone to malfunction resulting from kinking of the catheters in their subcutaneous tracts, and from separation of the components at their connecting sites. Again, these problems are being solved by changes in design; nonkinking tubes are being introduced and connectors are being improved or eliminated.

The ventricular ends of shunts may become occluded by entanglement with choroid plexus or by overgrowth of ependyma where catheter tips rest against ventricular walls. Improvements in design have been directed toward the elimination of these complications.

With the utilization of the most modern devices incorporating improvements in concept and design, and with careful surgical technique, it is reasonable to expect that shunt procedures will be more effective and will continue to function for longer periods of time.

Second to malfunction, the most common complication of shunt procedures is infection. This includes wound infection, ventriculitis, and meningitis, which may occur with all kinds of shunts. More specific complications are endocarditis and septicemia occurring in patients with atrial shunts (Luthardt, 1970), and peritonitis occurring in patients with peritoneal shunts. These infectious complications are frequent and are especially serious because they occur in conjunction with an in-dwelling foreign body. There is evidence that the shunt itself becomes colonized with the infectious agent (Cohen and Callaghan, 1961; Holt, 1970), and once this occurs the infection is virtually impossible to eradicate permanently without removal of all the foreign material.

Improvements in design, technique, and management have decreased the incidence of infectious complications from 30% to less than 10%, and further improvements are anticipated. Prophylactic antibiotics have not proved useful in lowering the infection rate and are recommended only when specific indications exist. The incidence of complications, either from malposition of the various portions of the shunt or from infection, is greater when shunts are performed by junior residents or neurosurgeons who do not consider such procedures as serious or important. The value of experience and of consistent, careful technique cannot be overemphasized if good results are to be anticipated from shunt operations.

When infection does occur after a shunt procedure, new concepts in management of this complication have improved the outlook for infected patients and have markedly decreased the morbidity (McLaurin and Dodson, 1971; Perrin and McLaurin, 1967). Once the infecting organism is identified, specific antibiotics in appropriately high dosage can be used, with monitoring of antibiotic levels in blood and CSF. If ventriculitis is present or if there is colonization of the ventricular end of the shunt, intraventricular instillation of appropriate antibiotics may be indicated; this can be done through the shunt itself. After 48 hours of appropriate systemic and intraventricular antibiotic therapy, the infected shunt device may be removed and a new shunt installed at the same setting. This regimen has been remarkably effective in the treatment of infected shunts. Severe ventriculitis can and should be managed by the direct intraventricular instillation of appropriate antibiotics; this can be done safely if adequate precautions are taken concerning dose regulation and dilution of the antibiotic agent prior to injection within the ventricle.

Long-term complications peculiar to ventriculo-atrial shunts (Erdohazi, Eckstein, and Crome, 1966; Emery and Hilton, 1961; Noonan and Ehmke, 1963; Nugent et al., 1966) include subacute endocarditis, cardiac valvular damage and vegetations, embolization of the catheters into the heart and lung, occlusion of the superior vena cava and the superior mediastinal syndrome, right heart failure, and the septicemia mentioned above. Certainly, bacterial endocarditis and systemic sepsis are the most common complications, and these must be treated by removal of the foreign body within the right atrium and appropriate high levels of systemic antibiotic therapy.

Ventriculo-peritoneal shunts have fewer and less serious long-term complications, with pseudocyst formation, intestinal obstruction, and perforated viscera occurring rarely (Wilson and Bertan, 1966). This decreased potential for serious long-term complications and the ability to provide more adequately for growth of the patient lead us to favor the ventriculo-peritoneal shunt in the management of infantile hydrocephalus.

A complication which may occur with any type of shunt procedure is the development of subdural hematomas. A functioning shunt permits the possibility of a relative decrease in intracranial pressure, so that the surface of the brain itself may fall away from the dura, tearing bridging veins and causing development of subdural hematomas. This is one of the reasons why we discourage parents from routine pumping of the shunt device. This complication is rare, and occurs more frequently in older children who have closed sutures, so that the skull cannot adjust to changes in intracranial volume.

PROGNOSIS

The most crucial factor in the outlook for patients with meningomyeloceles is their potential for normal mental development. Current figures (Lorber, 1971) indicate that in meningomyelocele patients who develop hydrocephalus which is diagnosed and treated properly, two-thirds have a potential for a "normal" (80–130) IQ. This figure for patients with hydrocephalus and meningomyeloceles is lower than in patients with hydrocephalus alone. However, since most children with meningomyeloceles and hydrocephalus have the potential for a near-normal intellect, we are encouraged in our attempts at comprehensive, organized, enthusiastic, and meticulous care of these patients.

BIBLIOGRAPHY

Ames, R. H. 1967. Ventriculo-peritoneal shunts in the management of hydrocephalus. J. Neurosurg. 27:525.

Anderson, F. M. 1959. Ventriculo-auriculostomy in treatment of hydrocephalus. J. Neurosurg. 16:551.

Barry, A., B. M. Patten, and B. H. Stewart. 1957. Possible factors in the development of the Arnold-Chiari malformation. J. Neurosurg. 14:285.

Bruce, A. M., J. Lorber, W. I. H. Shedden, and R. B. Zachary. 1963. Persistent bacteremia following ventriculocaval shunt operations for hydrocephalus in infants. Develop. Med. Child Neurol. 5:461.

Cassinari, V., A. Migliore, and R. Villani. 1963. Le traitement de l'hydrocephalie par drainage extracranien. Observation d'àpres 113 cas. Neurochirurgie. 9:329.

Chiari, H. 1895. Über Veränderungen des Kleinhirns, des Pons und der Medulla Oblongata in Folge von congenitaler Hydrocephalie des Grosshirns. Denkschr. Akad. Wiss. Wien. 63:71.

Cohen, S. J., and R. P. Callaghan. 1961. A syndrome due to the bacterial colonization of Spitz-Holter valves. A review of 5 cases. Brit. Med. J. 2:677.

Delcour, J., P. Grunêwald, and P. Galebert. 1971. Notre experience en drainage ventriculo-peritoneal des hydrocephalies. Neurochirurgie 17:157.

Elkins, C. W., and J. G. Fonseca. 1961. Ventriculovenous anastomosis in obstructive and acquired hydrocephalus. J. Neurosurg. 18:139.

Emery, J. L., and H. Z. Hilton. 1961. Lung and heart complications of the treatment of hydrocephalus by ventriculoauriculostomy. Surgery 50:309.

Erdohazi, M., H. B. Eckstein, and L. Crome. 1966. Pulmonary embolism as a complication of ventriculo-atrial shunts inserted for hydrocephalus. Develop. Med. Child Neurol. Supp. 11:36.

Fischer, E. G., and J. Shillito, Jr. 1969. Large abdominal cysts: a complication of peritoneal shunts; report of three cases. J. Neurosurg. 31:441.

Foltz, E. L., and D. B. Shurtleff. 1963. Five year comparative study of hydrocephalus in children with and without operation; 113 cases. J. Neurosurg. 20:1064.

Foltz, E. L., and D. B. Shurtleff. 1966. Conversion of communicating hydrocephalus to stenosis or occlusion of the aqueduct during ventricular shunt. J. Neurosurg. 24:520.

Forrest, D. M., and D. G. W. Cooper. 1968. Complications of ventriculo-atrial shunts. A review of 455 cases. J. Neurosurg. 29:506.

Hammon, W. H. 1971. Evaluation and use of the ventriculo-peritoneal shunt in hydrocephalus. J. Neurosurg. 34:792.

Holder, T. M., and M. L. Crow. 1963. Free intracardiac foreign body; a complication of ventriculo-venous shunt for hydrocephalus. J. Thorac. Cardiovasc. Surg. 45:138.

Holt, R. J. 1970. Bacteriological studies on colonised ventriculo-atrial shunts. Develop. Med. Child Neurol. Supp. 22:83.

Jackson, I. J., and S. R. Snodgrass. 1955. Peritoneal shunts in the treatment of hydrocephalus and increased intracranial pressure: a four-year survey of 62 patients. J. Neurosurg. 12:216.

Laurence, K. M. 1959. The pathology of hydrocephalus. Ann. Roy. Coll. Surg. Eng. 24:388.

Lichtenstein, B. W. 1959. Atresia and stenosis of the aqueduct of Sylvius, with comments on the Arnold-Chiari complex. J. Neuropath. Exp. Neurol. 18:3.

Little, J. R., A. L. Rhoton, Jr., and J. F. Mellinger. 1972. Comparison of ventriculoperitoneal and ventriculoatrial shunts for hydrocephalus in children. Mayo Clin. Proc. 47:396.

Long, D. M., R. A. DeWall, and L. A. French. 1964. Unusual complication of ventriculoauriculostomy: report of two cases. J. Neurosurg. 21:233.

Lorber, J. 1969. Ventriculo-cardiac shunts in the first week of life. Results of a controlled trial in the treatment of hydrocephalus in infants born with spina bifida cystica or cranium bifidum. Develop. Med. Child Neurol. Supp. 20:13.

Lorber, J. 1971. Medical and surgical aspects in the treatment of congenital hydrocephalus. Neuropediatrie 2:239.

Luthardt, T. 1970. Bacterial infections in ventriculo-atrial shunts. Develop. Med. Child Neurol. Supp. 22:105.

Matson, D. D. 1964. Current concepts: hydrocephalus. New Eng. J. Med. 271:1360.

Matson, D. D. 1969. Neurosurgery of infancy and childhood. Charles C Thomas, Publisher, Springfield, Ill., 934 pp.

McConnell, A. A., and H. L. Parker. 1938. A deformity of the hind-brain associated with internal hydrocephalus. Its relation to the Arnold-Chiari malformation. Brain 61:415.

McLaurin, R. L., and D. Dodson. 1971. Infected ventriculo-atrial shunts: some principles of treatment. Develop. Med. Child Neurol. Supp. 25:71.

Murtagh, F., and R. Lehman. 1967. Peritoneal shunts in the management of hydrocephalus. JAMA 202:1010.

Noonan, J. A., and D. A. Ehmke. 1963. Complications of ventriculovenous shunts for control of hydrocephalus. Report of three cases with thrombo-emboli to the lungs. New Eng. J. Med. 269:70.

Nugent, G. R., R. Lucas, M. Judy, B. M. Bloor, and H. Warden. 1966. Thromboembolic complications of ventriculo-atrial shunts. Angiocardiographic and pathological correlations. J. Neurosurg. 24:34.

Nulsen, F. E., and D. P. Becker. 1966. Control of hydrocephalus by valve-regulated shunt: infections and their prevention. Clin. Neurosurg. 14:256.

Nulsen, F. E., and D. P. Becker. 1967. Control of hydrocephalus by valve-regulated shunt. J. Neurosurg. 26:362.

Overton, M. C., III, and S. R. Snodgrass. 1965. Ventriculovenous shunts for infantile hydrocephalus. A review of five years experience with this method. J. Neurosurg. 23:517.

Perrin, J. C. S., and R. L. McLaurin. 1967. Infected ventriculoatrial shunts. J. Neurosurg. 27:21.

Portnoy, H. D. 1971. New ventricular catheter for hydrocephalic shunts: technical note. J. Neurosurg. 34:702.

Pudenz, R. H. 1957. Experimental and clinical observations on the shunting of cerebrospinal fluid into the circulatory system. Clin. Neurosurg. 5:98.

Pudenz, R. H. 1966. The ventriculo-atrial shunt. J. Neurosurg. 25:602.

Russell, D. S., and C. Donald. 1935. The mechanism of internal hydrocephalus in spina bifida. Brain 58:203.

Sakoda, T. H., J. A. Maxwell, and C. E. Brackett, Jr. 1971. Intestinal volvulus secondary to a ventriculoperitoneal shunt: case report. J. Neurosurg. 35:95.

Scarff, J. E. 1963. Treatment of hydrocephalus: an historical and critical review of methods and results. J. Neurol. Neurosurg. Psychiat. 26:1.

Shick, R. W., and D. D. Matson. 1961. What is arrested hydrocephalus? J. Pediat. 58:791.

Sieben, R. L., M. B. Hamida, and K. Shulman. 1971. Multiple cranial nerve deficits associated with the Arnold-Chiari malformation. Neurology 21:673.

Sperling, D. R., J. R. Patrick, F. M. Anderson, and D. C. Fyler. 1964. Cor pulmonale secondary to ventriculoauriculostomy. Am. J. Dis. Child. 107:308.

Stickler, G. B., M. H. Shin, E. C. Burke, et al. 1970. Diffuse glomerulonephritis associated with infected ventriculoatrial shunt. Am. Heart J. 79:426.

van Hoytema, G. J., and R. van den Berg. 1966. Embryological studies of the posterior fossa in connection with Arnold-Chiari malformation. Develop. Med. Child Neurol. Supp. 11:61.

Wiess, S. R., and R. Raskind. 1969. Twenty-two cases of hydrocephalus treated with a silastic ventriculoperitoneal shunt. Int. Surg. 51:13.

Williams, B. 1971. Further thoughts on the valvular action of the Arnold-Chiari malformation. Dev. Med. Child Neurol. Supp. 25:105.

Wilson, C. B., and V. Bertan. 1966. Perforation of the bowel complicating peritoneal shunt for hydrocephalus: report of two cases. Am. Surg. 32:601.

8

Mild Forms of Spinal Dysraphism and Associated Conditions

George B. Udvarhelyi, M.D.

Much confusion has resulted from the use of different terminology for forms of spinal dysraphism other than meningomyeloceles. Some terms are partly descriptive, representing the anatomist and embryologist's point of view; others are partly functional, emphasizing certain aspects of the complex clinical picture. Terms such as "spina bifida occulta" have been utilized by British authors to distinguish this clinical entity from spina bifida cystica (meningomyeloceles). The association of spinal dysraphism with tumors in the lumbosacral area has prompted the use of terms such as "lumbosacral lipomas," "lipomeningocele," and "fibrolipoma of the filum terminale." Functional aspects of tethering of the spinal cord are responsible for terms such as "tethered cord" and "fixed filum terminale." Because skin manifestations occur quite frequently in this condition, with or without underlying sinus-tracts, descriptive dermatological phrases (hypertrichosis, pigmented nevi, dermal dimple) were added to the list, in addition to the term "congenital dermal sinus." Finally, different degrees of bifid state of the spinal cord, known as "diastematomyelia," may be present alone or in combination. We prefer to use the nonspecific term "minimal spinal dysraphism" to distinguish this condition from meningomyeloceles. The significance of these lesions to the child are far from minimal.

James and Lassman have been interested in this particular condition since the early 1950's, and their monograph published in 1972 contains a comprehensive survey of the problem, together with a detailed analysis of 100 case histories, including the pediatric, orthopedic, dermatological, neurological, and neurosurgical aspects.

Although the pathology of the condition was discussed as early as 1940 by Lichtenstein, and various aspects of the clinical manifestations have been pointed out by many authors (Brickner, 1918; Levi, 1926; Russell and Donald, 1935; List, 1941; Ingraham and Swan, 1943; Walker, 1944; Meredith, 1944; Reimann and Anson, 1944; Groff and Yaskin, 1947; Bassett, 1950; Garceau, 1953; Gross, Holcomb, and Swan, 1953; Alexander, Garvey, and Boyce, 1954; Jones and Love, 1956; Jackson et al., 1956; James and Lassman, 1958, 1960, 1962a, b; Campbell, 1962; Gryspeerdt, 1963; Dubowitz, Lorber, and Zachary, 1965; Till, 1965; Sharrard, 1966; Matson and Jerva, 1966; Fluckiger, 1967; Yashon and Beatty, 1966; Lassman and James, 1967; Till, 1968, 1969; Anderson, 1968; Lobo, 1968; Burrows, 1968), even recent comprehensive textbooks on pediatric neurosurgery do not emphasize the practical implications of this clinical entity (Matson, 1969; Rand and Rand, 1960; Jackson et al., 1959), with few exceptions (Bunch et al., 1972).

On the basis of a comprehensive review of literature and personal experience with 28 cases (including 22 children below the age of 15), this chapter describes the clinical presentation, diagnosis, and treatment of children with "minimal spinal dysraphism."

The importance of separating this group of children from the group with overt meningomyeloceles cannot be overemphasized. The clinical signs are related to the skin, spinal column, faulty development of the lower extremities, impaired locomotion, defective sensory and reflex systems, and the genitourinary system. Almost without exception, these children do not have other abnormalities along the neuroaxis; they are mentally normal and do not have hydrocephalus. Since the condition is congenital, early recognition is of paramount importance. Most of the symptoms are related to long-standing, progressive, secondary involvement of the musculoskeletal, peripheral, and/or central nervous system and of the urinary system as the children go through the growth process. Therefore, only early surgical intervention may return these children to a relatively normal life and prevent irreversible and sometimes fatal secondary complications.

To understand the significance of the clinical presentation of this condition, the careful studies of Emery and Lendon (1969) should be reviewed. They have studied 100 spinal cords and spinal columns of children with spinal dysraphism and have divided their findings into six groups (Fig. 8-1a and b). The lipomatous lesions are the most frequently occurring pathological entities in this group of patients, although dermoid tumors, epidermoid tumors, hamartomas, and inclusion cysts also may be present. The term "spinal dysraphism" represents a group of congenital abnormalities, including diastematomyelia, congenital intraspinal mass lesions, and abnormal development of the spinal cord and medullary clonus, usually associated with spina bifida or other vertebral anomalies and cutaneous lesions. The clinical manifestations, therefore, consist of abnormalities in the cutaneous, muscular, osseous, vascular, and neural tissues, occurring separately or together.

Children with spinal dysraphism often are seen by a variety of specialists

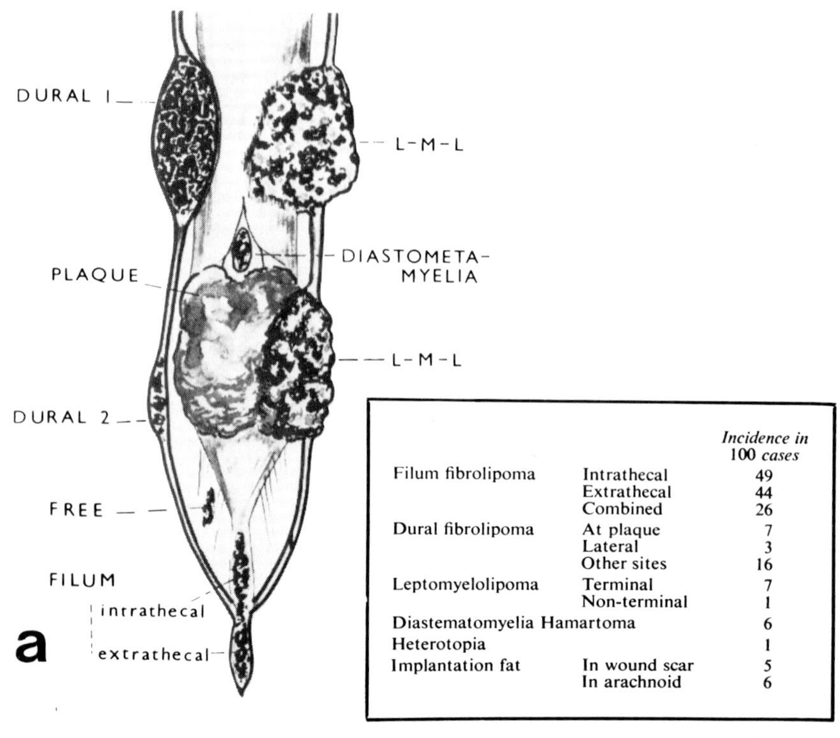

		Incidence in 100 cases
Filum fibrolipoma	Intrathecal	49
	Extrathecal	44
	Combined	26
Dural fibrolipoma	At plaque	7
	Lateral	3
	Other sites	16
Leptomyelolipoma	Terminal	7
	Non-terminal	1
Diastematomyelia Hamartoma		6
Heterotopia		1
Implantation fat	In wound scar	5
	In arachnoid	6

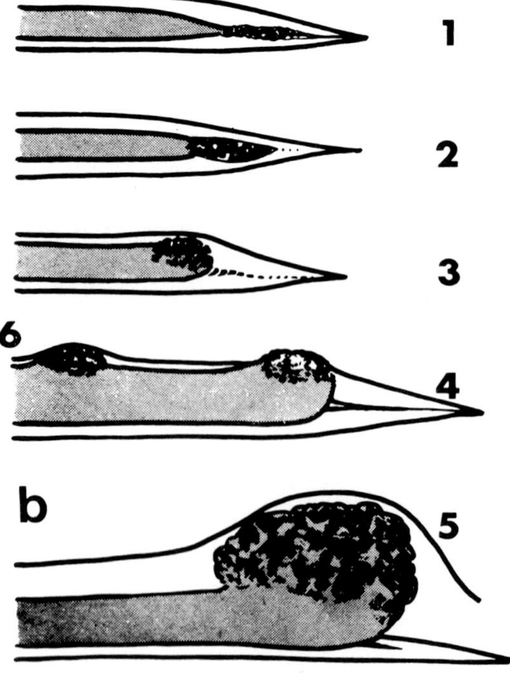

who concentrate on the particular aspects of their respective specialties, often treating the structural or functional aspects of this malformation without taking into consideration the possibility of a centrally originated disorder.

The local skin malformations are "treated" by pediatric surgeons, plastic surgeons, and dermatologists; the secondary involvement of the locomotor or urinary systems is treated by orthopedic surgeons, urologists, plastic surgeons, or radiotherapists. This unhappy ramification of incomplete work-ups and therapeutic approaches can be avoided if the etiology of the peripheral disorder is questioned and if the pediatric neurologist and the pediatric neurosurgeon are consulted before corrective measures are undertaken.

There are four principal modes of developmental error (Till, 1968). First, there may be simple incomplete fusion of a structure, such as that found in spina bifida. Second, there may be failure of separation of the germinal layers, ectoderm, mesoderm, and endoderm. A deep dermal sinus is an example of this mode. Third, there may be abnormal growth from what appear to be cell rests, i.e., cells from one germinal layer remain in the mesoderm and give rise to the familiar dermoid or epidermoid cyst. Fourth, there may be disturbance of growth of otherwise normal tissue, leading to the formation of intraspinal and even intramedullary lipomas. One view of the possible embryology of these lesions is discussed in Chapter 3.

The mechanism by which these lesions affect the neural elements can be divided into three groups.

1. Lesions causing pressure: these include intrathecal lipomas (intradural, extradural, or both); intrathecal dermoids; transverse bands of ligamentous origin, usually extradual; and inverted laminae (Fig. 8-2).

2. Lesions causing traction: these prevent the ascent of the spinal cord and cause traction by fixing the cord at a definite level in the vertebral canal. Since the rate of growth of the spinal cord is less than that of the vertebral column, as the length of the vertebral column increases the ascent of the spinal cord is prevented by traction on the cord (Figs. 8-3, 8-4). At birth, the distal end of the spinal cord normally is situated at or about the

---

Fig. 8-1 (a) Left, fatty tumors related to neurospinal dysraphism. Right, table shows a classification of fatty tumors found, together with the number of such lesions seen in a detailed study of 100 children dying with neurospinal dysraphism. In many children, more than one type of lesion was found. (b) Diagrammatic representation of different types of lesions found and the possible relationship between filar fibrolipomas and the large leptomyelolipomas: (1) the common intrathecal fibrolipoma; (2) the filar lesions incorporated into the conus; (3) the fibro-fatty tissue is now forming part of the conus and terminal cord (a separate filum may or may not be present); (4 and 5) progressive increases in size of the terminal cord lesions; (6) a similar type of lesion occurring in a more cephalad situation. Courtesy of Emery and Lendon, Develop. Med. Child Neurol. (Suppl.) 20:62, 1969.

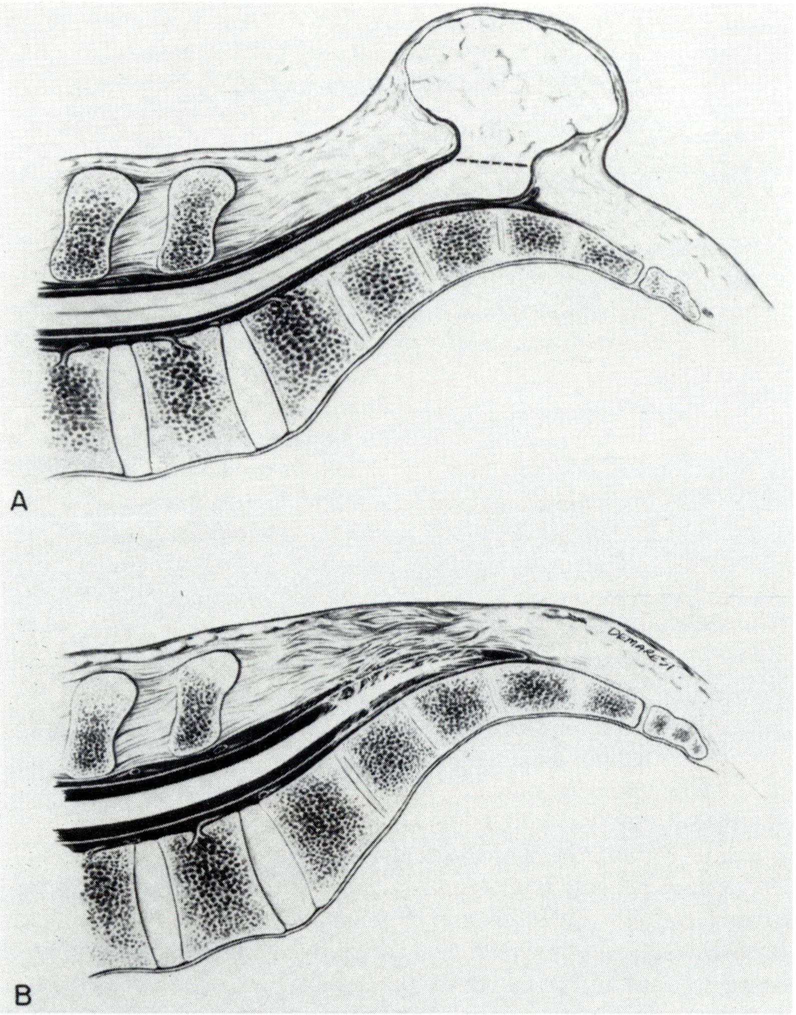

Fig. 8-2 Schematic drawings of the caudal portion of the neural axis. (A) Arrested ascent of the spinal cord as the result of confluence of the conus medullaris and an intramedullary lipoma with extension into the soft tissues overlying a spina bifida. Broken line, the site of amputation of the lipoma. (B) Retention of the conus medullaris at a low sacral level as the result of adhesions arising in conjunction with a meningocele. Courtesy of J. B. Campbell, Clin. Neurosurg. 10:133, 1962.

upper border of the body of the third lumbar vertebra, but by the end of growth it is located at the lower border of the body of the first lumbar vertebra. Diastematomyelia in which the spinal cord is bifid in part of its course and split by a bony or fibrous band, and fibrous bands which may tether the spinal cord of cauda equina to the bone or skin directly or through

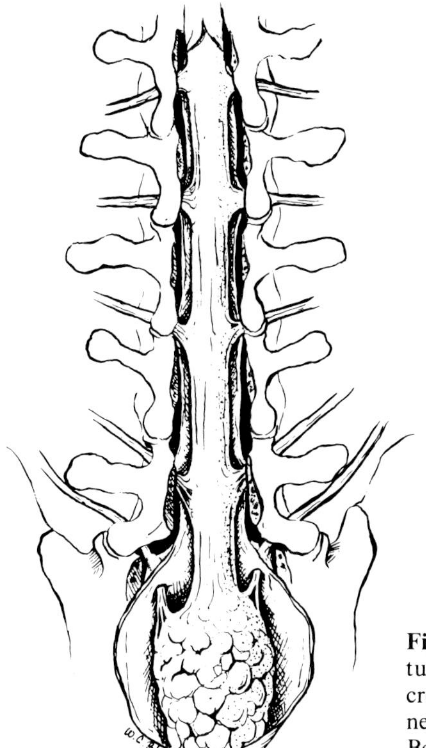

Fig. 8-3 Note the conus tethered by fatty tumor, upward-directed nerve roots, and increased distance between the more caudad nerve segments. Courtesy of Yashon and Beatty, J. Neurol. Neurosurg. Psychiat. 29:244, 1966.

attachment to the meninges are examples of lesions causing traction. A persistent, tense filum terminale also may produce traction on the spinal cord as the spinal column grows.

3. Lesions causing traction and pressure: combinations of the above lesions act together at the same time or separately at different times. It may be impossible to decide which is the cause of the damage.

All of these forms of interference with neural action, of course, are present in various degrees in children with meningomyeloceles. However, because of the exteriorization of the meningomyelocele, the condition is recognized early. The group of children discussed in this chapter, however, have the occult form of spinal dysraphism beneath a more or less normal skin. Although over 65% of the children will have some cutaneous sign, the significance of the skin manifestation often is missed (Tavafoghi, Hambrick, and Udvarhelyi, 1971). Recognition of the significance of midline lumbosacral skin changes is the first step in the appreciation of the underlying spinal dysraphism.

Before discussing the clinical manifestations, it seems to be of practical importance to divide these patients into two groups: (1) children less than 2

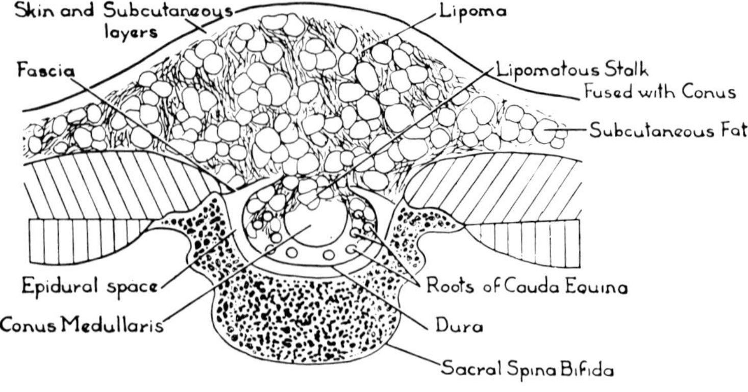

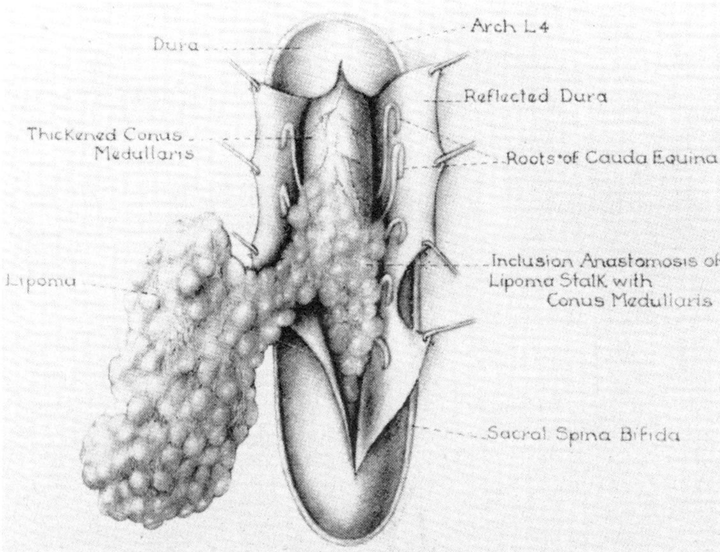

Fig. 8-4 Top, schematic cross-section showing relationship of lipoma to subcutaneous fat, deep fascia, dura, conus, and roots. Bottom, diagram showing mechanism of traction deformity of conus and roots of cauda equina. Courtesy of R. C. Bassett, Ann. Surg. 131:109, 1950.

years old and (2) children more than 2 years old (including adults). After age 2, certain aspects of the symptomatology, such as gait disturbances and increasing urinary incontinence, can be detected more easily. Other manifestations, such as delicate skin abnormalities or discrete sensory or motor deficit, require a careful evaluation in children less than 2 years old.

A careful scrutiny of small children allows an early recognition of this condition before neurological, urological, or locomotor disturbances become advanced or irreversible. While most authors (Till, 1969; Bruce and Schut,

1971; Dubowitz et al., 1965; Bassett, 1950) advocate operative intervention in the asymptomatic stage, others prefer to wait until symptoms appear. These arguments are discussed later.

CLINICAL MANIFESTATIONS

SKIN

The cutaneous manifestations are generally of five principal types which may occur singly or in combination. They include lumbosacral lipoma, hypertrichosis, small capillary hemangioma, dermal dimples, and dermal sinuses, and areas of atrophic skin. *Any midline lumbosacral skin abnormality should alert the physician to the possibility of underlying spinal dysraphism.*

Lumbosacral lipomas. These are superficial fatty tumors usually occurring in the lumbar or lumbosacral region in or near the midline (Fig. 8-5, 8-9C). They may be small and flat or quite large, measuring up to 15 to 30 cm in diameter. They are soft on palpation, can be moved gently from side to side, and occasionally have a tail-like configuration (Fig. 8-6). While they may be the only skin manifestation, there may be other associated skin abnormalities, such as a nevus, dimple, or a combination of the two. Tavafoghi et al. (1971) reviewed the literature of the cutaneous manifestations of

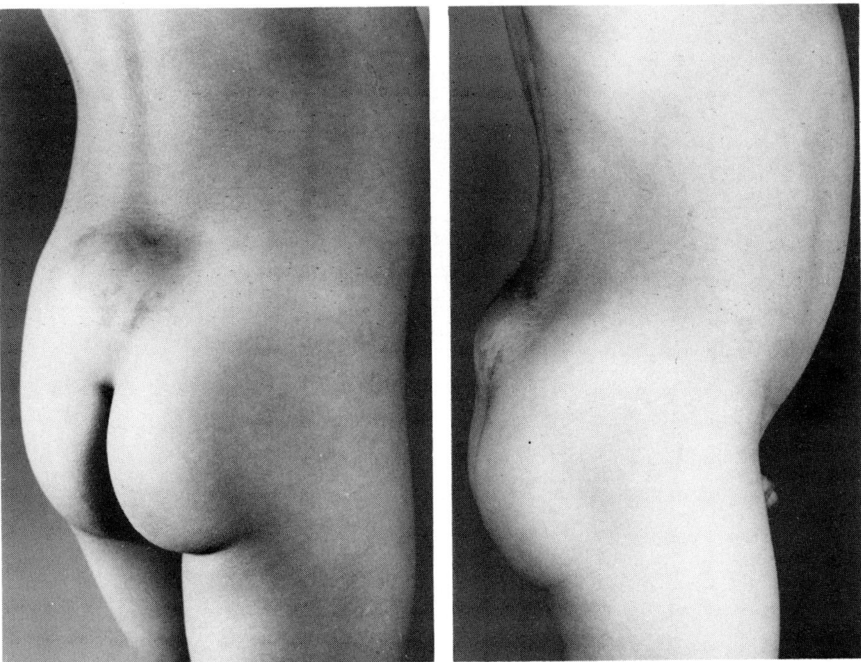

Fig. 8-5 Photographs showing the appearance of a lumbosacral lipoma. Note pigmented areas and marginal hypertrichosis.

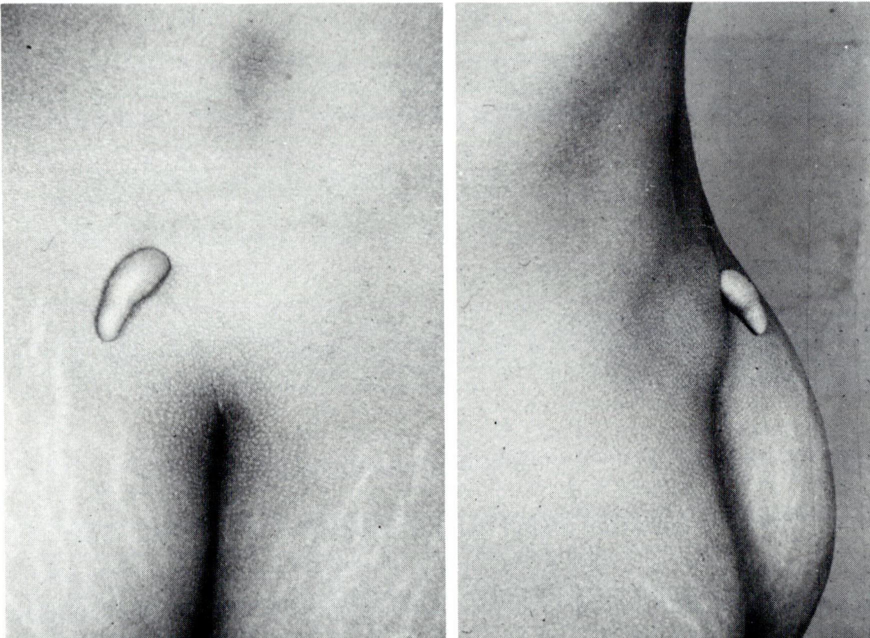

Fig. 8-6 Photographs showing a mild subcutaneous lipoma with a tail-like "appendix" in a girl of 20. Associated leg deformities and urinary incontinence were "treated" by orthopedic surgeons and urologists.

spinal dysraphism and found that in 200 clinically reported cases of spinal dysraphism, 102 had skin manifestations. The presence of subcutaneous lipomas with or without other skin manifestation should suggest strongly to the pediatrician the possibility of underlying bony or neural congenital abnormality. Many of the so-called superficial lipomas continue to the lumbosacral fascia and penetrate the dura with a small, neck-like structure ending inferiorly or laterally to the cauda equina, or they are in continuity with the conus medullaris (Figs. 8-7 and 8-8). It is important *not* to treat the superficial lipoma without the complete evaluation of intraspinal extension.

Hypertrichosis. This hairy patch on the skin is present in about one-third of the patients with spinal dysraphism (Fig. 8-9 A and D). The hairy patch may vary in its size and in length of hair. Pigmented patches of skin or hemangiomas in the midline may be present. Approximately one-half of the children with hairy patch and with underlying spinal dysraphism had a combination of cutaneous manifestations.

Skin abnormalities. Pigmented nevi may occur as a single area, rounded and about 5 cm in diameter or much larger, near the midline of the back, and usually near the lumbosacral area (Fig. 8-9 A and B). Oval-shaped scarred areas with hyperpigmentation and with a central, often white, and not pigmented area, where skin is much thinner, are called "apretic menin-

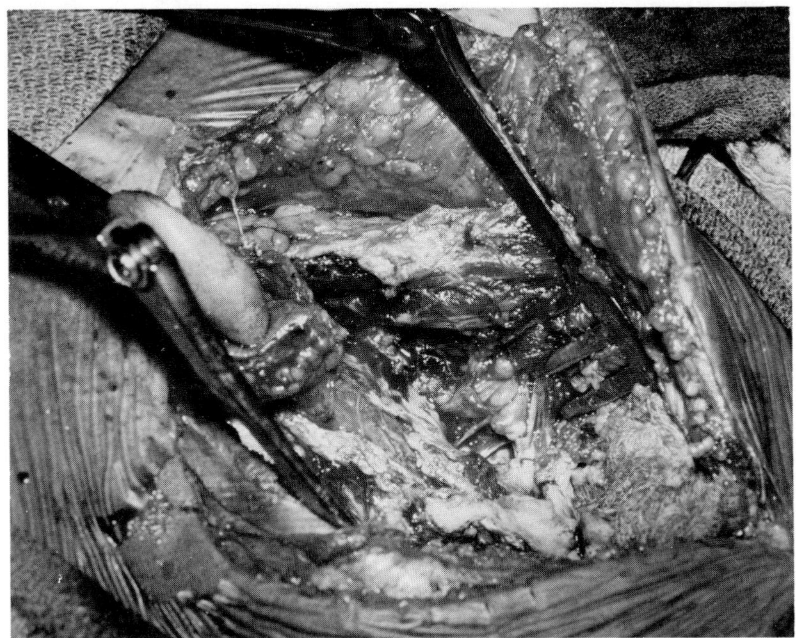

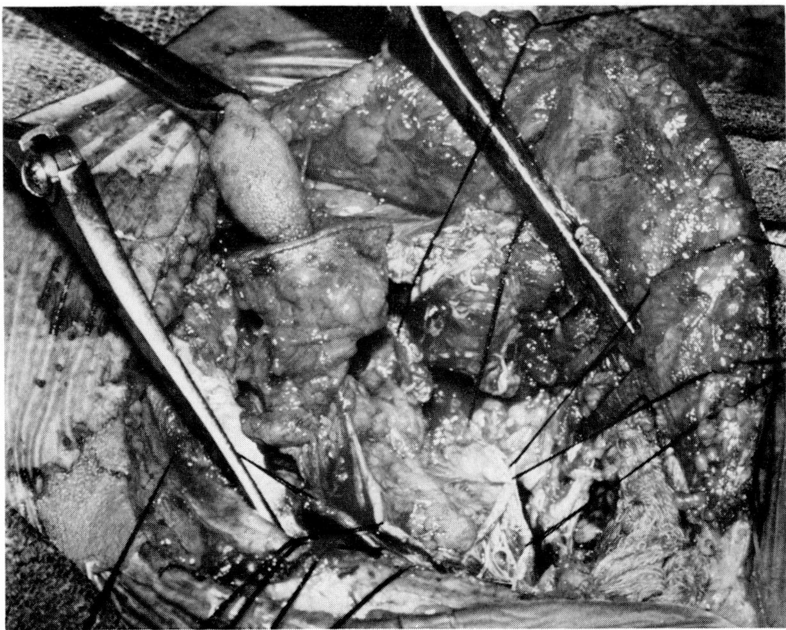

Figs. 8-7 and 8-8 Operative photographs showing the extension of the subcutaneous lipoma through the fascia and dura mater into the region of the cauda equina. Same patient as in Fig. 8-6.

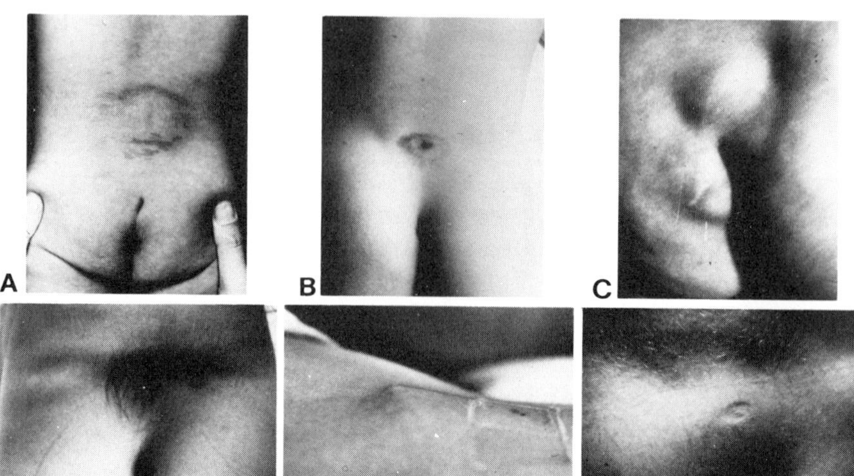

Fig. 8-9 Various skin manifestations: (A) pigmented nevus and peripheral hypertrichosis, dermal sinus; (B) nevus with membraneous center ("apretic meningocele"); (C) lipoma; (D) marked hypertrichosis; (E) bony spicule with fine pigmentation; (F) "apretic meningocele."

goceles" (Fig. 8-9 B and F). They probably represent small meningoceles which have atrophied and been absorbed *in utero*. The central area occasionally is slightly moist, indicating the earlier relationship of the thinned-out skin to underlying "fruste" meningocele. Quite often, the direct connection to the cauda equina or spinal cord can be traced at operation. Small midline vascular nevi also may indicate dysraphism.

Dermal dimples and sinuses. The dermal dimples are skin depressions near the midline, with fixation of the epithelium to the underlying layers (Fig. 8-9 A). Dermal sinuses resemble the dermal dimples, except that they are much deeper. They must be distinguished from pilonidal sinuses and coccygeal dimples. The former are regarded as being acquired rather than congenital and are rarely found in children; the latter are situated over the sacrococcygeal area and are of no significance unless they become infected and form abscesses. The dermal sinuses are, of course, important and potentially dangerous. They represent generally a direct contact from the surface of the skin to the meninges and to the cerebrospinal fluid. They may cause intermittent, recurrent meningitis and occasionally even formation of abscesses. Dermal sinuses and other skin manifestations (Fig. 8-9 E) often are associated with extra- or intradural lipomas (Walker and Bucy, 1934; Matson and Jerva, 1966).

Recognition of the significance of these skin manifestations is extremely important, especially in those less than 2 years old, since partial and incomplete removal results in serious complications. In addition, considerable technical difficulty will be present at a later stage if the underlying lesion necessitates further surgery. In our personal series of 28 cases, *all of them* had cutaneous manifestations. Some of the lipomas were extremely thin or small in size; the dimples occasionally were difficult to recognize; however, in some of our patients, the nevi were quite extensive. In one patient, a port wine-colored pigmentation was seen at age 2 months. Urinary incontinence, saddle hypoesthesia, and areflexia became manifest at age 5 months, and an intradural lipoma was removed, with significant postoperative improvement.

ORTHOPEDIC MANIFESTATIONS

The most common finding in those less than 2 years old is that one lower limb is underdeveloped in comparison with the other. The inequality may take the form of unilateral talipes or may show up as a reduction of the muscle bulk in calf or thigh (atrophy). The deformity can be very discrete or more marked, with rotation of the foot and decreased growth of the lower extremity. In older children, the motor deficit generally is manifested by the evidence of a limp and gait disturbance. In the beginning, the gait disturbance may be almost imperceptible, consisting only of an elevation of the first metatarsal head, as though something like a verruca were underneath it, the great toe usually remaining flexed. If no attention is given to this very discrete alteration, the pes cavus observed previously only when walking could become fixed. The arch becomes higher, the forefoot more abducted and more inverted, and the toes clawed. This is usually unilateral, and the result is not unlike the deformities seen in some late cases of poliomyelitis. The erroneous diagnosis of previous poliomyelitis frequently has been made in children with these symptoms. Orthopedic procedures have been performed repeatedly for the treatment of the foot deformity. In spite of the local operations, the situation usually worsens.

One of our patients presents the typical course of children with this entity. She presented with a limp and foot drop and was told that she had had polio, although neither the mother nor the child could remember it. Three operations on the foot were unsuccessful. When she was first seen by us at age 21, she had been incontinent of urine for 5 years and had a tail-shaped pendular skin malformation and mild subcutaneous lipoma in the lumbosacral area (Fig. 8-6). An x-ray of the lumbosacral spine showed severe sacral hypoplasia (Fig. 8-10). Examination of the back and some study of the *cause of progressive acquired orthopedic deformity* and urological symptomatology could have saved a lot of pain, discomfort, and unnecessary operations and frustration for this patient. Removal of her intraspinal lipoma after myelographic confirmation (Fig. 8-11) relieved her incontinence; operation at age 2 could have prevented her orthopedic problem.

In addition to the foot deformity, the shortened lower limb, and the gait disturbance, trophic changes may be present, together with disturbance of temperature because of peripheral circulatory deficiency.

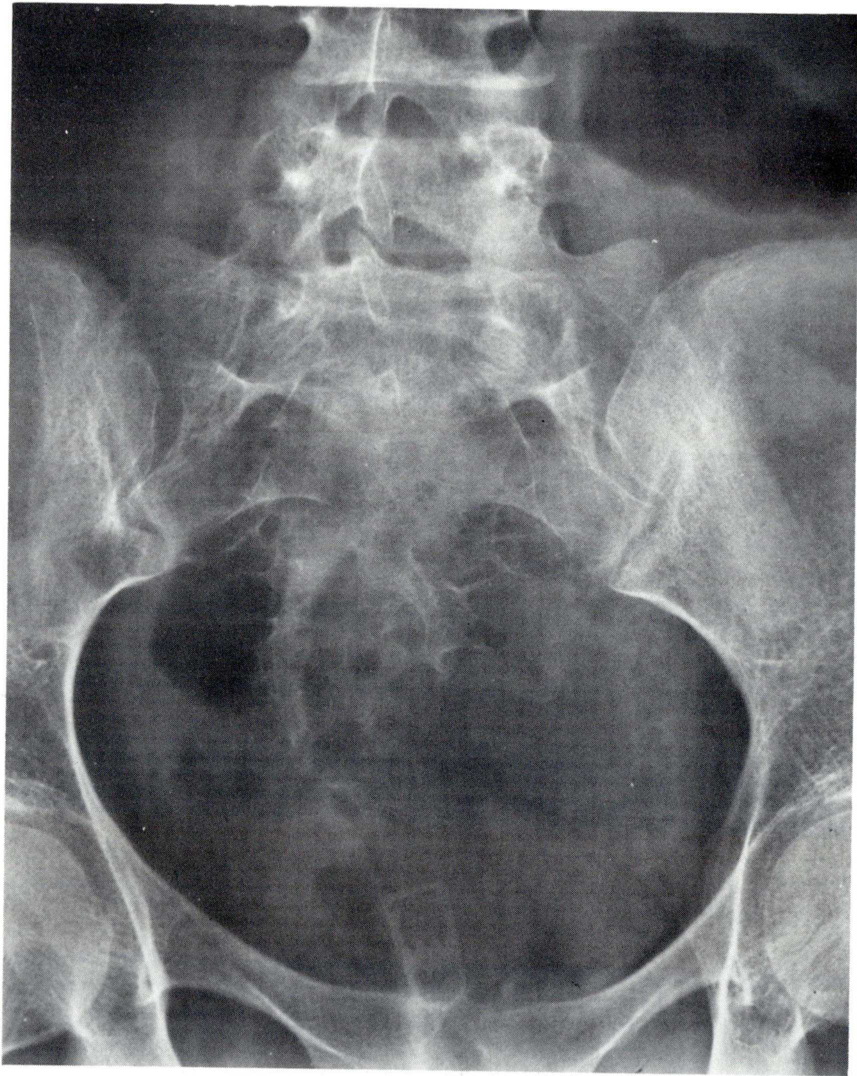

Fig. 8-10 X-ray of the lumbosacral spine showing extensive sacral hypoplasia and widening of the interpedicular distances. Same patient as Fig. 8-6.

UROLOGICAL MANIFESTATIONS

Intermittent incontinence with recurrent urinary trace infection is a most common presenting symptom. While it may be difficult to assess dribbling in children younger than age 2, older children either may not be toilet trained or may develop urinary and rectal incontinence. Treatment by the urologist often is local, including surgical intervention on the bladder

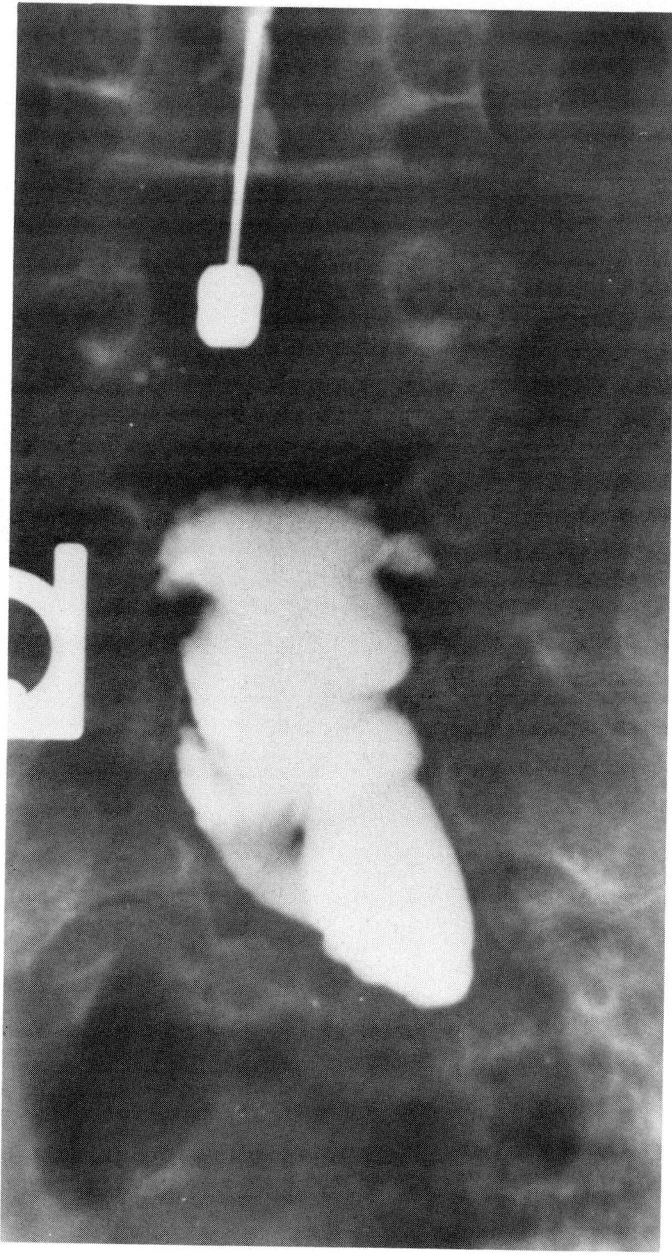

Fig. 8-11 Myelogram, anteroposterior view, showing the widened dural sac, the irregularly shaped lipomatous indentations, and a diagonal fibrous band, together with cranially directed course of some of the nerve roots. Same patient as Fig. 8-6.

neck, dilatation, and intermittent catheterizations. Urinary tract infection may progress and cause hydronephrosis and irreversible destruction of one or both kidneys. In one of our cases, a superficial lipoma was resected by a general surgeon, who paid no attention to the already present urinary incontinence in a girl 6 months old. The family did not keep a return appointment. Intermittent urinary tract infections and irreversible pyelonephritis developed in one kidney, necessitating nephrectomy; 50% destruction of the other kidney was present when the child was finally seen by us at age 6. She showed the classic evidence of spinal dysraphism, with skin manifestations, urinary incontinence, motor deficit, and underlying radiological changes. A partial removal of the intradural lipoma considerably improved her condition, but she had a single, severely damaged kidney for the rest of her life.

Although the importance of early recognition of urinary problems in this group of patients was emphasized by Campbell in the early 1960's, the fact that urinary incontinence with superimposed recurrent infections is a presentation of congenital lumbosacral abnormalities still is not recognized. Without exception, all of our 22 cases have had intermittent urinary problems, and approximately one-third of them finally were referred to us by urologists after the close relationship with the underlying treatable condition was emphasized. The management of the accompanying urinary tract involvement depends on the success or failure of neurosurgical therapy, and has been extensively discussed (Mertz and Smith, 1930; Gross et al., 1953; Morales, Deaver, and Hotchkiss, 1956).

RECTAL INCONTINENCE

This is much less common than urinary incontinence. Only two of our 28 children and none of James and Lassman's 100 cases had bowel dysfunction. However, Campbell (1962), Till (1968), and others describe the concomitant incontinence of both systems. In one of our own cases, a 12-year-old child was referred to a general surgeon for colostomy. X-rays showed widened interpedicular distances and mild sacral dysplasis (Fig. 8-12 a), and there was a history of a pigmented nevus treated by surgical excision at age 1. A discrete, subcutaneous lipoma, motor deformity of the foot with lower motor neuron involvement, and sensory disturbance in the sacral dermatomes suggested spinal dysraphism. Myelogram confirmed the clinical diagnosis (Fig. 8-12 b), and an extra- and intradural lipoma was partially removed and the tethered cord partially freed. The boy remained in control of his urinary and bowel function for the following 6.5 years, despite a rapid growth spurt.

NEUROLOGICAL SYMPTOMS

Since these lesions involve mainly the lower motor neuron, the most common neurological manifestations are areflexia, lack of muscle bulk, and discrete sensory disturbances. However, tethering of the cord or

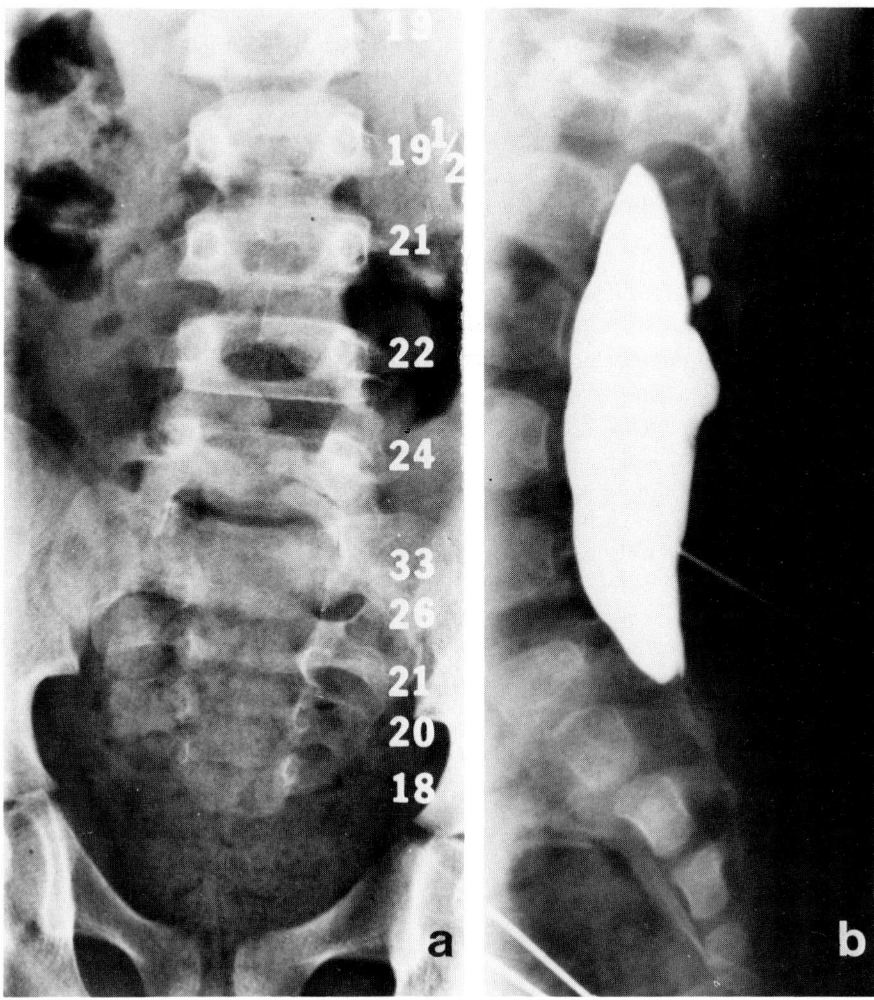

Fig. 8-12 (a) X-rays of the lumbosacral spine, showing spina bifida occulta, widening of the interpedicular distances at L5-S1-S2, and mild sacral hypoplasia. (b) Lateral view of the myelogram of the same patient, showing the irregular, posterior, lipomatous mass, widened dural sac with tethered cord.

lipomatous infiltration of the conus medullaris may produce upper motor neuron involvement. Spastic or tiptoeing gait and some hyperreflexia may be present alone or in addition to the lower motor neuron involvement. It should be emphasized that careful evaluation of the sensation in the lower sacral dermatomes together with meticulous examination of the reflexes (including the anal reflex) must be performed. Children with this condition often complain of a deep, pulling, radicular type of pain arising in the lumbosacral area radiating into one or both legs. This pain represents a combination of the orthopedic and neurological involvement. In those cases in which the spinal cord is tethered down by a lipoma, a fibrous band, or an enlarged filum terminale, the pain may be a more constant symptom.

The relative frequency of presenting signs and symptoms was tabulated by Till (1968) as follows: in 85 children, inequality of lower limbs was present in 55, reflex changes in the lower limbs in 54, limp in 46, reduction of muscle bulk in lower limb in 34, abnormal spinal curvature in 29, disorder of micturition in 27, trophic changes in toes in 11, backache in 8, and leg pain in 7. In the series by James and Lassman (1958, 1960, 1962 a, b, 1972), incontinence was present in 24% of the children, foot abnormalities and gait disturbance in 18%, weakness of the legs in 14%, paraparesis in 8%, and marked skin manifestation, including dermal sinus, in 25% of the patients; only 15% were "normal" out of the 100 patients operated.

Bruce and Schut (1971) point out that even in the larger group of so-called asymptomatic patients, two-thirds showed evidence of neurological or urological abnormality on careful clinical examination.

In our series (Table 8-1), all 22 patients showed evidence of urological involvement. The degree of incontinence was minimal in five patients; 17

Table 8-1A Presenting Clinical Manifestations in 15 Children Ages 2 to 15 Seen at Johns Hopkins Hospital

"Sacral mass" (subcutaneous lipoma)	15
with pigmented nevi	7
with hairy patch	4
with "dimple"	5
with sinus	2
X-rays	
spina bifida occulta	15
sacral hypoplasia	7
Urinary incontinence	15
Rectal incontinence	5
Foot deformity + atrophy (lower motor neuron)	13
Additional increased tone, hyperreflexia (upper motor neuron)	5
Sensory deficit	15
Previous surgery	6

Table 8-1B Surgical Results in Children Ages 2 to 15. Follow-up at Ages 4 to 9

Excellent (no functional deficit)	7
Good (mild deficit)	4
Unchanged	3
Worse	1

had repeated treatments by urologists and a history of recurrent infections, abnormal cistometrogram, and partial neurogenic bladder.

DIAGNOSIS

Diagnosis is based on the clinical manifestations: the presence of a combination of urinary dysfunction, mild neurological abnormality, and foot deformity with other evidence of lower limb involvement. A high suspicion of an underlying spinal dysraphism should occur even if only skin manifestations are present. A careful examination to discover the presence of involvement of one or a combination of various systems may uncover minimal neurological deficit. The pediatrician should consult the urologist, pediatric neurologist, and orthopedist before making a further decision with regard to diagnostic work-up and treatment. The danger exists, however, that "specialists" may submit these children to specific treatments or operative procedures without reaching the logical conclusion of a correct diagnosis. In the atmosphere of a Birth Defects Clinic, the various specialists are present at the same time, and an ample discussion is generated before the therapeutic decisions are made. This seems to be the best means to avoid the pitfalls of incomplete or erroneous diagnosis and unnecessary or insufficient treatment.

Once the clinical manifestations have been confirmed by careful examination, the next most important step in the diagnostic work-up is the study of the radiographs of the lumbosacral spine (Walker, 1944; Burrows, 1968).

Only rarely in patients with this condition is the x-ray of the spine normal. Slight degrees of spina bifida occulta with nonunion of either lamina or cleft between the fifth lumbar or first sacral lamina can be present in 30% of "normal" individuals. However, in children with clinical manifestations of spinal dysraphism, more significant abnormal x-ray findings will be present. The laminae may be deformed or fused with each other; there may be a split in the lateral bodies sagitally, or hemivertebrae may be present. The sacrum is very often dysplastic, or unilateral hypoplasia is present (Fig. 8-10) (Roller and Pribram, 1965).

Widening of the interpedicular distance indicates possible intraspinal component of a lipoma or dermoid, although cystic components of a lipomeningocele cannot be excluded (Fig. 8-12). The presence of a bony spur in diastematomyelia can, of course, be recognized on the x-ray. Unfortunately, only about 15 to 20% of the children with diastematomyelia will have radiographically visible bony spur (Burrows, 1968).

In most of our patients, simple radiographs of the child would have demonstrated the presence of serious abnormalities indicating a defect of midline fusion and would have led to the conclusion that the symptoms probably are related to a neurogenic condition within the spinal canal.

If the x-rays of the spine in the routine projections confirm the presence of bony abnormalities, we strongly suggest tomographic studies. These are especially important in the case of diastematomyelia, so that the bony spur with its anatomical variations (Fig. 8-13) may be defined.

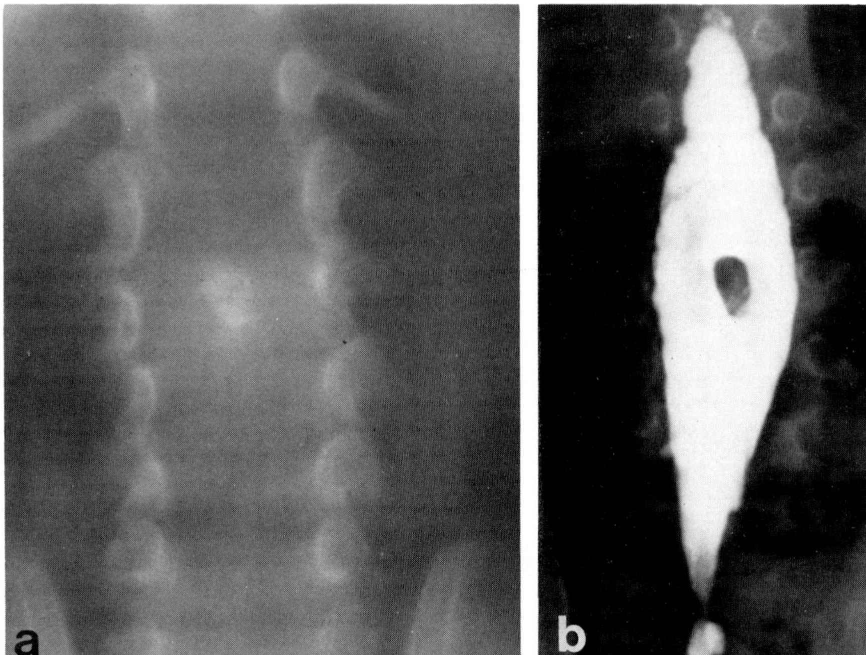

Fig. 8-13 (a) Tomographic cut in anteroposterior projection, showing the presence of a midline bony spur at L2. (b) Myelographic confirmation of diastematomyelia with duplication of cord-shadow.

The urological examination. A complete urological evaluation should be performed in all patients with evidence of spinal dysraphism, even without clinical evidence of urological involvement. Evaluation should include a cystometrogram, an intravenous pyelogram, and a voiding cystourethrogram. The cystometrographic examination may confirm the evidence of residual urine, decreased tone, or overflow incontinence and provide an *objective* evaluation of the patient's condition prior to any operative attempt to correct the condition. The intravenous pyelogram will objectively assess the amount of kidney involvement (retrograde flow, urether dilatation, etc.) (Campbell, 1962).

It should be stressed (Bruce and Schut, 1971) that it is the combination of the neurological examination, orthopedic abnormalities, and the urological evaluation which, together with the abnormal plain x-rays, makes the correct diagnosis a 90% probability.

Electromyography and nerve conduction tests. These tests may be of some benefit to assessment of the distribution and the involvement of the compromised nerve roots if and when the previously outlined steps support the diagnosis of spinal dysraphism.

Myelographic examination. The most important radiological examination is myelography. However, since the spinal cord may be lower than normal, the examination must be performed with care. Some (Gryspeerdt, 1963; Campbell, 1962; Swedberg, 1963) advise cisternal myelography, since Arnold-Chiari malformation is extremely rare in children with spinal dysraphism (Russell and Donald, 1935). However, there are cases in which this additional malformation did exist (DeLong and Schneider, 1966). Campbell (1962) does not think that myelography is necessary prior to surgery.

We believe that a myelogram is essential in the preoperative evaluation of spinal dysraphism. In the hands of an experienced neuroradiologist, the lumbar myelogram can be performed safely by using image intensification for control. We would utilize a cisternal myelogram only in those instances in which the lumbar myelogram is unsuccessful. In our 22 cases, lumbar myelography was performed without complication. We emphasize that these studies should be performed only by persons skilled in radiological techniques and the interpretation of results. In addition to the prone examination, films should be taken supine to outline the posterior aspect of the subarachnoid space, since it is usually the posterior aspect of the spinal cord or cauda equina which is fixed to dura and bone. Additional films in supine standing position may be required to obtain optimal information (Figs. 8-14, 8-15, 8-16).

While most studies are performed with positive contrast myelography (Pantopaque), air myelography also has been performed with considerable success and clarity in demonstrating these structures (Swedberg, 1963) (Fig. 8-17). However, the air myelographic examination requires more sophisticated tomographic equipment. A combination of positive contrast and air examination can be performed at the time of the routine myelographic study. We have found that this type of combined investigation allows a more three-dimensional assessment of the unusual anatomy and pathology of the lesion. With the patient in the prone position, the air will outline the posterior and upper parts of the potentially existing sac or enlarged subarachnoid space with the lipomatous component, while the positive contrast material will outline the anterior and inferior aspects of the same structures. With the patient in the supine position, just the reverse information can be obtained.

The *whole* neuroaxis must be examined. Although the statement has been made repeatedly that children with spinal dysraphism have no involvement of the cervico-occipital junction, Arnold-Chiari malformation and other types of dysraphism may occur.

The dye generally cannot be removed, and no attempt should be made to try to remove the dye at the time of the myelographic examination. Most of the injected Pantopaque will be recovered at the time of the operation.

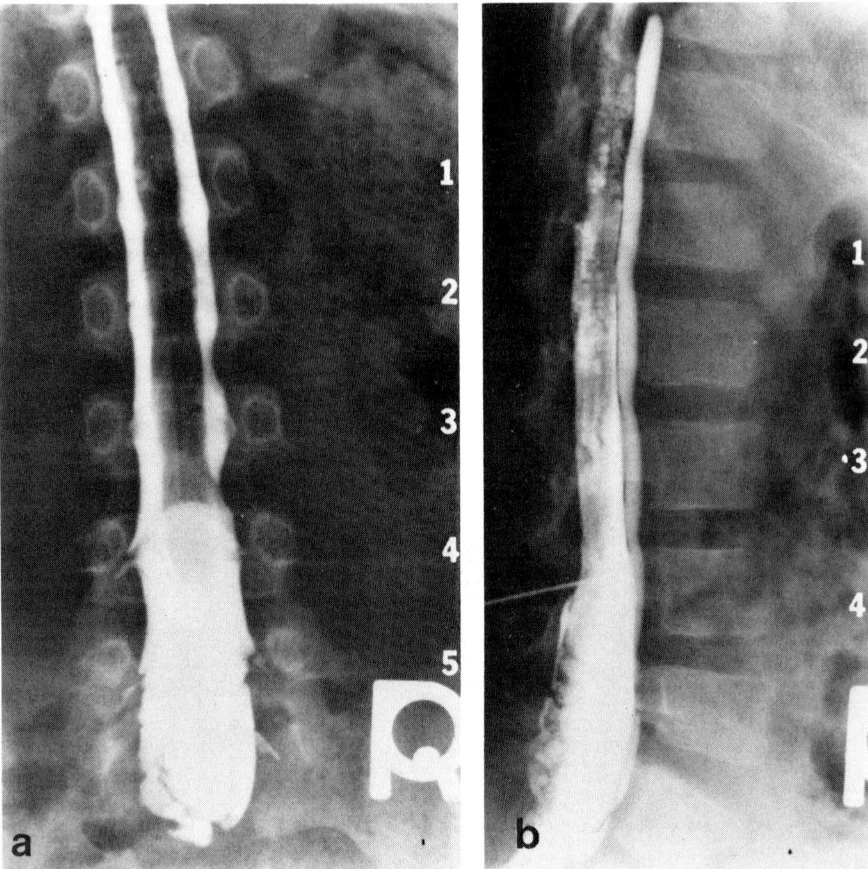

Fig. 8-14 Myelogram through lumbar puncture at L3-L4. Posteroanterior (a) and lateral view (b) showing the presence of a tethered cord and terminal lipoma.

DIFFERENTIAL DIAGNOSIS

The differential diagnosis of progressive neurological, orthopedic, or urological disability includes spinal cord tumors. In addition to the myelographic picture, the presence of skin manifestations or evidence of spinal dysraphism should enable a correct diagnosis. It is important to avoid diagnosis such as poliomyelitis, "old cord injury," or muscular dystrophy without attempting to rule out the presence of spinal dysraphism. Considerable harm can be done to children with spinal dysraphism if they are treated for such a presumptive diagnosis while a relatively benign process is allowed to cause irreversible damage.

The differential diagnosis of cerebral palsy affecting primarily or mainly the lower limbs may be difficult. In any child who presents the spasticity of one or both lower limbs and who has evidence of lower motor neuron involvement, a spinal cord lesion should be suspected. We have seen children in our clinic presenting with the diagnosis of "progressive cerebral palsy," one of whom proved to have an intraspinal epidermoid cyst at the conus medullaris and another of whom proved to have a cystic astrocytoma of the cervical cord with a progressive quadriparesis. *Cerebral palsy is not a progressive condition!*

TREATMENT

The ultimate treatment of children with spinal dysraphism is neurosurgical. These children are suffering from a progressive deterioration of many systems because of the involvement of the neural control by pressure, traction, or slow destruction of the motor, sensory, and visceral pathways. If an early

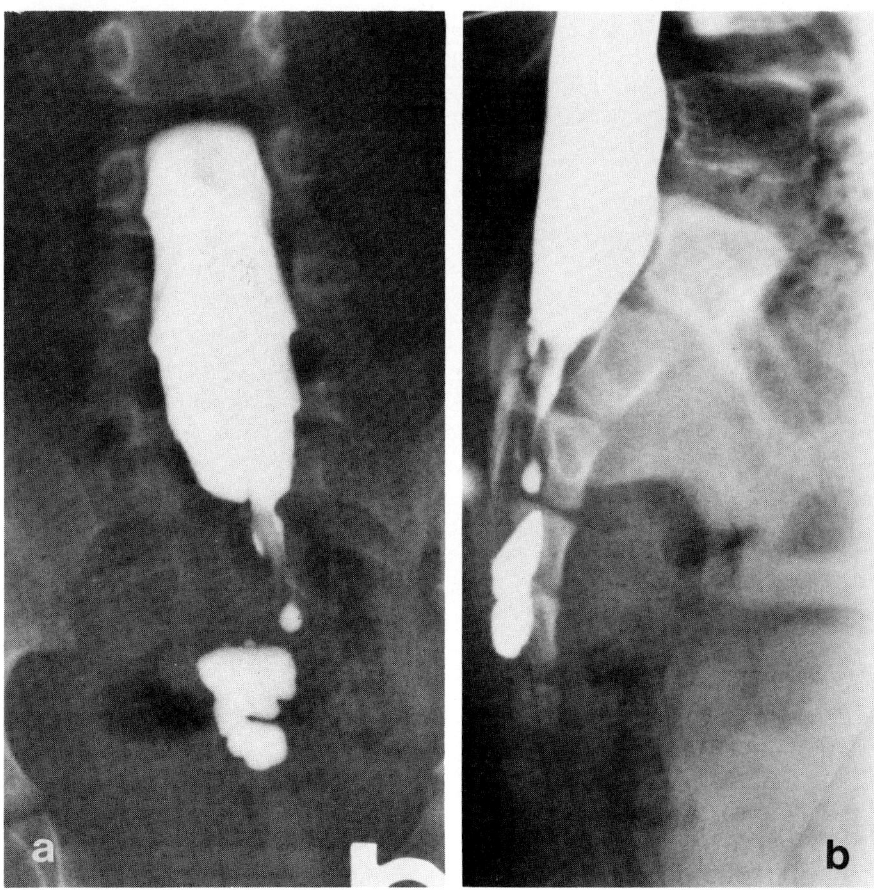

Fig. 8-15 Lumbar myelogram. Supine (a) and lateral (b) projection. Note the extremely low position of the dural sac (at S4-5), the presence of tethered cord, enlarged filum terminale, and an irregular, constricting mass (lipoma).

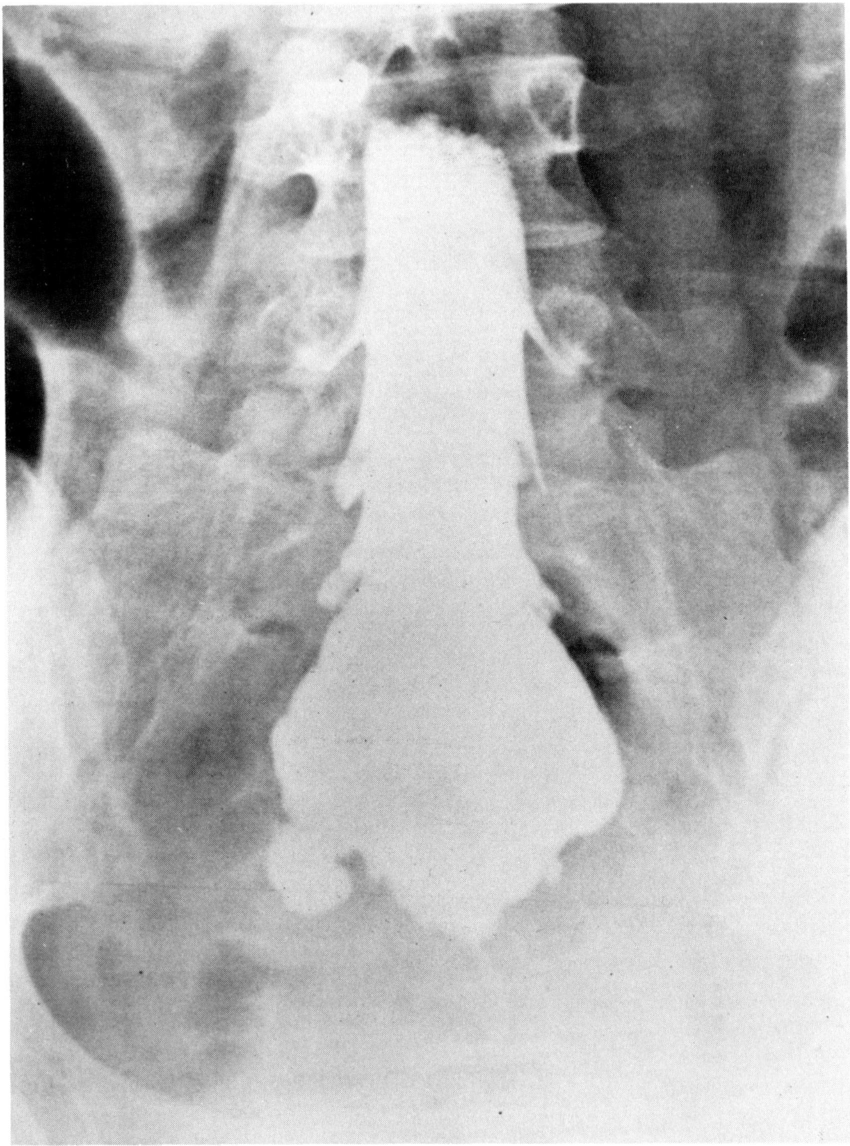

Fig. 8-16 Anteroposterior view of a myelogram showing huge dilatation of the dural sac with an irregular caudal mass (lipoma) attached to it.

diagnosis is made of this condition, the question is not *whether* surgery should be performed, but *when*. Surgical relief of the abnormal anatomy and judicious removal of the concomitant tissues (lipoma, epidermoid, etc.) offer the *only* hope for these children.

There is debate about the timing of surgery in those patients who have no evidence of deficit or who are so-called "asymptomatic." This is particularly

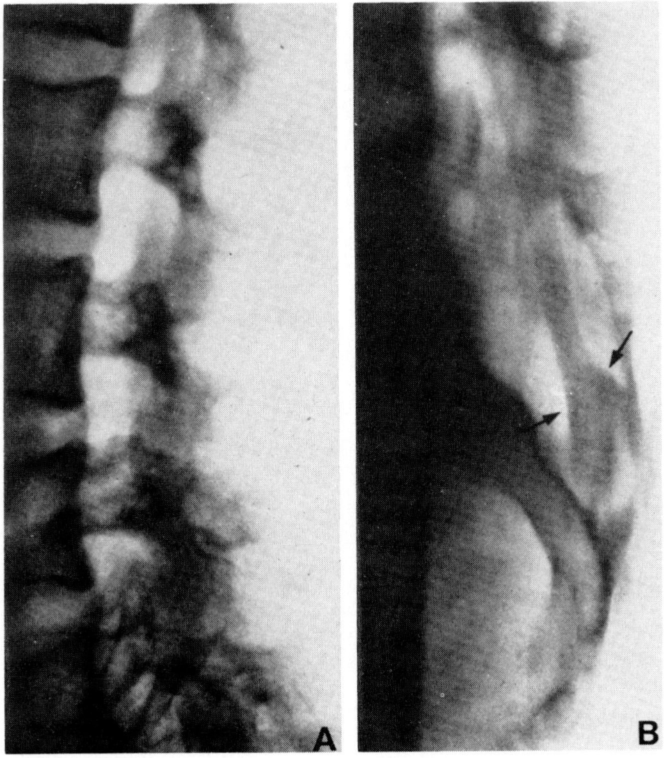

Fig. 8-17 Sacral meningomyelocele. (A) Lumbar region, lateral. The spinal cord does not end at the normal level but continues down through the whole length of the vertebral canal; total absence of lumbar intumescence. (B) Lateral tomography of sacral region. The sacral canal is abnormally wide and the subarachnoid space fills it completely (intrasacral herniation of the meninges); the spinal cord reaches as far down as the sacral hiatus, where it is attached to a tumor-like formation (arrows). Courtesy of Swedberg, Acta Radiol. Diagn. 1:796, 1963.

true in the group of children below age 2, as many of the findings become manifest only with future growth spurts.

Delay in operation may allow neurological deficit to appear. An apparently "normal" neurological examination may become abnormal within a relatively short period of time. Therefore, careful (monthly) neurological evaluation of those children under observation is mandatory. Sudden deterioration in the form of sensory loss, incontinence, or loss of reflex activity should prompt a more definitive diagnostic work-up. Even with careful observation, additional neurological deficit may develop within a relatively short period of time. Therefore, we feel that the complete evaluation is indicated in the asymptomatic patient, and a "prophylactic" operation should be performed before permanent neurological deficit ensues. In the hands of experienced pediatric neurosurgeons, the complication rate is minimal (Tables 8-1, 8-2). We have had two patients who have been fol-

Table 8-2A Presenting Clinical Manifestations in Seven Children under 2 Years of Age Seen at Johns Hopkins Hospital

"Sacral mass" (subcutaneous lipoma)	6
with pigmented nevi	2
with hairy patch	1
with "dimple"	2
with sinus	1
X-rays	
spina bifida occulta	7
sacral hypoplasia	2
Urinary incontinence	5(?2)
Rectal incontinence	1?
Foot deformity + atrophy (lower motor neuron)	5
Additional increased tone, hyperreflexia (upper motor neuron)	2
Sensory deficit	4
Previous surgery	0

Table 8-2B Surgical Results in Children Under 2 Years of Age at Surgery. Follow-up 6 Months to 6 Years

Excellent (no functional deficit)	4
Good (mild deficit)	2
Unchanged	1

lowed on a bimonthly basis without operation. One developed definite increase of saddle anesthesia and additionally, increased dribbling of the urine at age 6 months, findings which were not present 2 months earlier. Subsequent myelographic study confirmed the presence of a leptomyelolipoma with tethered cord. Surgery was performed, with incomplete removal of the lipoma and untethering of the cord. Four years after operation, there is intermittent stress incontinence and a borderline cystometric tracing. The saddle anesthesia remained unchanged, together with some weakness and atrophy of the right lower extremity with inversion of the right foot, signs which became more manifest when the child started to ambulate. Another child had a small area of skin pigmentation and no neurological deficit but marked sacral hypoplasia. On a follow-up visit, a decreased knee jerk, sensory blunting along the 3, 4, and 5 sacral dermatomes, and stress incontinence were found. Myelography confirmed a large extra- and intradural lipoma in addition to a tethered cord. At operation, the lipoma was subtotally resected, and the cord was freed. Postoperatively, the reflex activity and the sensation returned to normal. Although the infiltrating part of the lipoma into the conus medullaris could not be removed, the child has remained asymptomatic over a period of 2.5 years (Figs. 8-18, 8-19).

In a few instances, when a competent group of specialists can follow the asymptomatic child at *very* frequent intervals, a conservative attitude with careful observation may be justified. But even then, permanent neurological deficit may occur. However, under any other circumstances, early surgery should be advocated. In our patients, at least six out of the 22 had been told by their physicians to return for follow-up; however, for one or another reason, these patients did not return and the children were next seen with irreversible urinary tract involvement or neurological deficits.

Although early operation is urged once the correct diagnosis is made, it should be noted that remarkable recovery has been observed in a few patients who came to surgery late, at the ages of 12, 17, and 21. Recovery from urinary incontinence, marked improvement of sensation, and disappearance of "traction pain" were observed in five out of 28 of our own series. Long-standing motor deficit generally remained unchanged. It is clear that surgery definitely should be recommended in all these "late" cases once the diagnosis has been established.

The operative technique. All operations are performed with the patient in a prone position under general anesthesia. In small children, careful monitoring of temperature, careful replacement of blood loss, and administration of anesthesia with controlled respiration is mandatory. It is important to drape the patient with transparent plastic material in such a way that direct observation of the gluteal and perianal muscle contractions is facilitated. An intraoperative cystometrogram may help to identify the corresponding sacral roots at stimulation. Electrical stimulation is used routinely to identify functioning neural components. Bipolar coagulation,

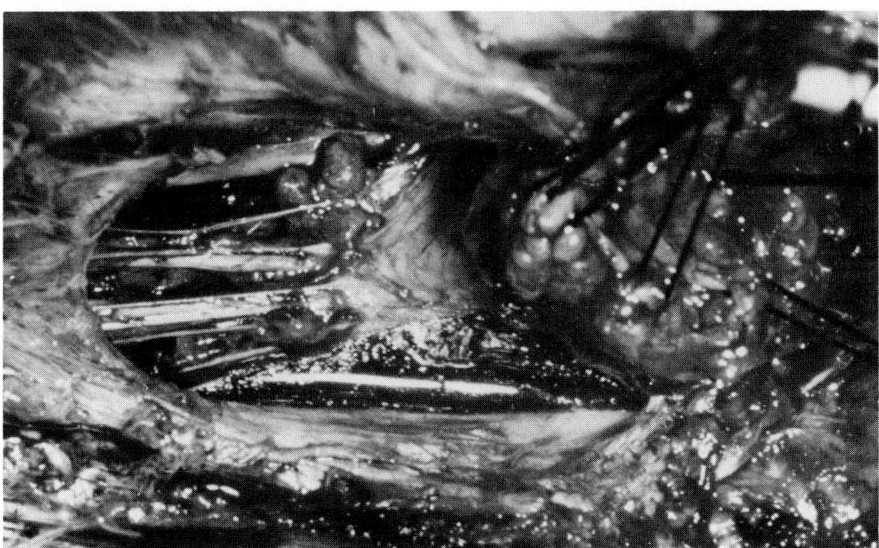

Fig. 8-18 Operative photograph showing the remaining lipomatous mass on the right side, after it has been dissected and removed from the sacral roots.

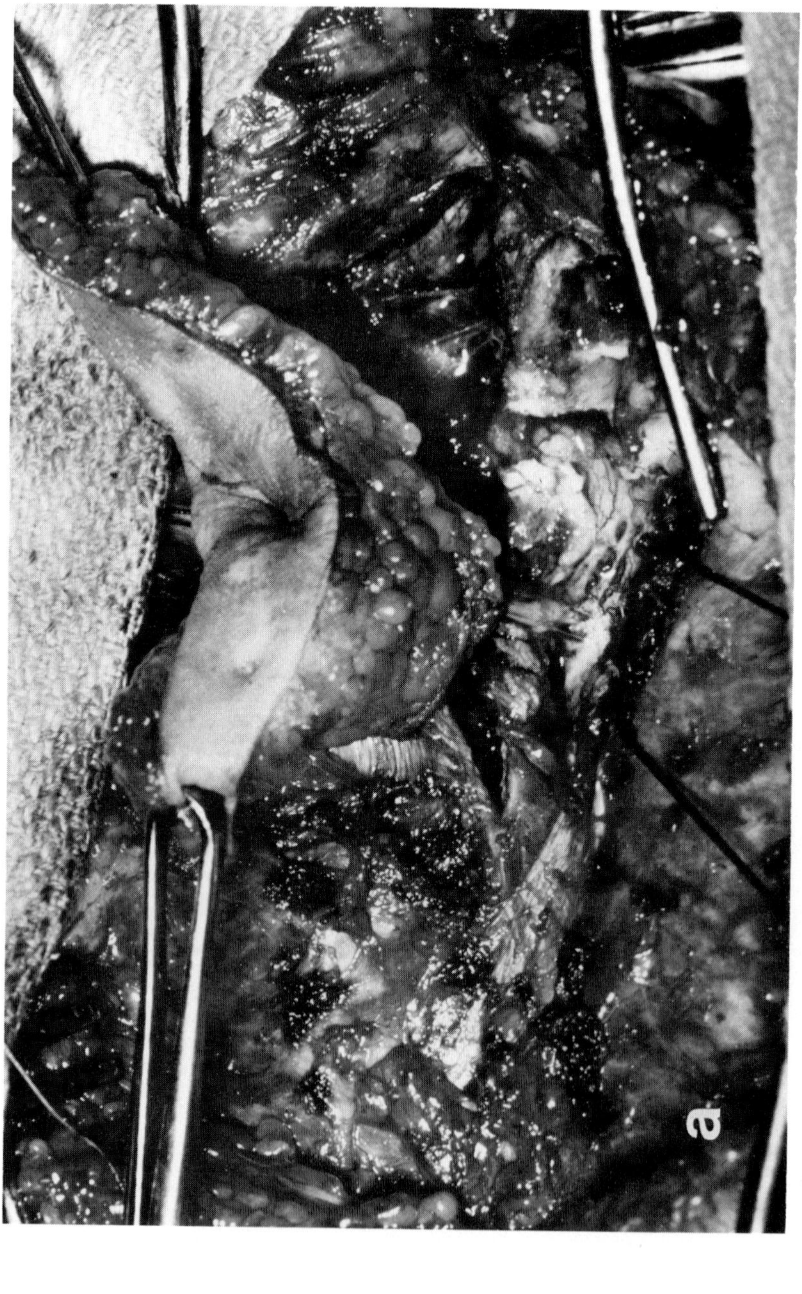

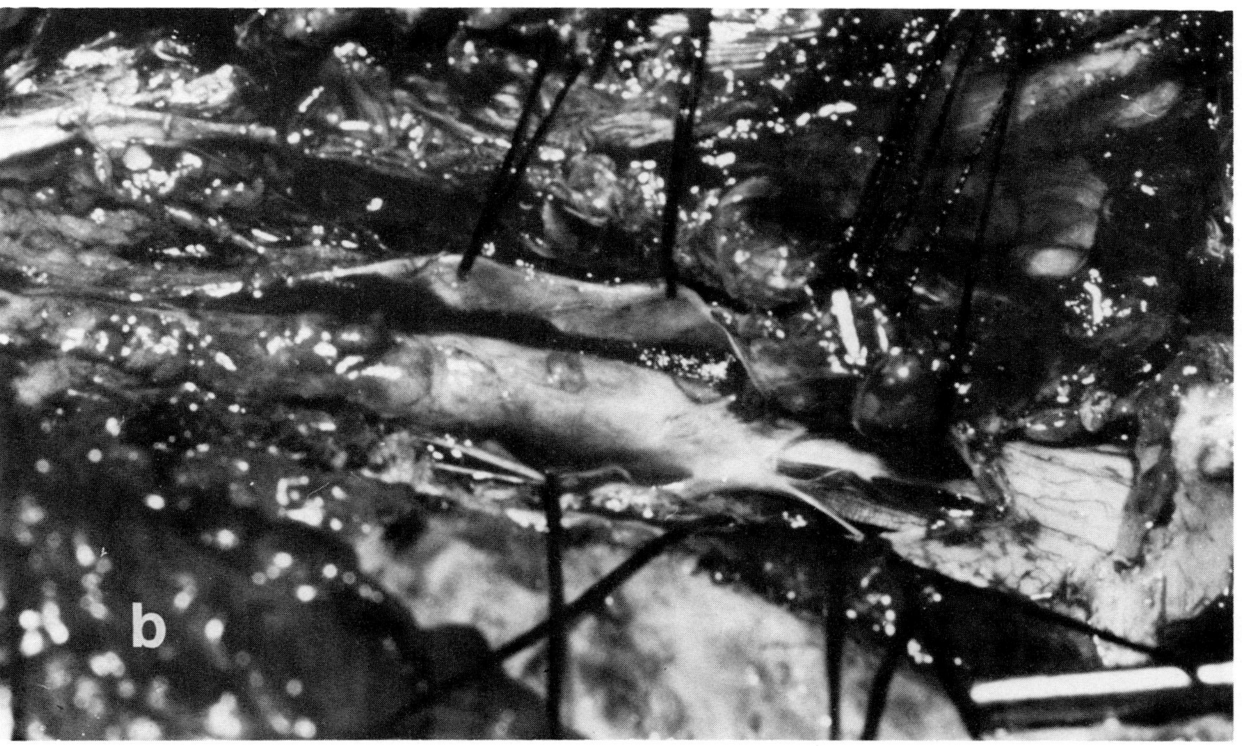

Fig. 8-19 Operative photographs. (a) Underneath the pigmented skin lesion, the subcutaneous lipoma is followed through the fascia and dura mater; attachment to one of the nerve roots can be seen. (b) showing the infiltration by intradural lipoma of the conus medullaris.

microsurgical instruments, and the use of the operative dissecting microscope allow meticulous and safe dissection of the adhesion and fibrous bands from vital neural structures. Even with this improved technique, the most important single factor for success is the judgment of the pediatric neurosurgeon. *Excessive zeal* in the removal of lipomatous tissue often results in increased neurological deficit.

Even though some infiltrating lipomatus tissue is left behind, if the tethering of the cord has been relieved, considerable improvement may occur and there may be no recurrence of symptoms.

Release of constrictive fibrous bands is extremely important. It is equally important to follow the filum terminale, because in many instances the lipomatous involvement is at the most distant portion of the filum, and continuation of the lipomatous tissue through the fascia and the subcutaneous tissue should not be missed. In many instances, it is feasible to sever the enlarged filum terminale and the adhesions around the cord. In a few cases, remarkable retraction (upward movement) of the cord could be observed on the operating table, measuring in one child almost 2 cm (Fig. 8-20). On the other hand, if viable roots are involved in the tethering mechanism of the cord, great care should be taken not to sacrifice important motor or sensory fibers for the sake of a mechanically "perfect undoing" of the tethered cord (Fig. 8-21).

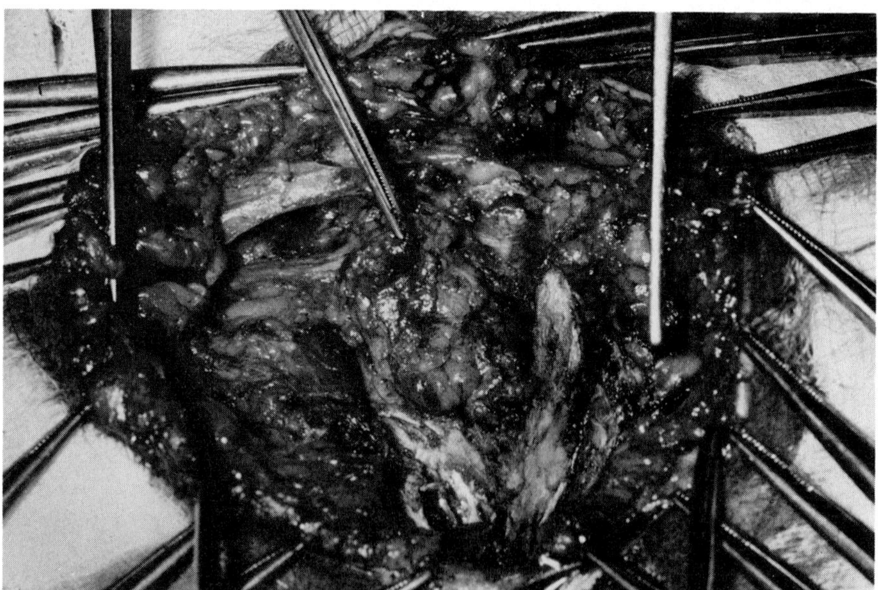

Fig. 8-20 Operative photograph showing the huge lipomatous mass attached to a widened and infiltrated filum terminale. After sectioning the latter and removing the lipoma, the tethered cord moved up an inch.

In most instances, it is extremely difficult to close the dura after the dissection is finished; this is especially true when the lipoma is extra- and intradural. It is our custom to patch the dura with fascia lata. Careful closure of the various muscular and fascial layers is important to prevent postoperative cerebrospinal fluid leaks and infections.

Although diastematomyelia can be diagnosed in many instances by plain x-rays and myelography, in at least 50% of the patients only fibrous bands were present and no bony spurs could be identified. There is usually evidence of incomplete duplication of the cord, nerve roots, or both. Complete removal of the bony spur may be difficult, but every effort should be undertaken to release the tethering effect of these spurs (Fig. 8-22). It is important that in addition to the removal of the spur, the fibrous adhesions and bands should be freed to allow the split cord to slide upwards. A careful closure of at least the dorsal dura is mandatory, and again, patching is recommended to avoid a cerebrospinal fluid leak.

Postoperative care. Absolute bedrest of 10 to 14 days is recommended to secure good healing of the operative area and to prevent the possibility of cerebrospinal fluid leak. The urinary catheter is generally left in place after operation for a period of 7 days, or longer if necessary. Antibiotics are administered intraoperatively and postoperatively. The child is seen at frequent intervals by the whole team, including the orthopedic surgeon, pediatric neurologist, psychologist, and neurosurgeon. Early rehabilitation is instituted by the physical therapy team. Psychological counseling and encouragement in order to reinforce and support the organic improvement are extremely important.

Long-term follow-up. This provides us with objective criteria with regard to the duration of improvement and possible recurrences. In our personal experience, we have reliable information up to 9 years after operation. Those children who showed improvement within the first 6 months after surgery retained the improvement or improved further.

SUMMARY

Children with spinal dysraphism form a well-defined clinical entity. The clinical manifestations are insidious and are signaled by skin lesions, discrete signs of urinary or rectal incontinence, motor reflex and sensory changes, gait abnormality, and occasionally, trophic changes. Many of these children are treated for their "peripheral" manifestations without the benefit of a correct diagnosis. The recognition of this entity based on the history, clinical manifestations, typical x-ray, and neurological findings should be facilitated by a team approach. Pediatrician, dermatologist, urologist, orthopedic surgeon, pediatric neurologist, and pediatric neurosurgeon, together with the rehabilitation staff, should coordinate their efforts to improve the early recognition of this entity. Early neurosurgical intervention can prevent irreversible deterioration of the urinary, motor, or sensory

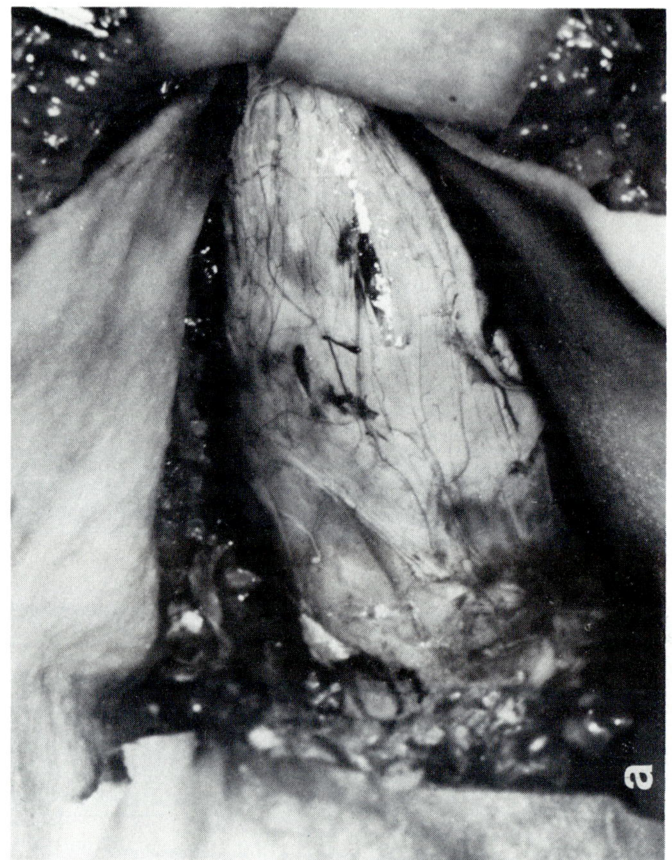
a

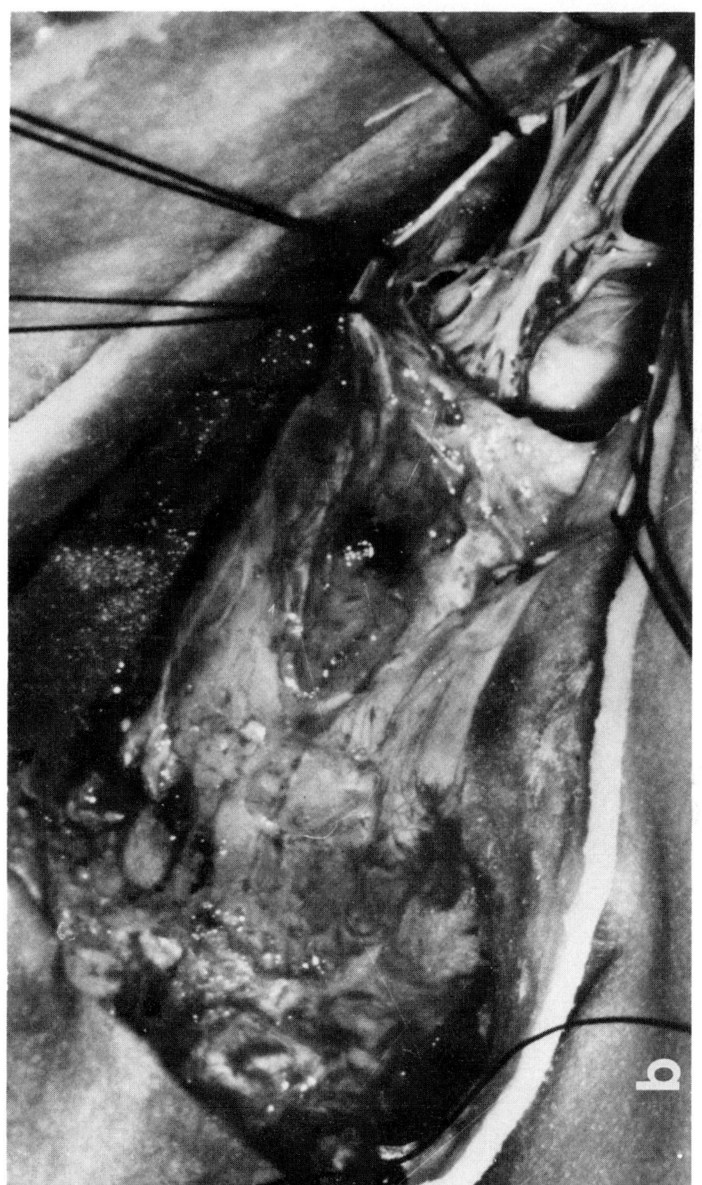

Fig. 8-21 Operative photograph showing (a) the extremely widened dural sac fused with a huge lipoma; and (b) the tethered conus medullaris with the cranially directed nerve roots. Some of the lipomatous mass had to be left behind. Fig. 8-16 shows the myelogram of the same patient.

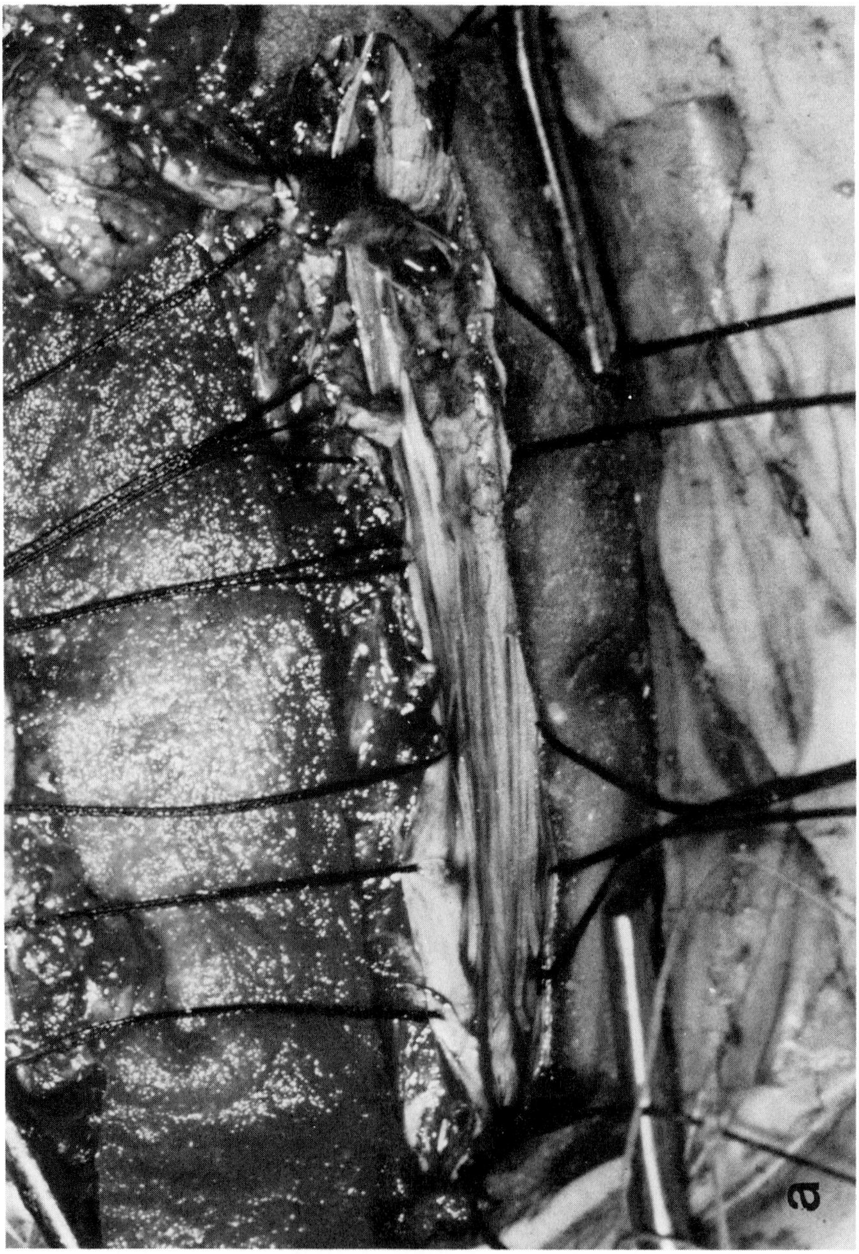

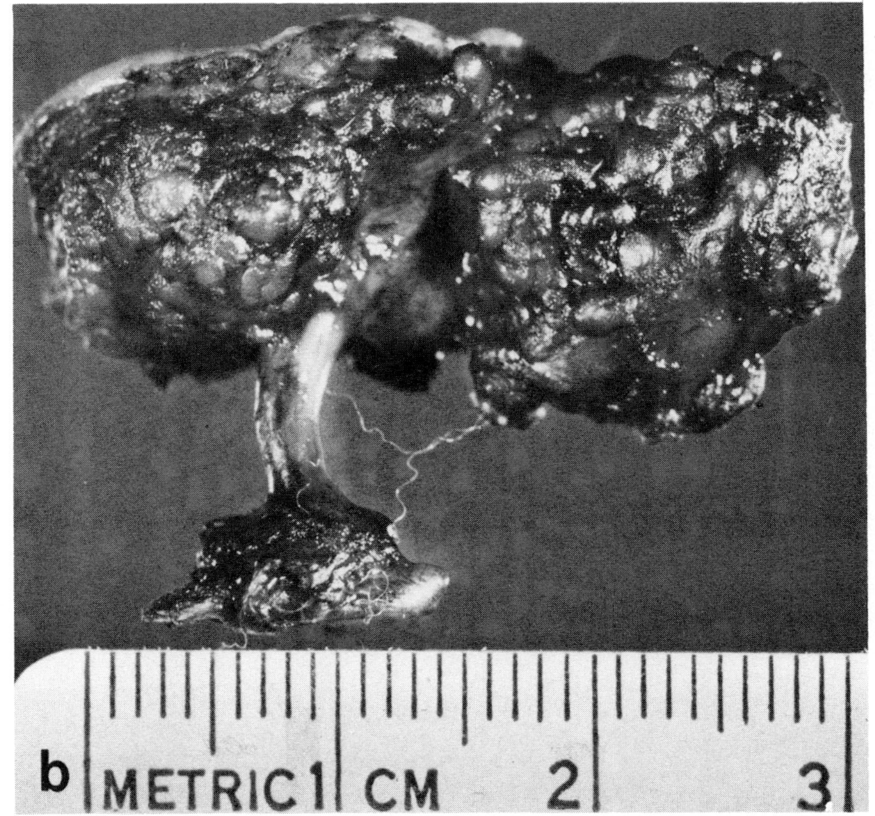

Fig. 8-22 Operative photograph of a 6-month-old child whose x-rays and myelogram are shown in Fig. 8-13. (a) The subcutaneous lipoma extends through the dura and the bony spur is located between the two halves of the split cord. The specimen can be seen (b) after *complete* removal of the lesion.

system. With appropriate careful technique, considerable improvement can be achieved in 50% of the patients who have acquired neurological deficit. Progressive deterioration is prevented in another 40% of the children. Less than 10% showed further deterioration or became worse after surgery. Early detection and operative intervention can prevent even this disability.

BIBLIOGRAPHY

Alexander, E., Jr., F. K. Garvey, and W. Boyce. 1954. Congenital lumbosacral myelomeningocele with incontinence: A contribution to the understanding of bladder physiology. J. Neurosurg. 11:183.

Anderson, F. M. 1968. Occult spinal dysraphism. J. Pediat. 73:164.

Bassett, R. C. 1957. The neurologic deficit associated with lipomas of the cauda equina. Ann. Surg. 131:109.

Bentley, J. F. R., and J. R. Smith. 1960. Developmental posterior enteric remnants and spinal malformations: The split notochord syndrome. Arch. Dis. Childh. 35:76.

Blockley, N. J., and J. Schorstein. 1961. Intraspinal tumours in the lumbar region of children. J. Bone Joint Surg. 43B:556.

Brickner, W. M. 1918. Spina bifida occulta. Am. J. Med. Sci. 155:473.

Bruce, D., and L. Schut. 1971. Spinal dysraphism and associated lumbosacral lipomata in childhood. Paper presented at the Annual Meeting of the American Association of Neurological Surgery, Houston, Texas, April, 1971.

Bryant, H., and A. D. Dayan. 1967. Spinal inclusion dermoid cyst in a patient with a treated myelocystococele. J. Neurol. Neurosurg. Psychiat. 30:182.

Bunch, W. H., A. S. Cass, A. S. Bensman, and D. M. Long. 1972. Modern management of meningocele. Warren H. Green, Inc., St. Louis.

Burrows, F. G. O. 1968. Some aspects of occult spinal dysraphism: A study of 90 cases. Brit. J. Radiol. 4:496.

Cameron, A. H. 1957. The Arnold-Chiari and other neuro-anatomical malformations associated with spina bifida. J. Path. Bact. 73:195.

Campbell, J. B. 1962. Neurosurgical treatment of bladder and bowel dysfunction resulting from anomalous development of the sacral neural axis. Clin. Neurosurg. 10:133.

Choremis, C., D. Economos, C. Papadatos, and A. Gargoulas. 1956. Intraspinal epidermoid tumours (Cholesteatomas) in patients treated for tuberculous meningitis. Lancet 2:437.

Cohn, G. A., and W. B. Hamby. 1953. The surgery of cranium bifidum and spina bifida. J. Neurosurg. 10:297.

Daniel, P. M., and S. J. Strich. 1958. Some observations on the congenital deformity of the central nervous system known as the Arnold-Chiari malformation. J. Neuropath. Exp. Neurol. 17:255.

DeLong, W. B., and R. C. Schneider. 1966. Surgical management of congenital spinal lesions associated with abnormalities of the cranio-spinal junction. J. Neurol. Neurosurg. Psychiat. 29:319.

DeRougement, R., R. Francois, M. Hermier, and P. Fournier. 1962. A propos d'une observation de tumeur epidermoide spinale de l'enfant d'origine traumatique. Pediatrie 17:691.

Dubowitz, V., J. Lorber, and R. B. Zachary. 1965. Lipoma of the cauda equina. Arch. Dis. Childh. 40:207.

Emery, J. L., and R. G. Lendon. 1969. Lipomas of the cauda equina and other fatty tumours related to neurospinal dysraphism. Develop. Med. Child Neurol. (Suppl.) 20:62.

Fisher, R. G., A. Uihlein, and H. M. Keith. 1952. Spina bifida and cranium bifidum: Study of 530 cases. Proc. Mayo Clinic 27:33.

Fluckiger, A. 1967. Les tumeurs lombosacrées associées au spina bifida occulta. Arch. Suisse Neurol. Neurochir. Psychiat. 99:201.

Garceau, G. J. 1953. The filum terminale syndrome (the cord-traction syndrome). J. Bone Joint Surg. 35A:711.

Gardner, W. J. 1964. Diastematomyelia and the Klippel-Feil syndrome. Relationship to hydrocephalus, syringomyelia, meningocele, meningomyelocele, and iniencephalus. Cleveland Clinic Quart. 31:19.

Groff, R. A., and J. C. Yaskin. 1947. Late occurrence of sphincter and other neurological disturbances associated with congenital malformations of the vertebral column. Trans. Am. Neurol. Assoc. 218.

Gross, R. E., G. W. Holcomb, Jr., and H. Swan. 1953. Treatment of neurologic urinary and fecal incontinence in children. Arch. Surg. 66:143.

Gryspeerdt, G. L. 1963. Myelographic assessments of occult forms of spinal dysraphism. Acta Radiol. (Diagn.) 1:702.

Ingraham, F. D., and H. Swan. 1943. Spina bifida and cranium bifidum. New Eng. J. Med. 228:559.

Jackson, I. J., I. M. Thompson, C. A. Hooks, and G. T. Hoffman. 1956. Urinary incontinence in myelomeningocele due to a tethered spinal cord and its surgical treatment. Surg. Gynec. Obstet. 103:618.

James, C. C. M., and L. P. Lassman. 1958. Diastematomyelia. Arch. Dis. Childh. 33:536.

James, C. C. M., and L. P. Lassman. 1960. Spinal dysraphism. Arch. Dis. Childh. 35:315.

James, C. C. M., and L. P. Lassman. 1962a. Spinal dysraphism. J. Bone Joint Surg. 44:828.

James, C. C. M., and L. P. Lassman. 1962b. Spinal dysraphism–The diagnosis and treatment of progressive lesions in spina bifida occulta. J. Bone Joint Surg. 44B:829.

James, C. C. M., and L. P. Lassman. 1972. Spinal dysraphism: Spina bifida occulta. Butterworth & Co. (Publishers) Ltd., London.

Jones, P. H., and J. G. Love. 1956. Tight filum terminale. Arch. Surg. 73:556.

Kahn, E. A. 1947. The role of the dentate ligaments in spinal cord compression and the syndrome of lateral sclerosis. J. Neurosurg. 4:191.

Lassman, L. P., and C. C. M. James. 1967. Lumbosacral lipomas: Critical survey of 26 cases submitted to laminectomy. J. Neurol. Neurosurg. Psychiat. 30:174.

Leveuf, J., I. Bertrand, and H. Steinberg. 1937. Étude sur le spina bifida. Masson et cie, Paris.

Levi, A. 1926. Études sur les affections de la colonne vertebrale. Masson et cie, Paris.

Lichtenstein, B. W. 1940. Spinal dysraphism–Spina bifida and myelodysplasia. Arch. Neurol. Psychiat. 44:792.

Lichtenstein, B. W. 1942. Distant neuroanatomic complications of spina bifida (spinal dysraphism). Arch. Neurol. Psychiat. 47:195.

List, C. F. 1941. Intraspinal epidermoids, dermoids, and dermal sinuses. Surg. Gynec. Obstet. 73:525.

Lobo, E. deH. 1968. Spinal dysraphism in children. Brit. J. Clin. Practice 22:423.

Loeser, J. D., and R. J. Lewin. 1970. Lumbosacral lipomas in the adult case report. J. Neurosurg. 29:405.

Matson, D. D. 1969. Neurosurgery of infancy and childhood. Charles C Thomas, Publishers, Springfield, Ill.

Matson, D. D., and M. J. Jerva. 1966. Recurrent meningitis with congenital lumbosacral dermal sinus tract. J. Neurosurg. 25:288.

Meredith, J. M. 1944. Unusual congenital anomalies of the lumbo-sacral spine (spina bifida) with a report of three cases. J. Nervous Mental Dis. 99:115.

Mertz, H. O., and L. A. Smith. 1930. Posterior spinal fusion defects and nerve dysfunction of the urinary tract. J. Urol. 24:41.

Morales, P. A., G. G. Deaver, and R. S. Hotchkiss. 1956. Urological complications of spina bifida in children. J. Urol. 75:537.

Peach, B. 1965. Arnold-Chiari malformation. Arch. Neurol. 12:613.

Rand, R. W., and C. W. Rand. 1960. Intraspinal tumors of childhood. Charles C Thomas, Publishers, Springfield, Ill.

Reimann, A. F., and B. J. Anson. 1944. Vertebral level of termination of the spinal cord with report of a case of sacral cord. Anat. Rec. 88:127.

Rogers, H. M., D. M. Long, S. N. Chow, and L. A. French. 1971. Lipomas of the spinal cord and cauda equina. J. Neurosurg. 34:349.

Roller, G. J., and F. W. Pribram. 1965. Lumbosacral and intradural lipoma and sacral agenesis. Radiology 84:507.

Russell, D. S., and C. Donald. 1935. The mechanism of internal hydrocephalus in spina bifida. Brain 58:203.

Saunders, R. L. 1943. Combined anterior and posterior spina bifida in a living neonatal human female. Anat. Rec. 87:255.

Sharrard, W. J. W. 1966. Occult spinal dysraphism. Develop. Med. Child Neurol. 8:464.

Shorey, W. D. 1955. Diastematomyelia associated with dorsal kyphosis producing paraplegia. J. Neurosurg. 12:300.

Streeter, G. L. 1919. Factors involved in the formation of the filum terminale. Am. J. Anat. 25:1.

Swanson, H. S., and J. C. Barnett, Jr. 1962. Intradural lipomas in children. Pediatrics 29:911.

Swedberg, M. 1963. Meningo and myelomeningocele studied by gas myelography. Acta Radiol. Diagn. (Stockholm), N.S. 1:796.

Tavafoghi, V., G. W. Hambrick, Jr., and G. B. Udvarhelyi. 1971. Cutaneous signs of spinal dysraphism: A tail-like lipoma. Presented at the Section of Dermatology, A. M. A. Meeting, Atlantic City, N. J.

Teng, P., and C. Papatheodorou. 1965. Arnold-Chiari malformation with normal spine and cranium. Arch. Neurol. 12:622.

Till, K. 1965. Spinal dysraphism. Turkish J. Pediat. 7:1.

Till, K. 1968. Spinal dysraphism: A study of congenital malformations of the back. Develop. Med. Child Neurol. 10:470.

Till, K. 1969. Spinal dysraphism: A study of congenital malformations of the back. J. Bone Joint Surg. 51B:415.

Walker, A. E. 1944. Dilatation of the vertebral canal associated with congenital anomalies of the spinal cord. Am. J. Roentgenol. 52:571.

Walker, A. E., and P. C. Bucy. 1934. Congenital dermal sinuses: A source of spinal meningeal infection and subdural abscesses. Brain 57:401.

Whitby, J. D. 1961. Spinal dysraphism and the anaesthetist. Anaesthesia 16:432.

Yashon, D., and R. A. Beatty. 1966. Tethering of the conus medullaris within the sacrum. J. Neurol. Neurosurg. Psychiat. 29:244.

Zachary, R. B. 1965. Early neurological approaches to spina bifida. Develop. Med. Child Neurol. 7:492.

9

Orthopedic Aspects of Meningomyeloceles

Steven E. Kopits, M.D.

Orthopedic care represents the major medical commitment in both time and money for the child born with a meningomyelocele. The role of the orthopedic surgeon is threefold: (1) to correct deformity, (2) to prevent the development of further deformity, and (3) to minimize the consequences of the neurological disability by providing skeletal support for ambulation. These goals are achieved by the judicious combination of surgery, bracing, and physical therapy.

Orthopedic handicap in these children may be divided into deformity and disability. Deformity includes contractures and dislocation of various joints, as well as spinal problems such as kyphosis and scoliosis. Disability is the result of muscle weakness which interferes with function. The type and degree of deformity and the amount of disability vary with the quality of care the patient has received. In the newborn period, deformity and disability exist concomitantly. In the older child, deformity and disability are discussed separately.

DEFORMITY AND DISABILITY IN THE NEWBORN

Although the orthopedist's therapeutic role does not start until later, he should evaluate the newborn as soon as possible after birth and preferably before closure of the back is begun.

In this first assessment, he should note the presence of deformities, the degree of motion present in the lower limbs, and the presence of associated birth defects. As a result of this evaluation, the orthopedist experienced in the management of this condition should be able to have an approximate idea of the prognosis regarding form and function of the patient in later life.

He should be able to give the prognosis for ambulation, as well as the therapeutic procedures necessary over the ensuing years. The examination at birth should include observation of both disability (neurological deficit) and deformity. It should be performed in a warm environment, since cold decreases the degree of response. Since there is no way to know what is "voluntary motion" in the newborn, one tends to equate it to spontaneous motion observed. The examiner therefore should observe patiently the spontaneous motion present before stimulating the newborn. Precise identification of the active muscles is often impossible and unimportant, but, even in the newborn, it is possible to identify active movement of joints and reach conclusions about the integrity of the muscle groups and nerve roots which provide that function.

Pelvic	control	T_{11}–L_1
Hip	flexion	L_1–L_2
	extension	L_5–S_2
	abduction	L_4–S_1
	adduction	L_2–L_4
Knee	extension	L_3–L_4
	flexion	L_4–S_1
Ankle	dorsification	L_4–L_5
	plantarflexion	L_5–S_2
Toe	extension	L_5–S_1
	flexion	S_1–S_2

The differentation between spontaneous and reflex movement is of major significance. According to Sharrard (1959), the activity which is spontaneous at birth usually will remain spontaneous and later become voluntary, while the reflex activity will remain such in later months, although exceptions to this rule are observed in both directions. Stimulation of the lower extremities with a pin may produce reflex movement which will have functional significance. However, stimulation above the level of the lesion may encourage an infant to make spontaneous movement which *can* be evaluated. Details of the neurological examination may be found in Chapter 5. We have found that diagnostic electrical stimulation adds little to the information gained by the clinical examination.

One should also gain an impression about the integrity of upper limb function because of its importance in ambulation.

In many cases, the level of the neurological deficit can be recognized readily by the typical pattern of lower limb deformity noticed at birth. Deformity affecting the lower limbs is usually symmetrical, particularly when there is a definite level of deficit with complete absence of neural function distally (Table 9-1).

Table 9-1 Joint Deformities at Birth

Last intact root	Hips	Knees	Feet
L_1	Flexion and external rotation	Completely paralyzed. Deformities are dependent on the intrauterine position	Completely paralyzed. Deformities are dependent on the intrauterine position
$L_{2\text{-}3}$	Moderate flexion and adduction	Extension or slight flexion	Dependent on intrauterine position
L_4	Flexion, abduction, external rotation	Extension or recurvatum	Calcaneovarus
L_5	Moderate flexion	Extension or slight flexion	Marked calcaneus
S_1	No deformity	No deformity	Calcaneovalgus; rocker bottom, foot convex pes planus, clawing of toes
S_2	No deformity	No deformity	Cavovarus and clawing of toes

The deformity arising in paralyzed lower limbs may be due to: (1) partial or unequal paralysis resulting from functioning muscle groups being unopposed by their paralyzed antagonists, causing joint deformity in the direction of the pull of the active muscle; (2) intrauterine posture acting on completely paralyzed limbs; or (3) a combination of both (1) and (2).

Asymmetrical deformity of the lower extremities usually is due to hemimyelia or unilateral involvement of the spinal cord. Asymmetrical deformity often will produce a chain of extensive and increasing orthopedic problems such as leg length discrepancy, pelvic obliquity with hip dislocation, and scoliosis (Fig. 9-1). Asymmetrical involvement therefore has a worse orthopedic prognosis than does symmetrical involvement.

The presence of segments of spinal cord with reflex activity distal to a nonfunctioning segment should be suspected when fixed foot deformities are present in a case with a high-level paralysis. Electromyography often will confirm such reflex activity with electrical inactivity between it and the level of neurological deficit proximally. Similar foot deformities, however, may also develop because of the posture adopted by the paralyzed lower limbs of the fetus against the uterine wall. In this case, electromyography will reveal no activity of the muscles of the foot.

Postural deformities which occur *in utero* in otherwise completely paralyzed lower limbs have an appearance quite similar to those seen in arthrogryphosis.

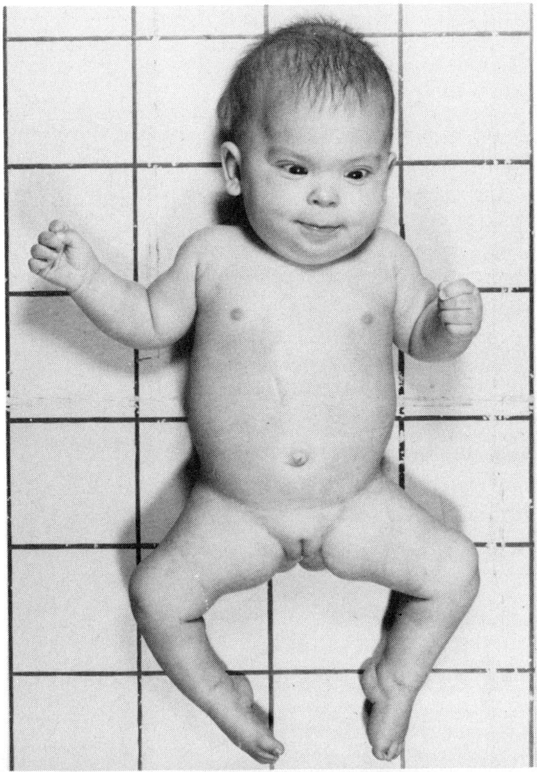

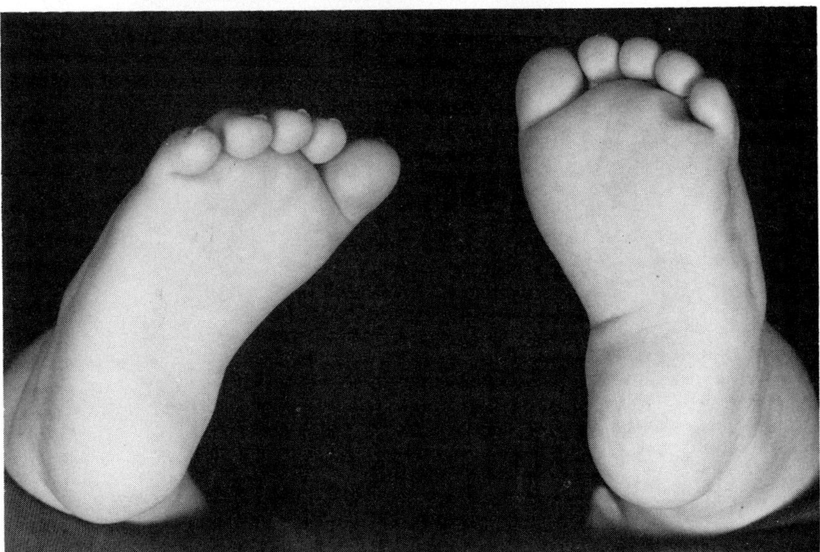

Fig. 9-1 Seven-month-old with fixed hip flexion-abduction, external rotation contracture, and knee flexion contracture bilaterally. The right foot is in a fixed equinovarus position, while the left is in a fixed cavus position.

It is important to establish whether the deformities are supple or fixed and to bear in mind that deformities which were originally supple may become fixed with time.

Deformity of the spine may occur at the level of the meningomyelocele. The most important of these spinal deformities is the fixed kyphosis which may occur within the confines of the meningocele sac. It is very important to diagnose this lesion during the first examination *prior* to closure of the back, because its correction should be done at this time. If left uncorrected at the time of closure, the result may be complete paraplegia distal to the apex of the kyphotic curve. The management of the kyphosis is further discussed below.

Deformities of the spine also may occur at levels other than that of the meningomyelocele caused by the same teratogenic agent. These include diastematomyelia, congenital scoliosis, and congenital kyphosis. Since the clinical diagnosis of such associated developmental defects of the spine in the newborn is almost impossible because of the absence of signs, anteroposterior and lateral x-rays should be obtained of the entire spine before closure of the back in *every* newborn infant.

Dislocation of the hip also may be present at birth, and although its diagnosis is made on the basis of the clinical examination, radiological examination of the hips may be done on the newborn by including the pelvis on the anteroposterior exposure of the spine.

The findings of the pediatrician, neurologist, neurosurgeon, and urologist should be taken into account when completing this first evaluation and before outlining a plan of orthopedic management.

INITIAL INTERVIEW WITH THE PARENTS

The first interview of the parents by the orthopedist is of paramount importance, since it sets the basis of a long-lasting relationship.

The orthopedist should identify himself as the physician whose function it is to help the child to stand and walk. He should keep in mind that the parents usually are dazed by the impact of the news about their baby and are unable to absorb detailed technical information at this time. Their interest usually is focused on what will happen to their child immediately, although they also expect a prognostic statement about his future possibilities of ambulation.

The temptation that one might feel at this point to outline the series of procedures which may have to be performed in the future to make the child ambulatory should be resisted. This is an unnecessary burden of added worry for the parents at this early stage. It is also advisable to keep in mind that the neurological picture is not yet stable. Function may be gained but also may be lost because of complications which may arise from the neurological procedures.

A broad statement has to be made to the parents, however, regarding ambulation (Table 9-2). In general, patients with good intelligence and

Table 9-2 Probable Prognosis for Ambulation
Related to the Level of Neurological Deficit (see "Ambulation")

Level of lesion	Joint control	Prognosis for ambulation
Normal to T_{12}	Trunk	Wheelchair
L_1	Pelvic	Exercise ambulation
L_3	Hip	Household ambulation
L_4	Knee	Community ambulation

normal upper limb function and a level of deficit between T_{11} and L_3 will walk while they are children and usually will become wheelchair ambulators in the teens. Those children with levels distal to L_4 will ambulate as adults, provided that everything else remains well. Those with $L_{3\text{-}4}$ may walk if the hips are stabilized and if they have full control of at least one knee, being able to get along with one above-knee and one below-knee brace (S. E. Stauffer, personal communication, 1972).

At the conclusion of this first interview, the orthopedist should be optimistically realistic. One should emphasize that these children will walk with varying degrees of assistance in childhood. The details of the degree of ambulation, the degree of assistance, and ultimate ambulation can be discussed further at a later time. Those who worry too much about leaving the parents with unreasonably high expectations about the child's future function and who therefore make the picture even bleaker than it is should realize that parents tend not to forgive the physician who breaks down their expectation below what turns out to be their child's ultimate level of function.

ORTHOPEDIC MANAGEMENT OF THE NEWBORN AND INFANT

The presence of spinal kyphosis requires a combined neurosurgical-orthopedic approach to the meningomyelocele. At the time of repair of the meningomyelocele sac, the orthopedist resects a segment involving several vertebral bodies from the apex of the curve (Sharrard, 1968). Not only does this facilitate the closure by eliminating the bony hump that tends to break through the fragile skin, but it also relieves the ventral compression on the neural structures.

In most instances, however, the therapeutic role of the orthopedist during the first 3 to 4 months of life is relegated to supervising the passive stretching and/or splinting of incompletely fixed deformities (Table 9-3). In the meantime, the neurosurgeon repairs the back and shunts the hydrocephalus and the urologist studies and follows the genitourinary system.

CARE OF THE HIP, KNEE, AND FOOT

NEWBORN

Paralytic dislocation of the hip is present in many children with meningo-

Table 9-3 Timing of Orthopedic Care (see text for details)

Age	Procedure
Birth	Examination Correction of kyphosis, if indicated
0–6 months	Hips: passive replacement and intermittent splinting Knees: splinting (if necessary) Feet: passive stretching, casts for holding only
6 months–1 year	Hips: Sharrard iliopsoas transfer Feet: surgical correction of deformities Standing with braces
1–2 years	Gait training
2 years+	Follow-up care of previously recognized problems Spine bracing and fusion, if indicated

myeloceles. These dislocations are due to imbalance of muscle power about the hip, with the usual predominance of the flexor-adductor over the extensor-abductor muscle groups. The treatment consists of surgical redistribution of available muscle power. Surgical treatment is not undertaken until the second half of the first year of life. The hips ought to be kept in the reduced position as much of the time as possible until then. Reduction can be achieved with relative ease in abduction, flexion, and external rotation. However, when the hips are splinted in this position permanently, a contracture may develop, complicating the future orthopedic problem considerably. We prefer to use hip splints only part of the time (McKibbin, 1973), and after teaching the mothers how to relocate the hips if they slip out, we ask them to perform a passive range of motion of the hips several times a day. This is only a holding procedure until surgical reconstruction can take place.

Knee deformities are seldom severe enough to require treatment during the first 6 months of life. Fixed deformities of the knees are manipulated and occasionally splinted in the opposite direction to the deformity.

The foot deformities are most frequently paralytic, adopting the equinovarus-adductus, the calcaneus, the calcaneovalgus, or the rocker-bottom patterns. These deformities are fixed in the majority of cases.

The prevalent opinion among orthopedists is to abstain from the use of the corrective casting technique applied to congenital clubfoot deformities, since with meningomyeloceles sensation is impaired and sizable pressure sores develop easily even in experienced hands. Manipulation of the foot and casting or splinting in the position which can be comfortably achieved has been recommended instead. The cast or splint is used in these cases not as a corrective but only as a holding device.

SIX MONTHS TO ONE YEAR

Surgical reconstruction of the dislocated hips is done in the second half of the first year. The goal is to reduce the dislocation and to balance the muscle power about the hip joint, so that the hips become and remain stable.

Surgical correction of the feet follows the recovery from hip surgery. Our goal here is to place the feet in plantargrade position so that they can be fitted with shoes and braces. The foot surgery is planned just before we think that the patient is ready to stand, and we utilize the bracing and the body weight to prevent recurrence of the foot deformity. The patient therefore is braced and ready to start standing and gait training by the time he is 1 year old.

Most experts recognize the benefits of bringing the patient to the standing position early. It provides better urinary drainage and prevents disuse osteoporosis by the physiological loading of the skeleton, thus preventing pathological fractures. Standing also keeps limbs in functional alignment and allows the patient greater interaction with his environment. In addition, it helps to improve the sense of balance and provides a positive emotional stimulus for patient and parents alike.

Some, such as Burr H. Curtis (personal communication, 1972), advocate passive standing for the 6-month-old, provided that the child has good head control. To provide a support for these young children, a lightweight, laminated plastic splint molded to the contour of the back and posterior aspect of the extended lower limbs has been designed at the Newington Children's Hospital. The splint has no joints at first, but a hinge is added at hip level when the patient is ready to sit.

Another form of exoskeleton is the Parapodium brace, designed by Motloch (1971) and used at the Ontario Crippled Children's Center. This brace supports the child in the standing position on a platform, permits some mobility in the room, and frees the child's hands for manual activities.

The brace used by us at the Birth Defects Clinic at Johns Hopkins Hospital also has the advantages of allowing free use of the hands while the patient is standing and all patterns of ambulation.

Whereas most of those who advocate very early standing start the standing before the time of reconstructive hip surgery, we prefer to perform hip surgery (see below) first and begin the standing afterwards at about one year of age, provided that the child has sufficient neurological maturity.

We advise against splinting the hips in extension, such as in a standing brace, when a tight psoas is present, because the increased tension on the psoas muscle may lever the femoral head out of the acetabulum and also may lead to the early development of a lumbar lordosis. In this situation, it is best to release the hip flexion contracture before bracing is begun. This is particularly true with an L_2 lesion.

We begin standing and gait training with bilateral long leg braces with a pelvic band, hips and knees locked at first, even in a child with a relatively low level of neurological deficit. The hips then are unlocked for sitting and for walking only if hip control is adequate and the patient is taught reciprocal gait. Depending on the degree of knee control, braces are unlocked at the knees considerably later. Probably by that time the patient already has shed the pelvic band.

The strength, coordination, and general control of the upper limbs is essential for ambulation in a paraplegic. We have limited use of the parallel bars, because although they provide stability, their prolonged use as a gait training device renders the child too dependent on an aid which is fixed to his environment. Parallel bars are used by our therapist mainly to teach standing, balance, and reciprocal gait. We prefer the use of weighted pushcarts in toddlers, followed by quadcanes or by Canadian crutches (Lofstrand) for ambulation because they move with the patient, thus making him more independent.

Any child who has reached some degree of ambulation with braces and crutches should be taught to fall, retrieve the crutches, and stand up again. This is a difficult task, but once it is accomplished it makes the gait more secure, effective, and safe and the patient more confident.

DEFORMITY AND DISABILITY IN THE OLDER CHILD

The differences between those children followed by our Center from birth and those whom we see for the first time at a later age are striking.

Most of the children we have followed from birth according to our timetable are past their major operative procedures and are standing or ambulatory in one way or another by 18 months of age. In the long run, they have required fewer operative procedures and less bracing and are more functional than later patients.

As our Center has gained impact in the community, many older children have been referred to us by neurologists, neurosurgeons, or orthopedists who perhaps have given adequate neurosurgical or orthopedic care but neglected the treatment of areas outside their competence. Occasionally, we are asked to see an older child who has been kept at home without benefit of medical care. It is through these patients that we are kept aware of the natural course of the deformities and the disability caused by the meningomyelocele.

We have been able to relate the progressive impairment of their deformities to the following factors.

Poor positioning habits. The importance of posture in a paraplegic cannot be overemphasized. The deforming role of posture increases with the higher levels of deficit and the greater degree of paralysis. Also, the higher the neurological level, the more dependent is the child on his environment for proper passive positioning. Any posture in which the paralyzed limb (or back) is allowed to remain during a prolonged period of time will become fixed (Fig. 9-1). Once the limb is fixed in the posture of deformity, surgery is usually the only solution.

Deformity at one joint can cause a chain of deformities at other joints. For instance, a hip flexion-abduction contracture may cause an ipsilateral knee flexion contracture, pelvic obliquity, contralateral hip flexion-adduction contracture, leg length discrepancy, and scoliosis (Fig. 9-2).

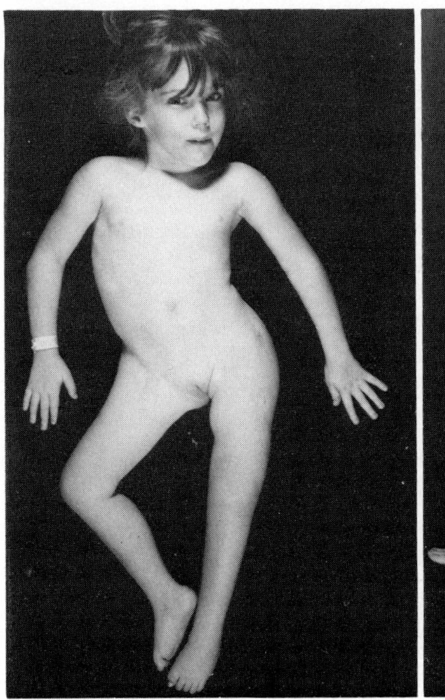
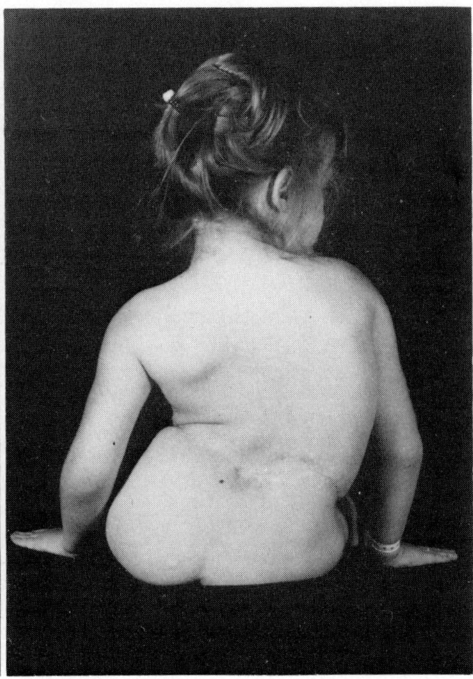

Fig. 9-2 Five-year-old with marked asymmetrical involvement. Scoliosis, pelvic obliquity, flexion-abduction-external rotation contracture of the right hip, flexion-contracture of the right knee, and adduction of the left hip are all interconnected deformities causing severe disability.

The functional position of the hip joint is of extension, neutral between internal and external rotation and between abduction and adduction. For the knee it is that of extension. The ankle should be at a right angle to the leg, and the plane of the sole of the foot also should be at right angles to the axis of the leg in the sagital and frontal planes. The spine should be straight during sitting and standing.

However, it is less important to keep this posture at all times than to carry the joints through a full range of motion several times a day. This prevents capsular adhesions and fixed deformities.

The mother or the family member in charge of the patient's daily routine has to be carefully instructed in these techniques, which should be rehearsed with this person at subsequent visits. Our goal is to keep the joints in the position of function or that of our choice for about 6 waking hours a day, making the position informal or elective the rest of the day, with controlled position for the sleeping hours. The joints should be put through a full passive range of motion two to four times a day.

In any child with capabilities for both sitting and standing, we emphasize standing over sitting, because the hips are extended and the bones of the lower limbs loaded in the standing position. Standing, even with braces and support, puts the whole lower extremity in the functional position.

Growth under muscle imbalance. Under normal circumstances, the muscle-tendon units crossing a given joint gradually lengthen as growth takes place in the bones. When paralysis affects some muscles but spares their antagonists, the active muscles, lacking opposition, will bend the joint in the direction of their pull. When these muscles are not stretched out actively, they will fail to lengthen adequately with growth, and contractures and deformity will result. The contracture ultimately may affect the rate of growth of the growth plate by establishing a differential of pressures, causing the bones slowly to bend and deform. This problem can be prevented by early recognition, passive stretching or bracing of the active muscle-tendon unit, surgical tendon release, or transfer, as indicated by the circumstances.

Overall stature is thwarted in the patient with meningomyeloceles because the affected segment of the spine does not grow properly (congenital kyphosis or scoliosis) and the paralyzed trunk collapses in the upright position. Also, the paralyzed lower limbs fail to grow adequately. This results in a preponderance of the upper over the lower segment. The ultimate height reached is an average of 4 feet and rarely 5 feet. It should be pointed out to parents who worry about this aspect of their child's future that the relative differences in length of the upper limbs (normal) and the lower limbs (shorter) is to the advantage of their child regarding his ambulation in coming years. Not only is the center of gravity nearer to the ground, but it has to be lifted through a lesser vertical distance. Also, a child's relatively longer upper limbs give him a better leverage to do so.

Iatrogenic factors. Medical intervention often creates more new problems than it was called to solve. A flexion-abduction-external rotation contracture which develops in a hip splinted for several months in abduction is a greater problem than the paralytic dislocation for which the splint was applied. The extensive pressure sores which develop as a consequence of surgical correction of a fixed paralytic clubfoot deformity can be as great a problem as the original deformity. In addition, the deformity may recur during the management of the pressure sores.

In the first instance, the orthopedist applied a method indicated for the treatment of the congenital dislocation of hip; in the second case, the operation performed is the operation of choice for the treatment of a resistant case of congenital clubfoot deformity. The orthopedist did not take into account the difference between the congenital and the paralytic deformities of the hip and the foot.

Management of a patient with meningomyeloceles cannot be extrapolated from one's experience with poliomyelitis, other types of congenital deformities, or varied types of scoliosis. Since the etiologies are different, the solutions also must be different. The orthopedic surgeon should make an effort to keep the number of operations down to a minimum and to *choose the simplest procedure*. It is important to keep the number of scars to a minimum, since surgical scars, particularly about the hip and the foot, act as fibrous bands in much the same way as an unopposed active muscle and cause deformity with growth. The surgeon must utilize the procedure with the least amount of morbidity, even though the end result may be less than could be obtained with a more involved operation. The goals have to be assessed, realistically fitting the orthopedic problem and planned solution into the overall clinical picture.

As we proceed to describe the specific deformities affecting the spine and the lower limbs, we will do so by following the concept of levels of neurological deficit whenever applicable. We want to point out, however, that many cases have a random pattern of paralysis and of deformities, with segmental loss and interspersed spared roots. We include in this group those patients who have reflex activity in some area of the cord distal to the level of neural damage. Some patients, have, in addition, upper motor neuron involvement, which further complicates the clinical situation. Thus, we come to realize that in spite of the fact that the concept of neurosegmental levels of deficit is attractive from a didactic standpoint, it is only truly realistic when talking about isolated joints.

ORTHOPEDIC MANAGEMENT OF THE OLDER CHILD: DEFORMITIES AFFECTING THE SPINE

There are three major categories of spinal deformity: (1) congenital kyphosis, (2) congenital deformities at other levels, and (3) paralytic deformities.

CONGENITAL "OPEN" KYPHOSIS

This is the most frequent and severe spinal deformity present at birth (Hoppenfeld, 1967). The lumbar spine curves out with the sac, with its prominence surpassing the surface level of the back (Fig. 9-3). The transverse processes, pedicles, and what is present of the neural (posterior) arches are located in the same plane with the vertebral bodies. The vertebrae within this curve are usually larger and those of the apex may be wedged anteriorly, the curve usually exceeding 80°. The lateral displacement of the arches displaces the paraspinal musculature virtually to the facet joints. The action of this important muscle group changes from one of trunk extension to one of flexion of the lumbar spine, producing severe and progressive kyphosis (Drennan, 1970) (Fig. 9-4). The presence of this bony curve compresses the spinal cord and nerve roots from anteriorly, and this compression is increased if the sac is surgically closed on top of it. Therefore, resection of two to three vertebrae from the apex of the curve should be performed at the time of closure of the meningomyelocele (Sharrard, 1968). This is the only chance that the patient has to preserve some neurological function distal to the apex of the curve. Subsequent to the operation, the child is nursed in an incubator in the prone Trendelenburg position for 3 to 4 weeks, the expected healing time of the spine osteotomy. While there is

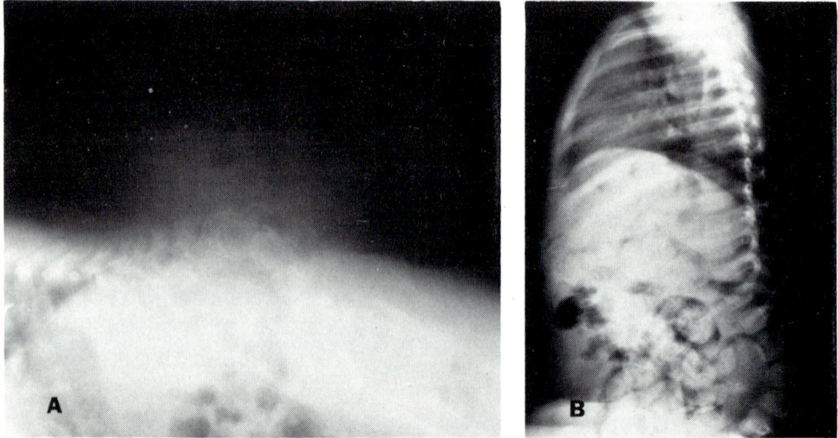

Fig. 9-3 (A) Lateral x-ray of the thoracolumbarsacral spine taken of a 4-month-old patient in the prone position. Head is oriented toward the left. Observe the lumbar spine curving out dorsally within the meningomyelocele sac. The sac is seen distended with some air bubbles within it. (B) A sitting lateral of the spine of the same patient at 4 years of age. Since the pelvis is flexed because of the kyphosis, the hips are partly extended during sitting. Note that the vertebrae within the kyphotic curve are somewhat larger.

an increased mortality rate when performing the spinal osteotomy and closure of the sac as a combined procedure in the newborn, those who survive have a far better functional result.

When this kyphosis is allowed to persist into the later years, not only will it usually cause a complete, high-level paraplegia, but it will also be a hindrance to proper sitting. The child sits with the pelvis buckled under and the hip in relative extension, since the flexion needed for sitting takes place at the level of the kyphos, not at the hips (Fig. 9-5). This posture results in a decreased distance between the sternum and the pubis and buckles the abdominal wall into many folds. The latter creates serious problems of maintenance of the ureteroileostomy, with obstruction and reflux, maceration and bleeding of the stoma, and frequent detachment of the ileostomy bag.

In addition, the lateral tips of the splayed-out neural arches are sharp and prominent subcutaneously and will cause repeated breakdown of the skin covering them.

The treatment of the kyphotic curve in the older child is in essence the same as that described above for the newborn. The correction of the curve is achieved by resection of several vertebral bodies and fusion of the spine at the level of the osteotomy. The two most common complications observed when using the technique described by Sharrard (1968) are the inability to achieve complete correction and the lack of bony fusion of the osteotomized vertebrae. Since the morbidity of the procedure in the older child is usually

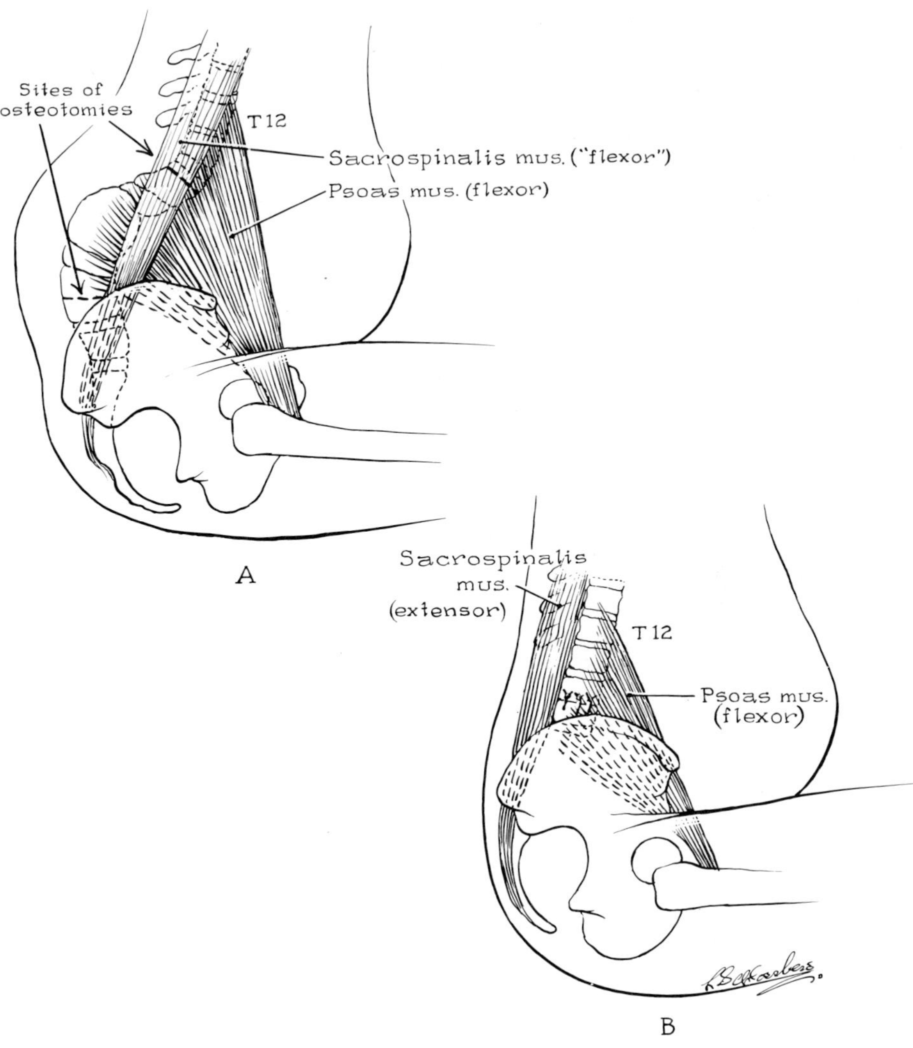

Fig. 9-4 (A) Schematic lateral view showing the kyphotic lumbar spine, with consequent flexion of the pelvis and extension at the hip during sitting. It also shows the displacement of the paraspinal musculature anterolaterally to the kyphos, acting as trunk flexor instead of extensor musculature. (B) The aim of the osteotomy which involves the resection of one and two half-vertebral bodies is to correct the spinal and pelvic alignment, restoring the paravertebral musculature to its extensor function.

great and complications are the rule rather than the exception, it should not be undertaken in anyone whose life expectancy is limited by other reasons or in those who will not be able to take full advantage of the improved sitting position. Occasionally, the spinal deformity at the level of the sac is a scoliotic curve (Fig. 9-6).

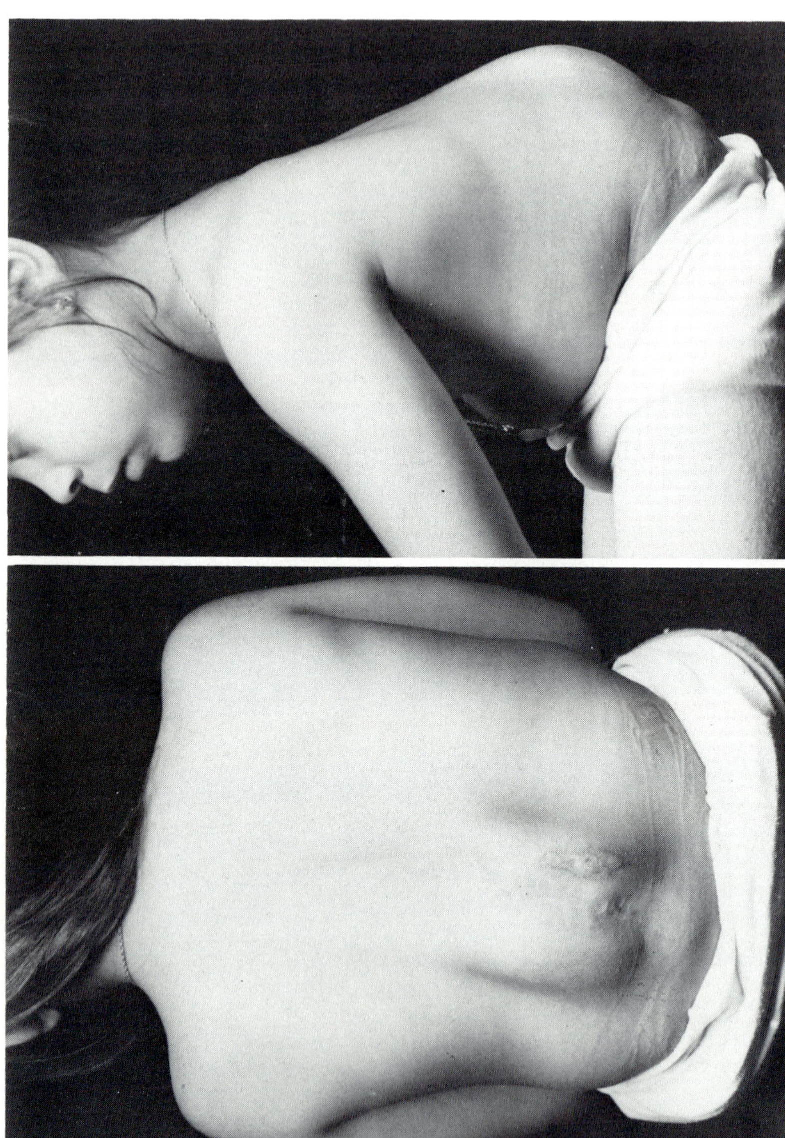

Fig. 9-5 The child with an uncorrected kyphosis breaks down frequently at the level of the prominent lateral masses. The trunk is collapsed; the xyphoid-pubic distance is decreased; the respiratory function is markedly limited as the abdomen bulges forward in several folds, often interfering with the successful application of an ileostomy bag or with the urinary drainage itself.

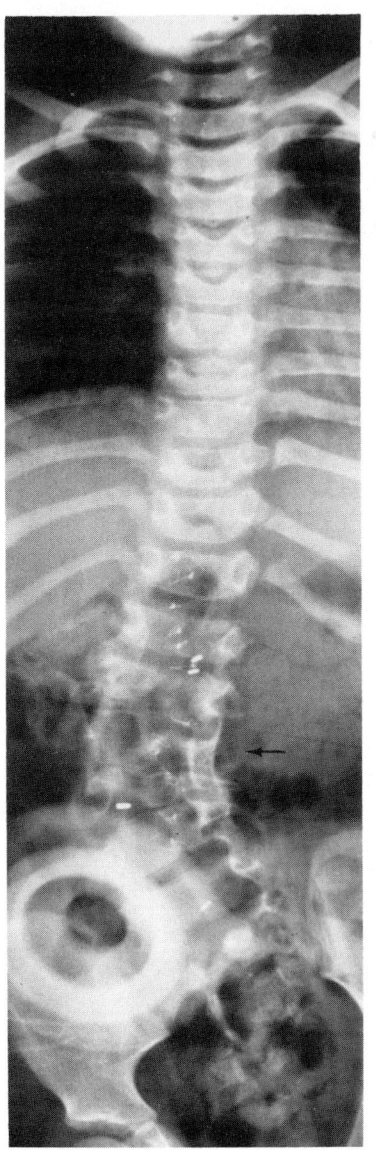

Fig. 9-6 Congenital scoliosis at the level of the meningomyelocele caused by the left-sided lack of vertebral segmentation (unilateral bar) between L_2 and L_4.

CONGENITAL DEFORMITIES AT OTHER LEVELS OF THE SPINE

Frequently, a defect in the proper development of the spine at one point is associated with defects at other levels. It is not unusual to observe an associated congenital scoliosis (Winter, Moe, and Eilers, 1968) caused by hemivertebra or unilateral lack of segmentation, or both (Fig. 9-7). At other times, the presence of a high thoracic kyphosis, a Klippel-Feil deformity

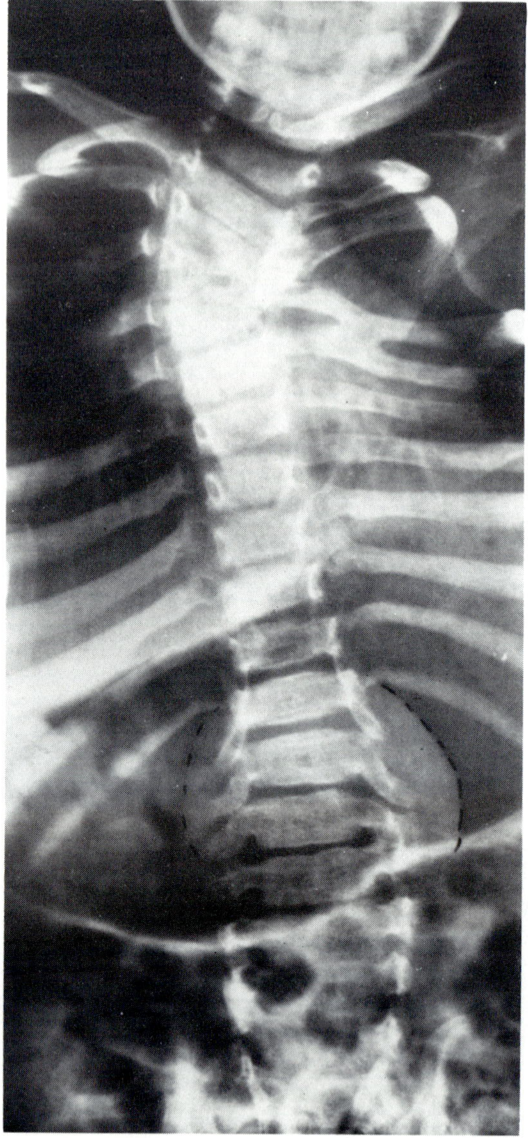

Fig. 9-7 Child born with a lumbosacral meningomyelocele (sac is visible on this anteroposterior film) and with a progressive high thoracic scoliosis caused by both a hemivertebra and a left unilateral lack of segmentation of the vertebrae involved in the curve.

of the cervical spine, or a diastematomyelia complicates the spinal problems of a child with meningomyeloceles.

Decisions regarding the treatment of the associated lesions have to be made in the light of the circumstances created by the meningomyelocele.

The difficulties which may be expected usually surpass those encountered in the normal course of treatment of each condition separately.

PARALYTIC DEFORMITIES OF THE SPINE

In the case of paralytic deformities, the vertebrae are not deformed at birth, in contrast to the congenital lesions, in which deformity is always present. With paralytic deformities, the spine is usually straight at birth (Fig. 9-8), and the deformity does not appear until weight bearing on the spine is started in the sitting or standing position. The paralytic deformity may be either a scoliosis or a lordosis.

Paralytic scoliosis. Paralytic scoliosis is due to paralysis of the abdominal, paravertebral, flank, or hip musculature; it creates a pelvic obliquity (tilt) with secondary deformity of the hips. The lateral curvature of the spine usually progresses to a pronounced deformity if no treatment is initiated. Gravity alone will rapidly increase curves of more than 60°. This type of scoliosis in meningomyeloceles is usually, but not always, related to high lesions. The curves are ample, involving many vertebrae, and are largely correctable with the patient in the horizontal position.

Treatment consists of holding the progression of lesser curves with bracing and by fusing the greater curves in a corrected position. This fusion should, if possible, be deferred until the growth of the spine is terminated.

Bracing of these patients presents special problems. Often the skin around the iliac crests is anesthetic and unable to take the pressures of a corrective brace. The skin is even less able to tolerate corrective casting. We use either an upward extension of the pelvic band, such as a Bennet type of brace, or a lightweight, laminated plastic back brace, adequate to hold mild to moderate curves. Only rarely do we use the Milwaukee brace in paralytic scoliosis caused by meningomyeloceles. The latter brace, which extends from the occiput and chin to the pelvis, tends to immobolize completely a patient already braced in the lower limbs. Also, the paralytic patient lacks sufficient muscle power to work against the brace and achieve the correction which this "active" brace could offer.

Operative correction of the scoliosis with posterior spinal fusion is indicated if the patient has reached the end of spinal growth with a curve of more than 35° or if at any time the progression of the curves cannot be halted with bracing. Since growth does not take place within a fused segment of spine, it should be delayed for as long as possible, with the provisions stated above.

Paralytic curves, which are supple in young children, have a tendency to become relatively fixed in the teens. The correction of such curves can be obtained by several methods:

(1) Preoperative traction is used for several weeks by the Cotrel method (soft tissue traction rig) or by halofemoral (skeletal) traction. A localizer (corrective) body cast is applied with the limitations described above.

(2) Intraoperative correction occasionally is performed by the Harrington instruments (Crenshaw, 1971), although the steel hooks have a tendency to

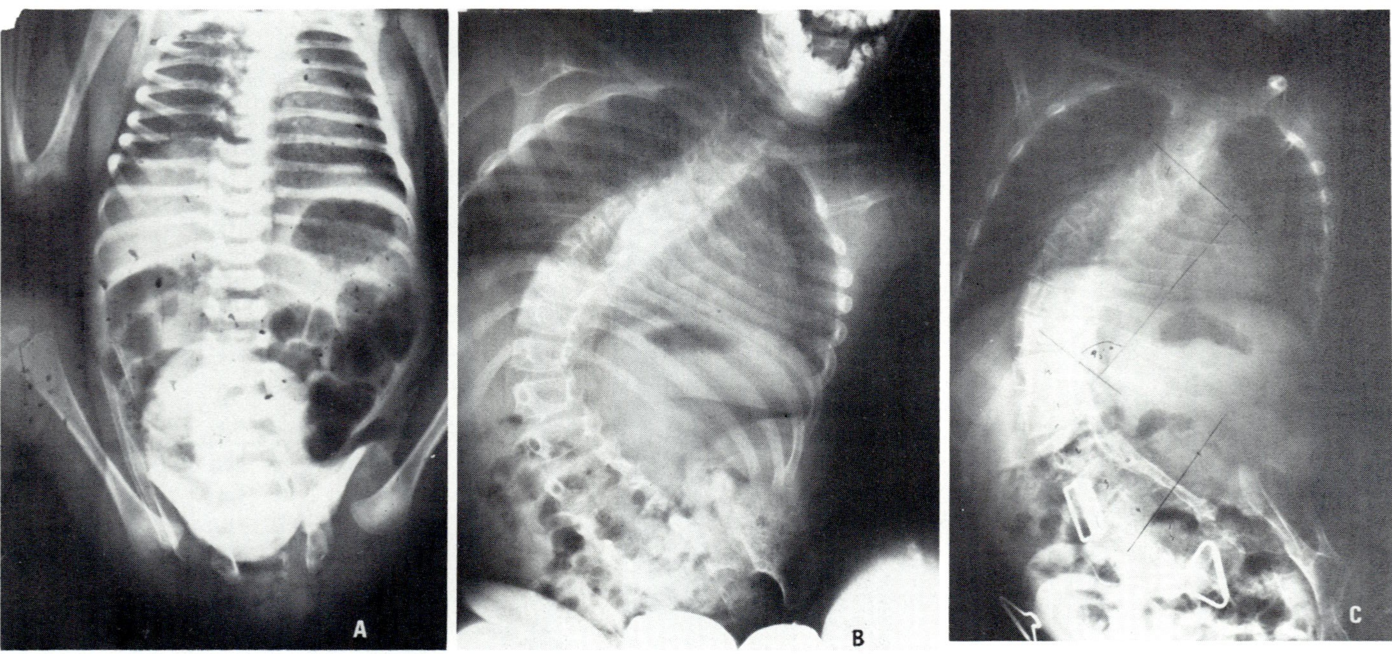

Fig. 9-8 (A) On an anteroposterior view, the spine is straight at 16 days of age. (B) Shows the same patient at 4 years of age with a 70° right-sided paralytic scoliosis which developed because of the influence of gravity on the spine in the sitting position. (C) Notice the progression by 7 years of age. The curve measures 95° and there is a greater degree of vertebral rotation at the thoracolumbar level.

cut out of the laminae because of the osteoporosis commonly observed in these patients. This limits the usefulness of the Harrington instrument in treatment of meningomyeloceles.

(3) Postoperatively, there are special technical difficulties in fusing the spine at the level of the meningomyelocele because of the absence of posterior bony elements. In the case of absence of neural function distal to the bony defect, the nonfunctioning cord and roots may be excised and a posterior fusion of the vertebral bodies performed. Normally, patients should be well immobilized in a body cast for 3 to 6 months following spinal fusion. This is extremely difficult to carry out without compromises to the anesthetic skin and the development of pressure sores. Because of all of these difficulties, the rate of nonunion is very high compared to the spinal fusions done for other conditions.

Paralytic lumbosacral lordosis. This is a particularly severe deformity for which there is no satisfactory treatment to date (Sharrard, 1968; Shiram, Bobechko, and Hall, 1972). It develops in "sitters" with active and/or shortened iliopsoas and weak abdominal, paraspinal, and gluteal musculature. The psoas, which originates on the transverse processes and the bodies of the first four lumbar vertebrae, attaches to the lesser femoral trochanter. It is supplied by the first two lumbar roots and is the major flexor of the hip. When it is unopposed by the weak abdominal muscles, the gluteus maximus, and the paraspinal erector muscles, it produces a lumbar lordosis. The sitting posture increases the deformity until the abdomen is opposed to the anterior thigh. As the patient brings his thoracic spine to the vertical position, a 90° lordosis may develop at the thoracolumbar junction. The hips may become dislocated because of the unopposed psoas pull.

The best treatment is to prevent this deformity by early psoas release and proper trunk support of the patient in the correct sitting position.

Once the deformity is established and becomes fixed during the teens, there is little one can do to improve it. Anterior wedge resection, anterior fusion, and posterior fusion with and without Harrington instrumentation all have been attempted with a high failure rate.

We have used the Siebens' brace in selected cases of paralytic spinal deformity where ischial pressure sores are a concomitant problem.

The Siebens back brace (Fig. 9-9) is attached to the wheelchair and suspends the patient by supporting his lower rib cage, so that the buttocks do not have to take the weight of the sitting body.

DEFORMITIES AFFECTING THE HIP

Paralytic scoliosis will result in pelvic obliquity (tilt) and secondary deformity of the hips. Similarly, asymmetrical deformity of the hips, such as that caused by a tight psoas, will result in pelvic obliquity and secondary scoliosis.

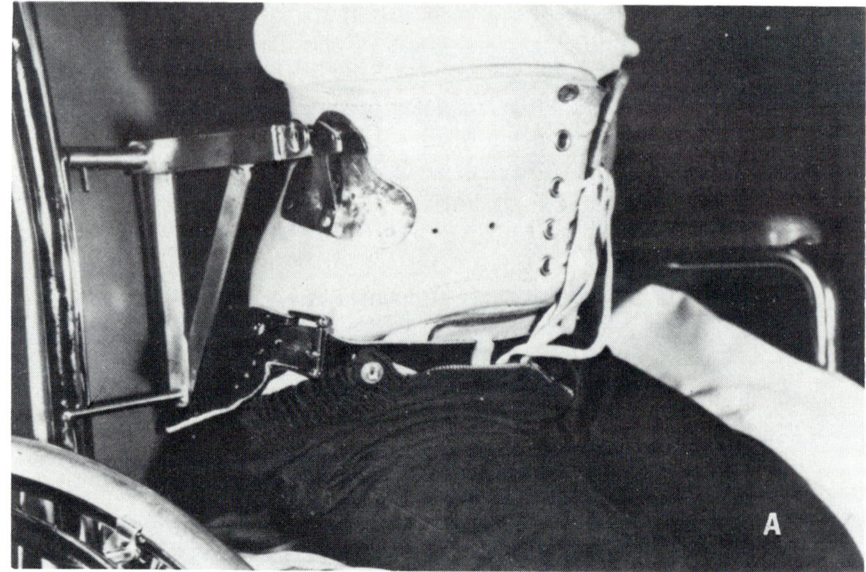

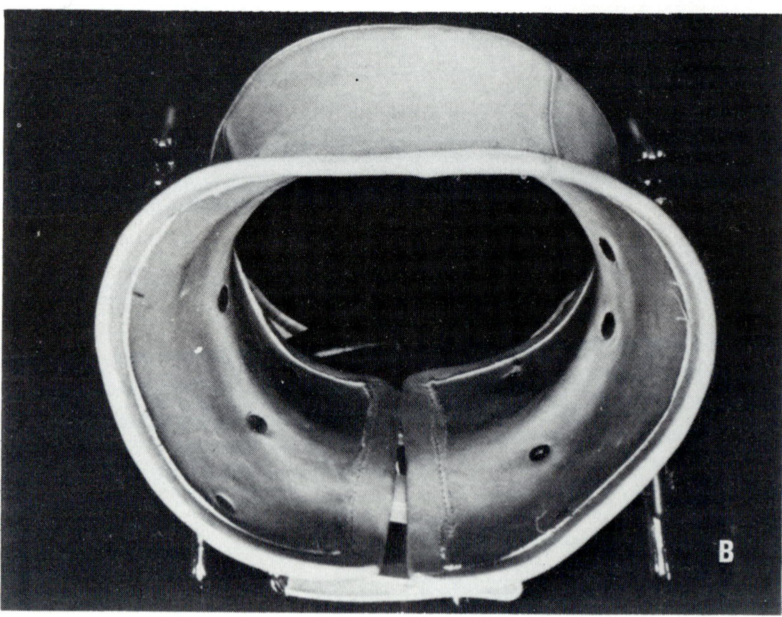

Fig. 9-9 The Siebens brace is attached to the wheelchair, and by conforming to the contours of the lower rib cage supports the patient by his ribs. It helps to straighten supple paralytic thoracolumbar or lumbar curvatures and prevents ischiatic pressure sores. (A) View from the side. (B) Viewed from above showing the inside contours (Courtesy of Dr. Arthur A. Siebens, reprinted with permission from the Hopkins Medical Journal).

PARALYTIC DISLOCATION OF THE HIP

Paralytic dislocation of the hip is one of the most disabling conditions in the patient with meningomyeloceles. It is due to the imbalance of muscle power controlling the hip joint, with predominance of the flexor and adductor over the extensor-abductor group (Sharrard, 1959). Its maximal incidence is in cases with an $L_{3\text{-}4}$ level of neurological deficit. At this level the psoas (main hip flexor) and the adductors are strong and the gluteus maximus (main hip extensor) and medius (main hip abductor) are paralyzed. The psoas and adductors tend to lever the femoral head out of the socket, and the paralyzed gluteus is unable to hold it in place. Therefore, the hips are likely to be dislocated at birth in children with $L_{3\text{-}4}$ level of deficit. The hips appear markedly flexed, adducted, and externally rotated, and the knees are extended, because of functioning quadriceps. Most of those hips not yet dislocated at birth with an $L_{3\text{-}4}$ deficit will be dislocated by the end of the first year of life.

If the level of deficit is $L_{1\text{-}2}$, the psoas is present, although it may be weak, adduction is usually weak, and abduction and extension are absent. Since the quantitative difference of forces is not as great as with the $L_{3\text{-}4}$ lesion, the dislocation occurs more gradually over the first few months or even years. In some cases the hips remain in the subluxed position and a permanent flexion contracture is present.

If the level is L_5, the situation is similar to that at the $L_{1\text{-}2}$ level. Although the hip flexion-adduction is present at this level, there is weak hip extension and abduction. Therefore, the dislocation or subluxation will take place over an extended period of time.

If the level is T_{12}, all muscle power about the hip is abolished and dislocation does not occur. Similarly, if the level is S_1, all muscle power about the hips is present and dislocation does not occur. The effect of lesions at various levels on the hip is summarized in Table 9-4.

Occasionally, a patient is seen during the first few months of life with dislocated hips and no muscle power in the hips to explain it (Fig. 9-10). In

Table 9-4 Forces Affecting Dislocation at the Hip

Motor deficit	Flexor-adduction (psoas)	Extension-abduction (gluteus maximus and medius)	Hip
T_{12}	0	0	No dislocation
$L_{1\text{-}2}$	2+	0	Gradual dislocation
$L_{3\text{-}4}$	4+	0	Dislocate at birth or early
L_5	4+	2+	Gradual dislocation
S_1	4+	3–4+	No dislocation

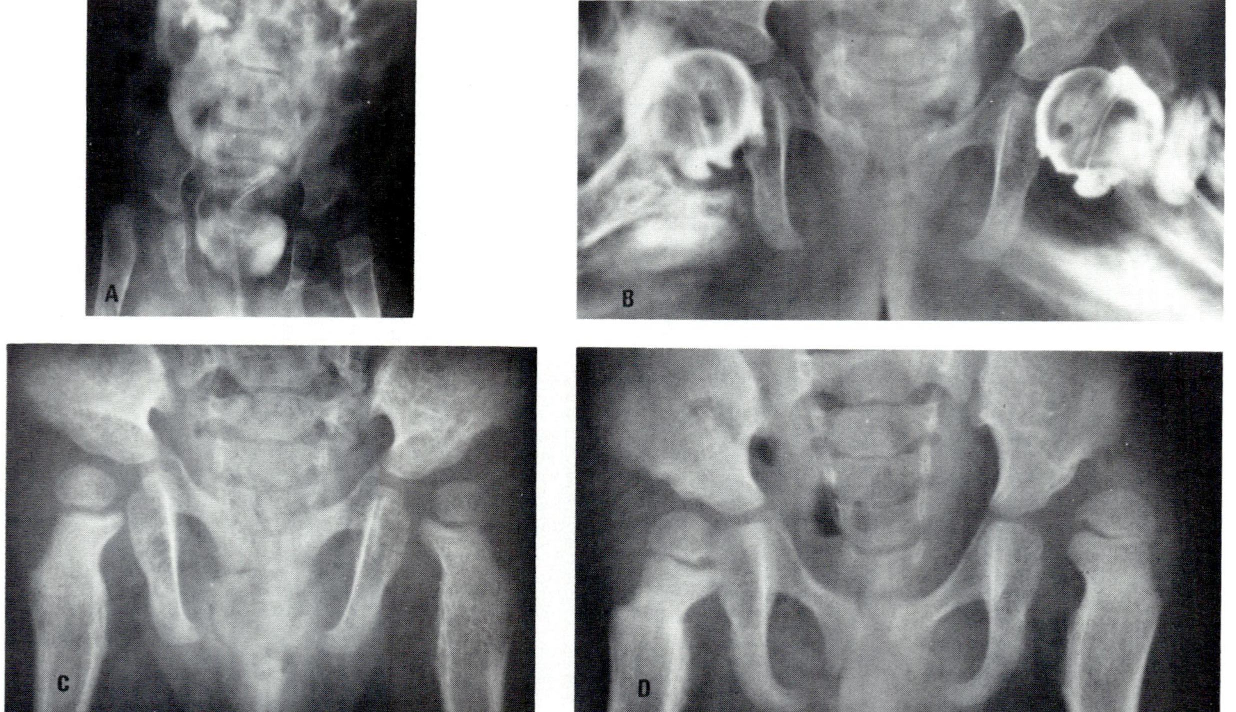

Fig. 9-10 The same patient as in Fig. 9-3, born with a high lumbar meningomyelocele, was said to have some active hip motion at birth. (A) Hip x-rays taken at 4 months of age in 1967 reveal bilateral paralytic hip dislocation. The child had no hip motion at this time. Notice the oval shadow of the sac on this film. (B) Manual reduction was easily accomplished and arthrograms reveal round femoral heads, well reduced in the abducted position. The cartilaginous portion of the left acetabulum is clearly outlined. (C) In the absence of muscle function, the hips were still well located in 1969. (D) As some psoas function returned, the left hip slowly went on to dislocate by 1971.

such a case, one has to postulate loss of muscle power subsequent to the dislocations.

The mechanism of dislocation is shown in Fig. 9-11. The psoas muscle attaches to the lesser trochanter and as a flexor tends to pull the femur toward the pelvis. In combination with the adductors it tends to lever the head out of the acetabulum. The action of the psoas and adductors normally is countered by the gluteus maximus, which extends the hip, and the medius, which abducts the hip. These muscles stabilize the hip within the acetabulum.

If dislocation occurs gradually, the proximal femur will undergo structural changes, increasing its neck-shaft angle (coxa valga) and its degree of anteversion prior to the subluxing or dislocating.

The *clinical appearance* of the child with paralytic hip dislocation is usually that of the hip flexion-adduction-external rotation in the first year of life and of hip flexion-adduction and either external or internal rotation in later years. However, we have seen dislocated hips that coexist with almost any type of postural deformity and even with no deformity at all.

It is most important to recognize that the *paralytic dislocation of the hip is a completely different entity from congenital dislocation of the hip*, with a different pathogenesis and treatment.

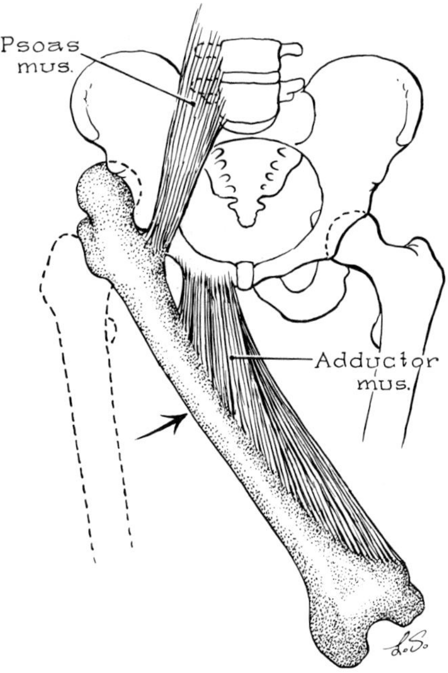

Fig. 9-11 The combined pull of the psoas and the adductors, unopposed, attributable to paralysis of the glutei muscles, causes increased anteversion femoral and an increase in the neck-shaft angle (coxa valga) and leads to dislocation of the hip.

In the paralytic dislocation, the patient has a recognizable neurological deficit, the hip reduces easily, in most cases by doing the Ortolani maneuver, and the acetabulum appears normal. Arthrograms reveal a lax joint capsule but no interposition of soft tissues between femoral head and acetabulum, as occurs in many cases of congenital dislocation of the hip.

With time, the old untreated paralytic dislocation and the congenital dislocation may become radiologically indistinguishable from each other. The acetabulum turns shallow and fills with fibrofatty tissue. The capsule narrows proximal to the dislocated femoral head and the head, which is pressed against the lateral aspect of the ilium, flattens and becomes deformed.

The contracted psoas and adductors prevent abduction and extension of the hip, and if the paralytic dislocation is unilateral, an important leg length discrepancy results. This discrepancy is partly real, because of the loss of skeletal length attributable to the dislocation, and partly apparent, because of the pelvic obliquity created by the dislocated hip which is in flexion and adduction. The opposite hip becomes abducted and the limb appears to be relatively longer. Secondary scoliosis develops.

It is important to point out that whereas in the vast majority of cases the paralytic dislocation involves both hips, only about 20% of congenital dislocations are bilateral. Therefore, it is important to rule out a neurological deficit in any newborn or infant who apparently has bilateral congenital dislocation. An anteroposterior roentgenogram of the lumbosacral spine showing *increase* in the interpedicular distances can be helpful in diagnosing a hidden lesion, such as an intrathecal lipomyelocele, responsible for the hip dislocation.

The bases of modern treatment of paralytic dislocation of the hip in meningomyeloceles were established by Sharrard (1959, 1964). Previously, surgeons treated paralytic dislocations with casting and at times with operative replacement as if they were congenital dislocations. Most hips promptly redislocated because of the failure to correct the muscle imbalance.

Sharrard insisted that stability of the hip could be reached only by balancing the existing muscle power about the hip. He achieved this by an open adductor tenotomy and a posterior iliopsoas transfer.

According to his technique, the adductor tenotomy is indicated whenever abduction is not possible to 80°. In the same operation, the iliopsoas is detached from the lesser trochanter and dissected proximally in the retroperitoneal space, and the origin of the iliacus is detached from the inner aspect of the iliac wing. A hole is then made through the iliac bone just lateral to the sacroiliac joint, and the iliopsoas is passed through it and then tunnelled down to and through the gluteal muscle mass and attached to the greater trochanter from posterior to anterior, replacing the pull of the paralyzed gluteii (Fig. 9-12). Frequently, an open reduction of the hip is also necessary in older children, in which case it is done simultaneously with

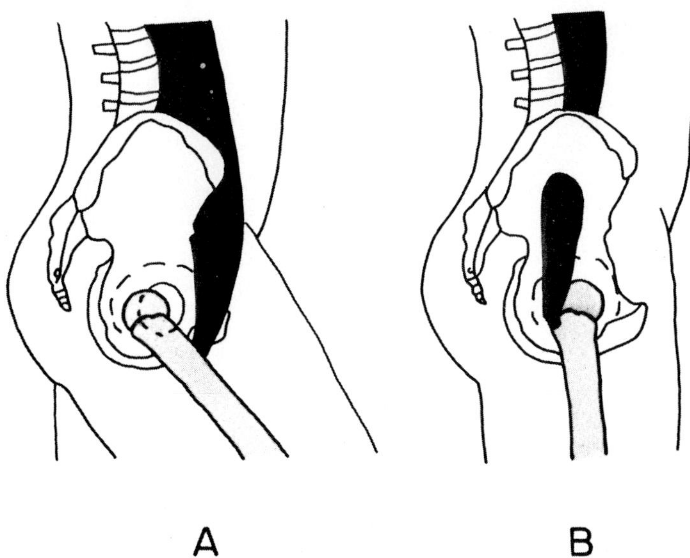

Fig. 9-12 Mechanics of the posterior iliopsoas transfer. (A) The unopposed psoas levers out the femoral head from the acetabulum. (B) The psoas, transferred through a window in the iliac bone and attached to the posterior aspect of the greater trochanter, stabilizes the hip in the reduced position.

the iliopsoas transfer. A hip spica cast is applied for 3.5 to 4.5 weeks. This operation converts the psoas from a flexor and adductor to an extensor and an abductor of the hip. It then stabilizes the femoral head in the socket (Fig. 9-13).

We have empirically protected our transfer by placing the child in long leg braces and a pelvic band for up to 1 year after removal of the cast.

In separate studies, Raycroft and Close (personal communications, 1969) demonstrated by following the electromyographic patterns of the transplanted iliopsoas that it gained antigravity action between 8 and 12 months following the transfer. In some of our early experience, as we applied the Sharrard procedure to older children, whose hips had been dislocated for a considerable length of time, the shallow acetabulum and the coxa valga and anteversion of the proximal femur allowed redislocation to occur. Since then, when operating on older children with previously untreated hip dislocation, we have established an adequate relationship between the socket and the head either before or simultaneously with the Sharrard procedure.

Results. Numerous studies have confirmed Sharrard's early experience (Freehafer, Vessely, and Mack, 1972; Sharrard, 1964, 1971) that the posterior iliopsoas transfer succeeds in attaining hip stability. In many cases the transferred tendon acts only as a passive tenodesis or checkrein; in others, there is variable active strength in the transfer which acts as either a predominant hip extensor or abductor of the hip. Stability seems to be

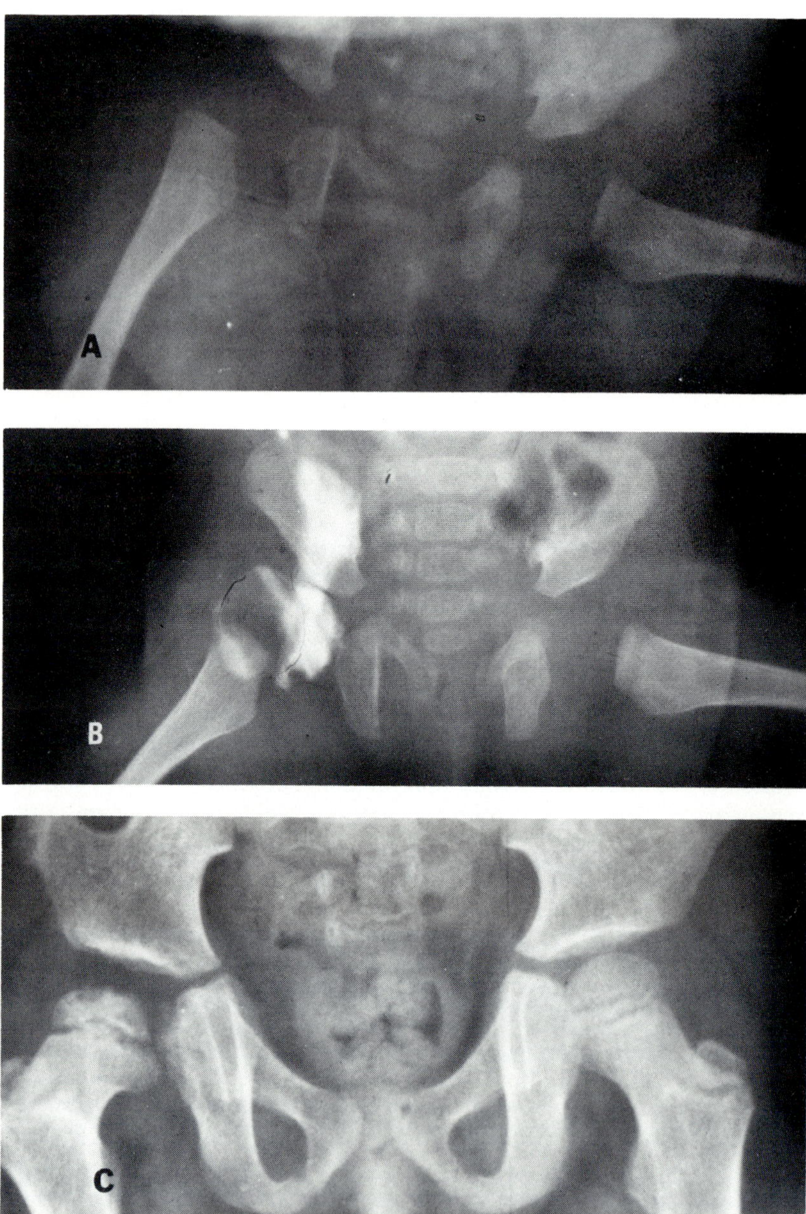

Fig. 9-13 (A) Illustrates the paralytic dislocation of the right hip in a newborn with an $L_{3\text{-}4}$ deficit and predominantly right-sided involvement. (B) The arthrogram of the right hip shows an ample joint capsule without inversion of the limbus and hourglass stricture of the capsule. (C) Four and a half years after a Sharrard posterior iliopsoas transfer on the right, the hip is well located and stable. Note the partial view of the "window" in the right iliac wing.

caused by the extensor action of the transfer. In time, and because of the stability achieved in the hip by the procedure, patients walk with only short leg braces instead of the long leg braces with pelvic band which would be needed otherwise. That is to say, that with all the other factors being equal, this operation often makes the difference between nonfunctional and functional ambulation by the achievement of hip control.

Complications. The secondary hip flexors (rectus femoris, sartorius, pectineus) remaining after the psoas is transferred are usually insufficient to flex the hip enough to allow the patient to walk stairs. For this reason, we try to avoid performing the Sharrard procedure bilaterally, if at all possible. Another secondary effect is a marked out-toeing gait, caused by the action of the sartorius which, besides being a secondary hip flexor, is also an external rotator of the lower limb. This can be bothersome at times and is a problem of difficult management.

Pathological fractures of the lower limbs frequently complicate the recovery from the operation. Fractures may be prevented by standing the patient repeatedly while he is in the cast, applying braces as soon as possible after the removal of the cast, not permitting the patient to roll in bed when he is out of the cast or brace, and turning the child in the air with a sufficient number of helpers.

Pathological fractures in these children are usually painless and may be suspected when local pain, swelling, and heat develop, as well as fever, sometimes up to 39°C. The fractures are treated by splinting the children in their own braces and standing them up in their braces as soon as the swelling starts to subside.

Indications for surgery of the paralytic hip. An $L_{3\text{-}4}$ level of neurological deficit with dislocation or subluxation of the hip, caused by strong flexor-adductors and paralyzed extensor-abductors, is an absolute indication for the posterior iliopsoas transplantation. When the muscle imbalance is not too great (some of the cases with L_2 and L_5 lesions and particularly in bilateral cases), dislocation or redislocation can be prevented by a subtrochanteric varus osteotomy, thereby avoiding the Sharrard procedure. If the hip slowly redislocates, a Sharrard procedure is unavoidable.

We perform the Sharrard procedure as soon as we feel that the anatomical structures are large enough to work with, usually at 6 to 12 months of age.

FLEXION-ABDUCTION–EXTERNAL ROTATION DEFORMITY OF THE HIP

This is a less common deformity primarily affecting hips which at one point were splinted in this position. The tensor fascia lata is usually an active deforming force in these cases. The proximal and distal release of the fascia is occasionally insufficient, and if the contracture is longstanding, a more extensive procedure, including opening the anterior capsule of the hip joint and release or proximal transfer of the psoas, is needed. Since recurrence is the rule rather than the exception, mainly because the patients adopt the same posture postoperatively, in selected cases we prefer a simple oblique osteotomy of the proximal femur. The proximal fragment is left in the original position and the distal fragment (the limb) is brought into the weight-bearing position. Our long-term results have been uniformly good. We compensate for the leg length discrepancy created by our intervention with appropriate lifts. This deformity probably can be prevented by avoidance of constant abduction splints.

DEFORMITIES AFFECTING THE KNEE

HYPEREXTENSION DEFORMITY OF THE KNEE (GENU RECURVATUM)

This is a commonly observed deformity at birth caused by the presence of active knee extensors (quadriceps, $L_{3\text{-}4}$) and paralyzed knee flexors (hamstrings, L_5). An even greater degree of hyperextension deformity occasionally is observed at birth in the absence of active knee extensors in newborns who have only active hip flexors ($L_{1\text{-}2}$ level) and who are born in the breech position. The hyperextension deformity in these cases is due to the intrauterine posture and represents a passive deformity.

Treatment of the hyperextension deformity is mandatory and has to take place as soon as possible after birth to prevent stiffening of the knee in this position. It consists of gently straightening the knee and splinting it in the extended or slightly flexed position.

On rare occasions, the hyperextended knee will resist attempts at manipulation into the corrected position and radiographs may reveal dislocation of the knee. The treatment of this rare condition is surgical, as outlined by Curtis (1969). In the case of the hyperextended knee caused by an unopposed active quadriceps, early correction and splinting obviously does not solve the problem by itself because the knee will tend to return to that position when the splint is removed. However, the splinting will have prevented the permanent shortening of the quadriceps and the development of a fixed deformity.

After 7 to 10 days, we advocate part-time splinting and gentle passive manipulation through a range of flexion several times a day until weight bearing is begun in braces. The manipulation has to be gentle because the bones are brittle, and preferably it should be carried out by the same person.

While the patient wears long leg braces, the knees are obviously under control; however, difficulties may arise again as one tries to utilize short leg braces. None of the surgical methods designed for the treatment of "back-knee" in other conditions, such as polio, are really satisfactory for this problem. A compromise solution can be reached with the use of the Saltiel below-knee, one-piece, lightweight, laminated plastic brace (Saltiel, 1969). This brace was developed to help lock the knee in extension when the physician is dealing with a weak quadriceps. However, it can be adapted to prevent back-knee deformity by making minor changes in its construction.

Fortunately, most cases with paralytic back-knee deformity have some active hamstring power (L_4–S_1) which tends to decrease the magnitude of the problem.

FLEXION DEFORMITY OF THE KNEE

This is rarely a paralytic deformity, since the lower neurological level of the medial hamstrings (L_4–S_1) presupposes the presence of a functioning quadriceps (L_3–L_4). The level of the biceps femoris (lateral hamstring) is even lower (L_5–S_1). Most frequently, knee flexion occurs in response to hip flexion and becomes a fixed deformity in time if that posture is not corrected. We see this in patients who were kept under a "custodial" type of care for a prolonged period of time or as a consequence of a distal femoral fracture which united in flexion and which may give the clinical appearance of flexion contracture of the knee joint.

Except for the last instance, we recommend part-time splinting or bracing as outlined above. We tend not to perform surgery for flexion contractures of up to 30° if the patient will use a long leg brace on that extremity, but do not accept more than 15° if he is going to wear a below-knee brace. Depending on the circumstances surrounding the contracture, the procedure will be on soft tissues and/or bone. Sometimes the simplest solution is a supracondylar femoral osteotomy. This may circumvent a complicated problem, and is adequate enough in this case because the goals of the orthopedist are limited to achieving a knee which is stable in the extended, functional position.

DEFORMITIES AFFECTING THE FOOT

Since the foot is innervated by the lowest motor roots, it is affected by deformities in over 90% of the patients with meningomyeloceles.

The deformity usually will be due to either the unopposed action of a muscle or the intra- or extrauterine position adopted by a paralyzed foot.

Our goals and methods of treatment tend to be limited, commensurate with the general condition of the patient. We are satisfied to achieve a plantargrade weight-bearing foot with its muscle-tendon units balanced around it as well as possible. Whenever possible, we choose the simplest surgical method, the one with the least morbidity.

Although there are many different types of foot deformities, we are going to describe in some detail only the following types.

CALCANEUS FOOT

The foot appears acutely dorsiflexed at birth because of the presence of an active anterior tibial muscle as the only active muscle below the knee (level L_4). The dorsum of the foot is usually touching the anterior surface of the distal leg (Fig. 9-14). In spite of the fact that the anterior tibial is an inversor of the foot and therefore would bring it in an inverted or varus position, the uterine wall, against which the foot rests during pregnancy, may force it into

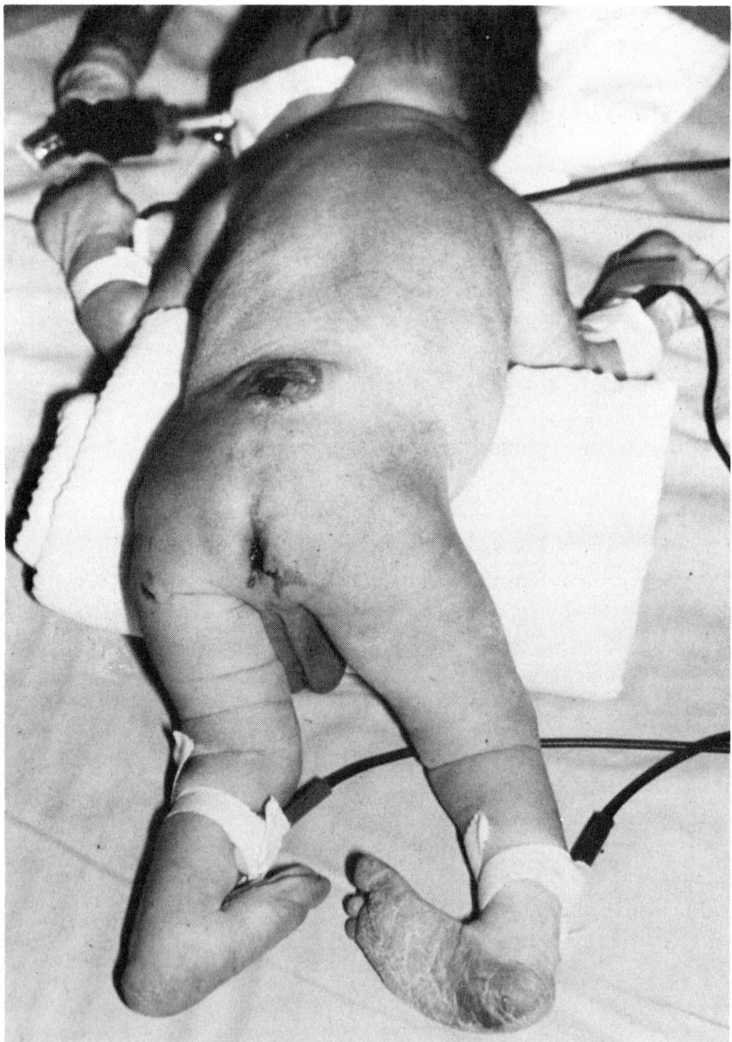

Fig. 9-14 Bilateral calcaneus feet in a newborn with an L_4 level.

some valgus. Therefore, we may see a calcaneovarus or a calcaneovalgus deformity. The deformity appears to be fixed at birth to the point that some advise simply dividing the tendon with manipulation repeated by the mother several times a day, so that the patient could be fitted with braces by the end of the first year of life. Some of these patients are heel-walkers and do not use their braces at home. Their toes may barely touch the ground.

When the spinal lesion is at the L_5 level, the appearance still may be the same but not as marked, modified by the presence of some posterior tibial, long-toe extensor, and minimal peroneal action. The predominant action is still that of the anterior tibial, and the patient walks on the heel but the entire sole touches the ground. The child will walk without the use of braces. The child with this type of lesion has no toe-push-off during gait and walks like a cross-country skier (Fig. 9-15). He is unable to walk fast.

We have performed the Peabody transfer (Peabody, 1949) in two cases of the L_4 and five cases of the L_5 level. This procedure consists of the transfer of

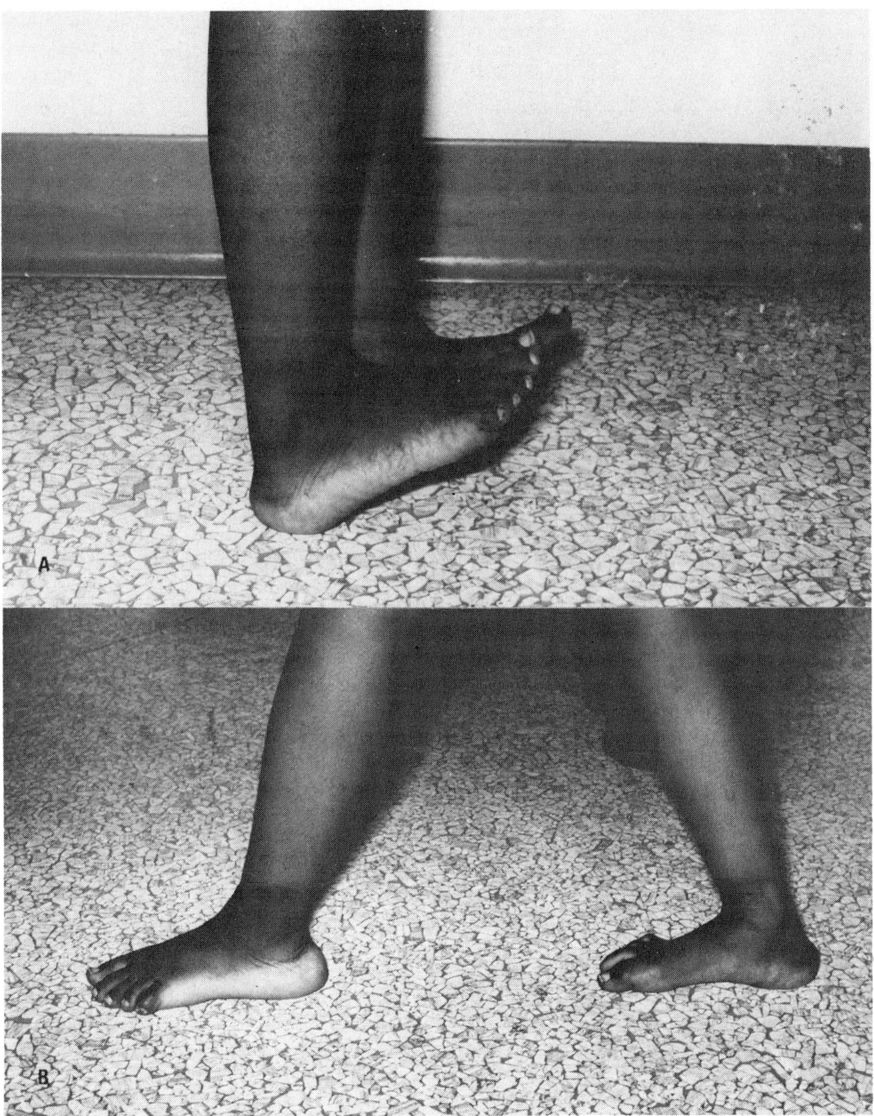

Fig. 9-15 Nine-year-old patient with an $L_{4\text{-}5}$ level. (A) He is able to stand on the heels but not on the toes. (B) Unable to push-off, he walks with the cross-country skier's gait.

the anterior tibial tendon through the interosseus membrane between tibia and fibula through the posterior compartment into the heel, transforming the anterior tibial muscle into a plantarflexor.

One patient with an L_4 level developed an intractable equinus deformity secondary to the transfer, and the transferred tendon had to be excised. In the other case of L_4 level, the transfer was too weak. Both patients had to wear short leg braces permanently. Of the five patients with level L_5, a definite improvement of gait occurred in the one who had good long-toe extensors, which acted as foot dorsiflexors during gait, replacing the action of the transferred anterior tibial. The patient walked without a brace before and after surgery. The remaining four had lesser degrees of success, depending on the postoperative strength of the transfer and of the long-toe extensors replacing it. Of the three who walked with braces before surgery, one did not have to do so afterwards. The remaining one who did not use braces before had to do so after surgery.

On the basis of this limited experience, we do not advocate the Peabody transfer in patients with an L_4 level, but are prepared to do a simple anterior tibial tenotomy if necessary to rid the foot of its deforming force and then fit the patient with a below-knee, fixed ankle brace.

We will advocate the Peabody transfer only in those patients with an L_5 level who have good to excellent strength in the anterior tibial muscle and good strength in the long extensors of the toes. Since we have noticed the appearance or an increase of previously existing valgus deformity of the heel, we foresee the need for subtalar fusion done either simultaneously with or subsequently to the transfer. In general, the procedure does not seem justified in a patient who has been walking functionally without braces before surgery if the child will have to be braced as a consequence of the operation, or if he may have to keep on wearing the same brace after surgery that he has worn before. In the absence of the above indications, we recommend treatment with below-knee braces with limited ankle motion.

CALCANEO-CAVUS DEFORMITY (CAVUS FOOT)

A cavus deformity, with an increase of the longitudinal arch of the foot, may appear concomitantly with the previously described deformity. It is due to the preserved activity of the intrinsic short flexors of the toes (L_5–S_1) unopposed by the short extensors of the toes (S_2) (Fig. 9-1).

If this deformity is diagnosed in the child before 4 years of age, before growth has created a permanent bony deformity, the operation described by Steindler (1920) is indicated. This is a simple procedure and consists of stripping the plantar fascia and the origin of the short-toe flexors from the plantar aspect of the greater tuberosity of the calcaneus. We prefer to perform this procedure just before the patient begins to stand so that weight bearing will be our best insurance against a possible recurrence. We have had uniformly good results with this operation.

An untreated cavus deformity can be a handicap for the older child because the lack of even weight distribution will predispose the foot to pressure sores under the metatarsal heads, and the shoe will cause the same problem over the middorsum of the foot.

In the presence of a normal hindfoot, and once a permanent fixed bony deformity in cavus has developed, such a foot is best treated by a midtarsal osteotomy as described by Japas (1968), with the same considerations as are described for the triple arthrodesis.

EQUINOVARUS FOOT (PARALYTIC CLUBFOOT)

The hindfoot is plantarflexed in equinus, inverted into varus, and the sole curves with the toes pointing toward the midline of the body (metatarsus adductus). The inner border of the foot is shorter. In other words, the deformity is identical to the congenital clubfoot (Fig. 9-16). This should be recognized as a different entity because it clearly occurs in paralyzed extremities which in addition have variable degrees of anesthesia. This anesthesia is the single most important factor influencing our thinking regarding the treatment of the paralytic clubfoot.

When considering the paralytic clubfoot, we have to dissociate ourselves from the concept of levels of deficit. This deformity is the result of the intrauterine position on a paralyzed foot, rather than of muscle imbalance. It is observed either in completely denervated limbs or where reflex activity exists in some muscle groups. We also see it in cases of scattered loss of function, where a definite level cannot be recognized.

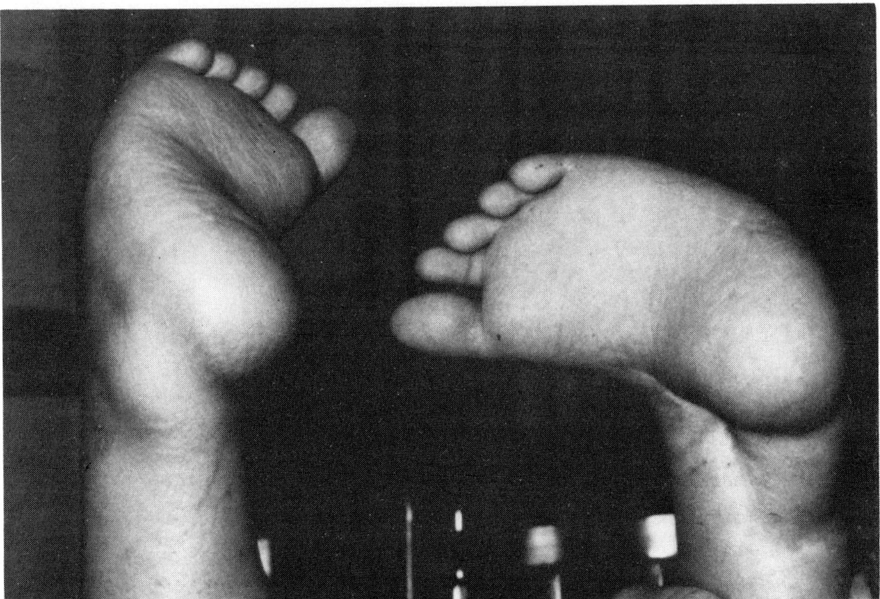

Fig. 9-16 Fixed paralytic (equinovarus) clubfoot deformity in a child with an L_1 defect.

The deformity is fixed in most cases and the treatment is primarily surgical. Serial corrective casting used for the treatment of congenital clubfoot should *not* be used in paralytic anesthetic clubfeet because of the possibility of pressure sores. However, major degrees of correction often can be obtained by passive manipulation. We use the cast as a splint *only to hold* feet in a position which can be reached comfortably by manipulation. We do not persist with manipulation of those feet which are obviously rigid, but rather wait until the patient is ready for weight bearing and then perform surgical correction.

Only as an exception do we use a surgical technique similar to that described by Turco (1971) for the correction of resistant cases of congenital clubfoot, because we consider the dissection involved in this technique excessive and potentially too hazardous (Fig. 9-17) to use in anesthetic feet, and prefer simpler methods to achieve our more limited goals for correction.

The talectomy (excision of the talus) is a simpler procedure with less operative morbidity and is quite satisfactory in the correction of the fixed paralytic clubfoot. However, the talectomy leaves the incongruous articular surfaces of the distal end of the tibia and the upper surface of the calcaneus in contact with each other, which in a neuropathic foot may lead to the development of a Charcot type of joint. Instead, we have been using the opera-

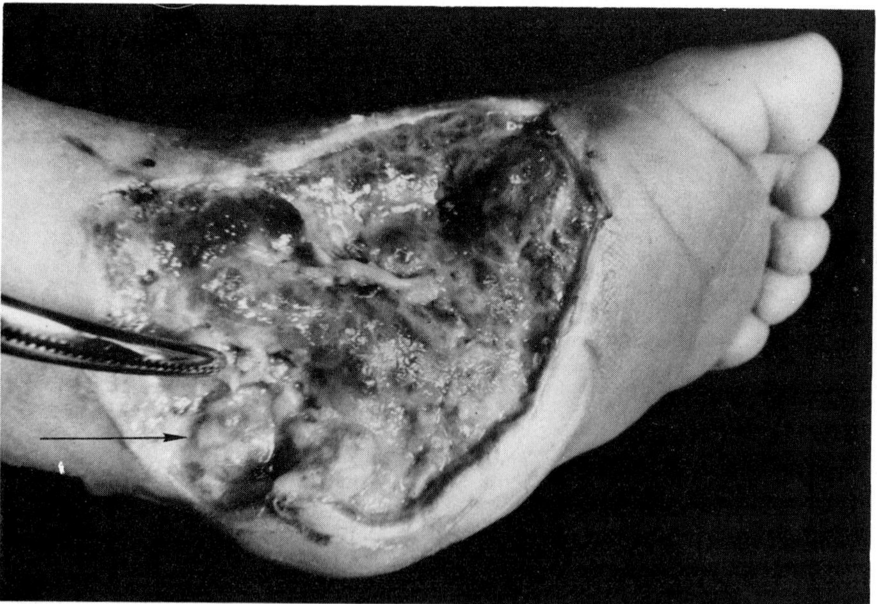

Fig. 9-17 Large slough on the posteromedial aspect of the anesthetic foot of an infant 10 days following a radical posteromedial release for the correction of a fixed paralytic clubfoot deformity. The tip of the clamp points to the posterior tibial neurovascular bundle and the arrow to the exposed greater tuberosity of the calcaneus. The deformity recurred completely during the healing of the tissue defect.

tion practiced by Laszlo Verebélyi, Sr. (Kopits and Kopits, 1942) at the end of the last century and somewhat later by Ogston (1902) for the treatment of the congenital clubfoot.

These surgeons curetted out the talus and the cuboid, reducing them to empty shells, then manipulated the foot and corrected both the varus of the hindfoot and the adductus of the mid-forefoot by collapsing the emptied talus and cuboid, respectively (Fig. 9-18, 1 to 6). A percutaneous Achilles tenotomy may be performed *after* the manipulative correction of the foot for the correction of the equinus deformity. This operation has distinct advantages over the excision of these bones or over the Codivilla or Turco radical posteromedial soft tissue release, not only because it causes much less surgical trauma and demands very little dissection, but also because it leaves the joints of the foot undisturbed. At the expense of only minimal operative morbidity, a braceable plantargrade foot is achieved. It is an ideal procedure for the 6- to 12-month-old infant whose fixed foot deformities prevent him from being fitted with a brace. The procedure does not preclude the possibility of subsequent tendon transfers. The only disadvantage is that the obtained correction may be occasionally less than that which may be obtained with the other more radical procedures. Then again, our goals are more limited than with the congenital clubfoot.

We have performed this procedure in six feet, on patients under 2 years of age, with excellent results in three, good in two, and satisfactory in one. Our longest follow-up is of 2 years and 8 months.

Triple arthrodesis (Crenshaw, 1971) (resection and fusion of the subtalar, talonavicular, and calcaneocuboid joints) has been used for the correction of paralytic clubfoot and other complex paralytic foot deformities for many years, but with less than satisfactory long-term results in neuropathic feet. The operation corrects the deformity but the subsequent swelling easily may cause necrosis of the flaps unless exceptional postoperative vigilance and care are applied. Non-union has been the rule, and some joints go on to a "Charcot-joint" type deformity. The prospects of a pantalar fusion (including, in addition to the former three, that of the ankle joint) are even worse.

PARALYTIC VERTICAL TALUS OR ROCKER-BOTTOM FOOT

This deformity is similar to its congenital counterpart. It is a mixed paralytic-postural deformity. The head of the talus points toward the sole of the foot, forming an angle of 60 to 90° between it and the axis of the calcaneus on a lateral x-ray of the foot (Fig. 9-19). Its treatment is surgical and consists of establishing a normal relationship between the talus, the calcaneus, and the navicular. The deformity must be corrected as early as possible, preferably before the first birthday.

PARALYTIC VALGUS FOOT

This is a supple deformity which appears with weight bearing in a fairly

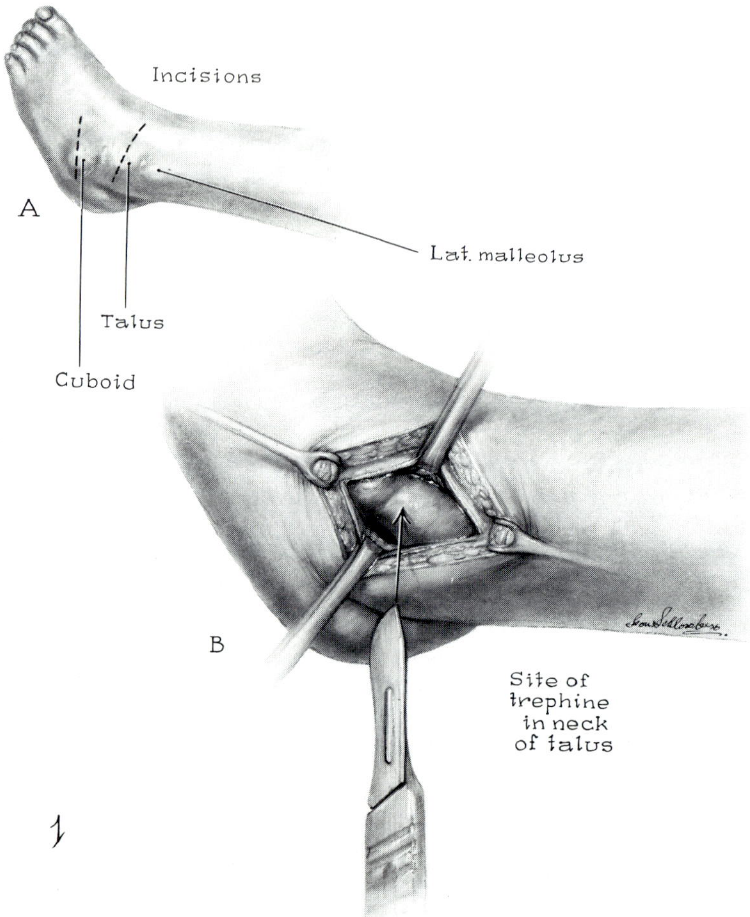

Fig. 9-18 The Verebélyi-Ogston procedure consists of the enucleation of the talus and the cuboid, and heel cord lengthening for the correction of the heel, varus midfoot adduction, and equinus deformities, respectively. The foot is in a cast for 6 weeks, then braced. (1) Oblique incisions are made on the dorsolateral aspect of the foot to expose the talar neck and the cuboid. Exposure of the neck of the talus is demonstrated. (2) Curetting of the talar ossification center is shown. (3) The cartilaginous lateral wall is incised longitudinally to facilitate its collapse as manipulation is applied to correct the heel varus. (4) Calcaneocuboid curettage is performed for correction of the midfoot adduction. (5) Correction is obtained by collapsing the empty shells of the talus and the cuboid. (6) Since the resistance of the tight heel cord is used to affect the manipulation of the hind- and midfoot, the heel cord lengthening is left for last. It is performed either percutaneously or by exposing it surgically.

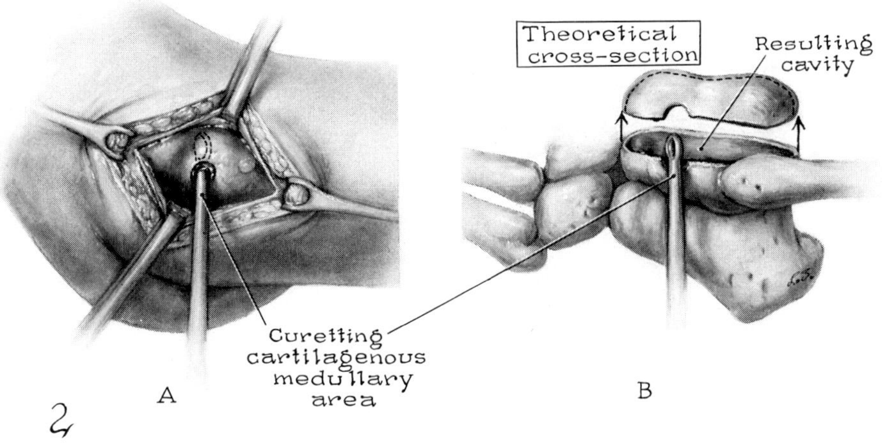

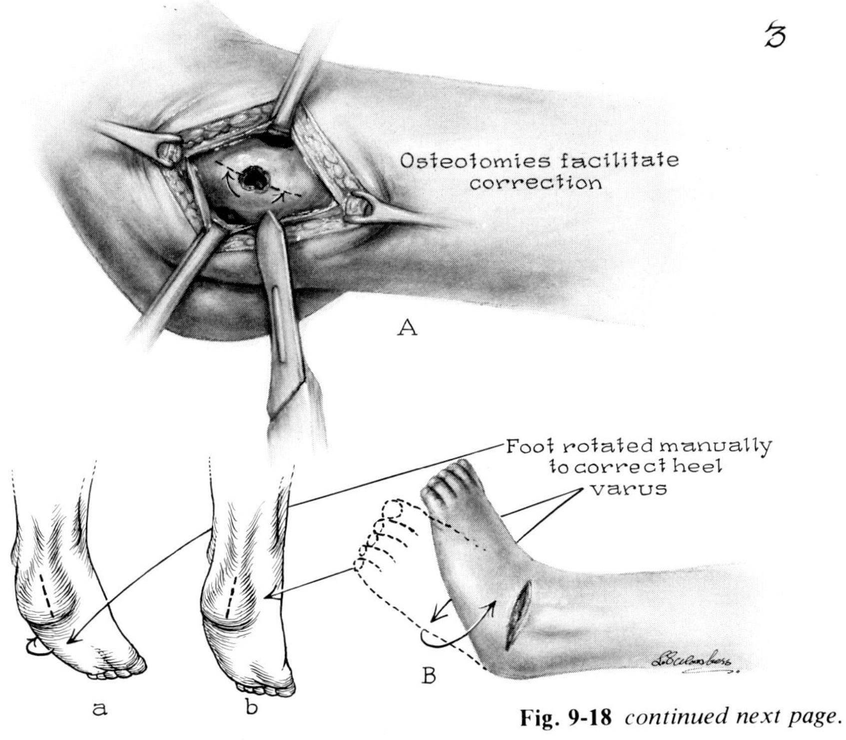

Fig. 9-18 *continued next page.*

Fig. 9-18 *continued.*

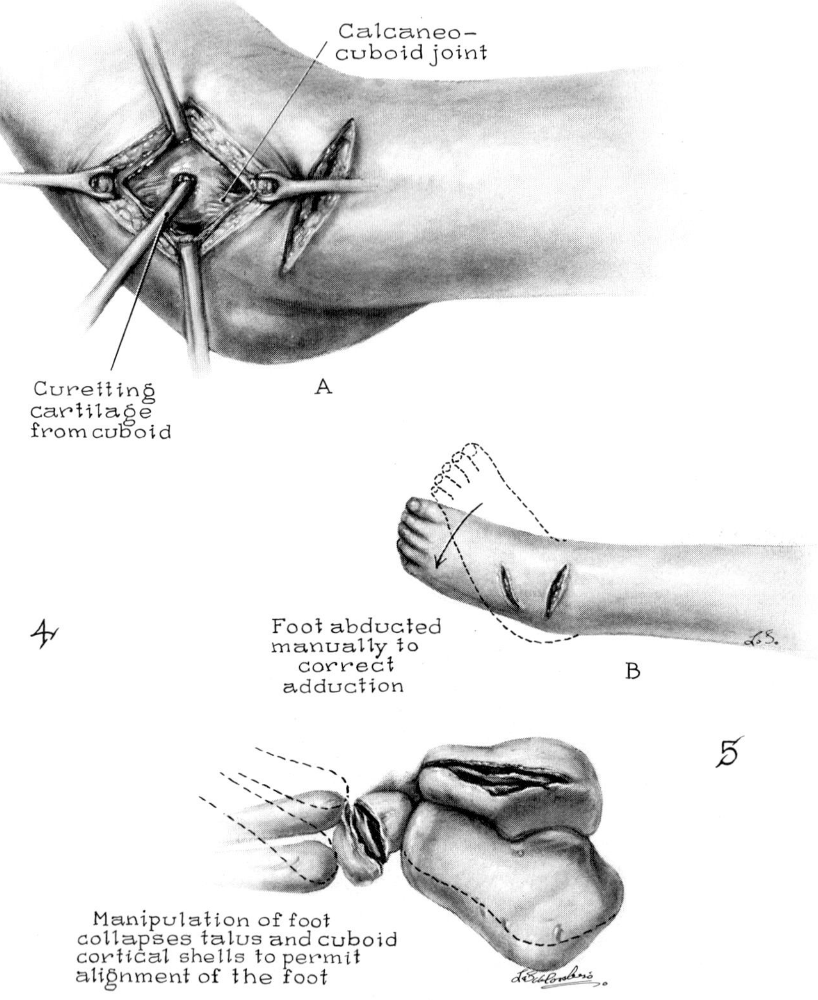

well-inervated foot and is due to weakness of the anterior and posterior tibial muscles (Fig. 9-20). No single muscle transfer is able to correct this deformity. In mild to moderate cases, the foot can be corrected with the help of laminated plastic antivalgus heel molds which fit inside the shoes (Yates, 1968) (Fig. 9-21). In more severe cases, a subtalar fusion is recommended. Disenchanted with the Grice technique (Grice, 1952), we have been using the operation described by Brown (1968) and attributed to Batchelor. The operation is performed by inserting a 5-cm long segment of fibular shaft through a 0.5-cm hole drilled through the talus into the calcaneous, with both of them in corrected alignment (Fig. 9-22).

Fig. 9-18 *continued.*

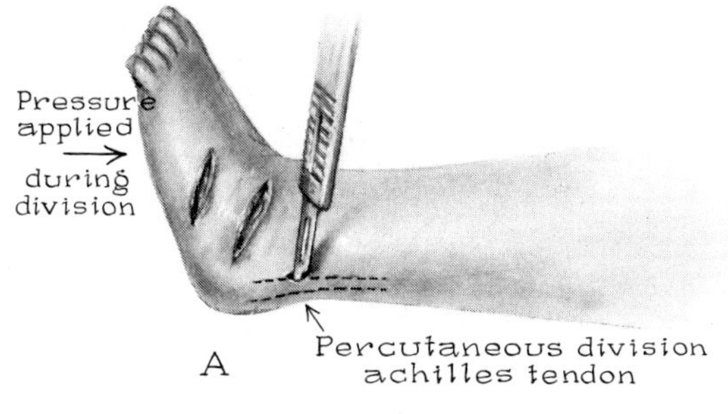

6

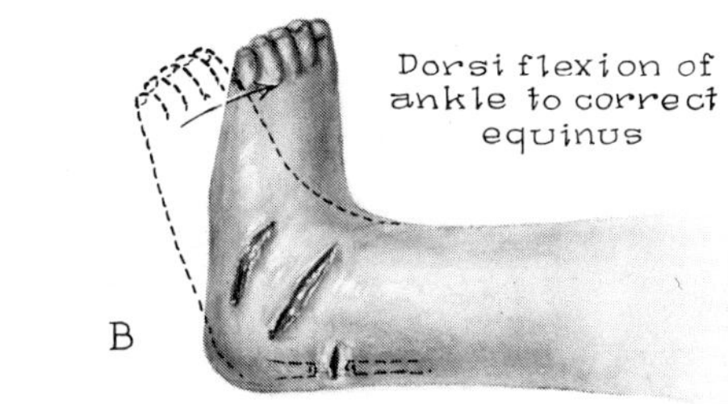

We modified the period of postoperative immobilization recommended by the authors to 6 months (6 weeks in below-knee plaster with nonweight bearing, 6 weeks in same plaster with weight bearing, and 3 months in short leg brace). In spite of this, our failure rate in 22 feet in 16 children with paralytic valgus feet caused by meningomyeloceles is 50%. Graft breakage and reabsorption may occur as late as 8 months after operation. The high failure rate seems to be due more to the fact that we operate on neuropathic feet than to operative technique itself, because in 12 additional feet done for valgus deformity from other causes, we had only one failure. We have reoperated some of our failures with good subsequent results. In others, the corrections obtained at surgery held up in spite of the fracture or resorption of the fibular graft.

AMBULATION

Ambulation is the process by which a person displaces himself from one point to another in his environment by *his own will* and, to an extent, under *his own power.*

Whether a child with meningomyeloceles will ambulate and what type of ambulation he may develop will depend on the level of denervation, the presence of spasticity, the condition of his upper limbs, and the presence of contractures. The presence of hydrocephalus and associated brain damage and the degree of motivation to ambulate also are determining factors.

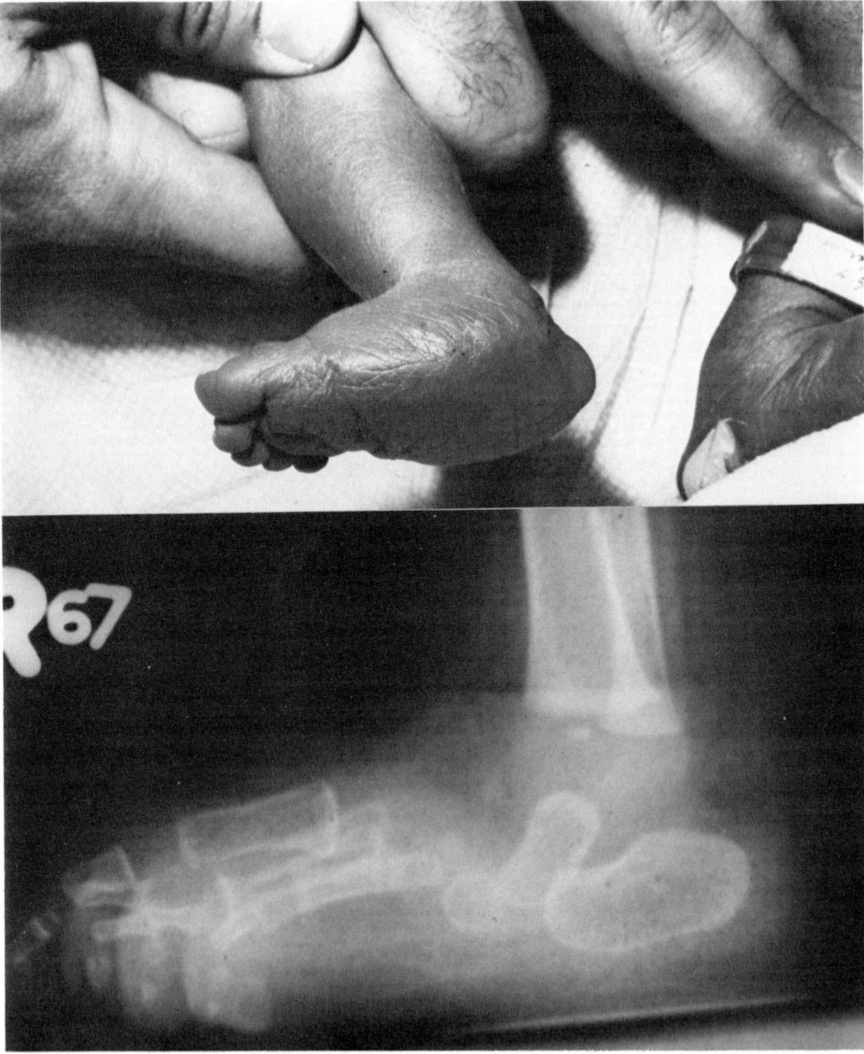

Fig. 9-19 The paralytic rocker-bottom foot gained its name from the shape of its plantar surface. The prominence of the midfoot on its plantar aspect is given by the equinus of the heel, the dorsiflexion of the forepart of the foot, and the prominence of the head of the talus in the vertical position (Courtesy of Dr. Kenneth C. Gertsen).

Most of these patients need orthotic devices (wheelchairs, external braces, crutches, canes, etc.) to facilitate their ambulation. Hoffer and associates (1973) have graded ambulation functionally into four levels:

1. *Community ambulators* are able to use walking for most functional activities. They walk indoors and outdoors for most of their activities, although they may require orthotic devices (braces, canes) to do so. In addi-

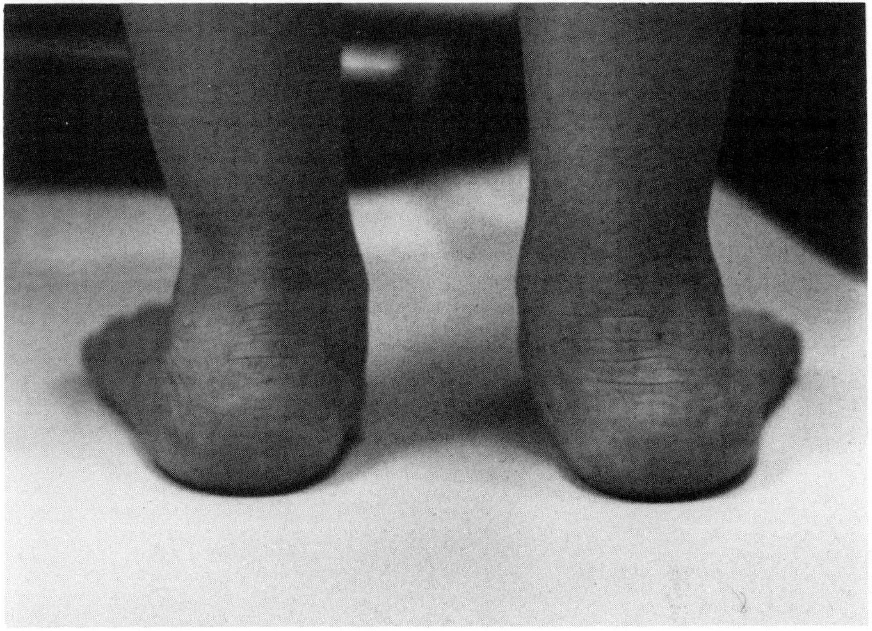

Fig. 9-20 Moderate valgus heel deformity in an 8-year-old girl with a spina bifida occulta and diastematomyelia at the $T_{8\text{-}11}$ level. Note the inversion of the heel. The patient bears weight predominantly on the medial border of the foot.

tion to good pelvic and hip control, they need fair to good knee control and usually have some degree of foot control.

2. *Household ambulators* are able to walk only very limited distances. They walk indoors with the help of orthotic devices and are nearly independent within their homes for their physical needs, but need a wheelchair when going into the community. As children, they may manage with two long leg braces, but as they grow in the teens, about half of them will become wheelchair ridden unless they have sufficient control of both hips.

3. *Exercise ambulators* (nonfunctional ambulators) use ambulation only for exercise, not for function. They reach the standing position usually with help and walk a few lengths in physical therapy, in the school, or at home, as a therapy session, but use the wheelchair to satisfy transportation needs both indoors and outdoors. Pelvic control and good upper limbs are a minimum requirement for this type of ambulation. These patients walk with a swing-to swing-through gait, braced with long leg braces and a pelvic band, and only rarely do they progress to household ambulation. Unless they develop some degree of hip control, they become wheelchair bound by the time they reach adolescence.

4. *Wheelchair ambulators* (nonambulators) rely on the wheelchair as their only means of transportation. They are usually able to transfer be-

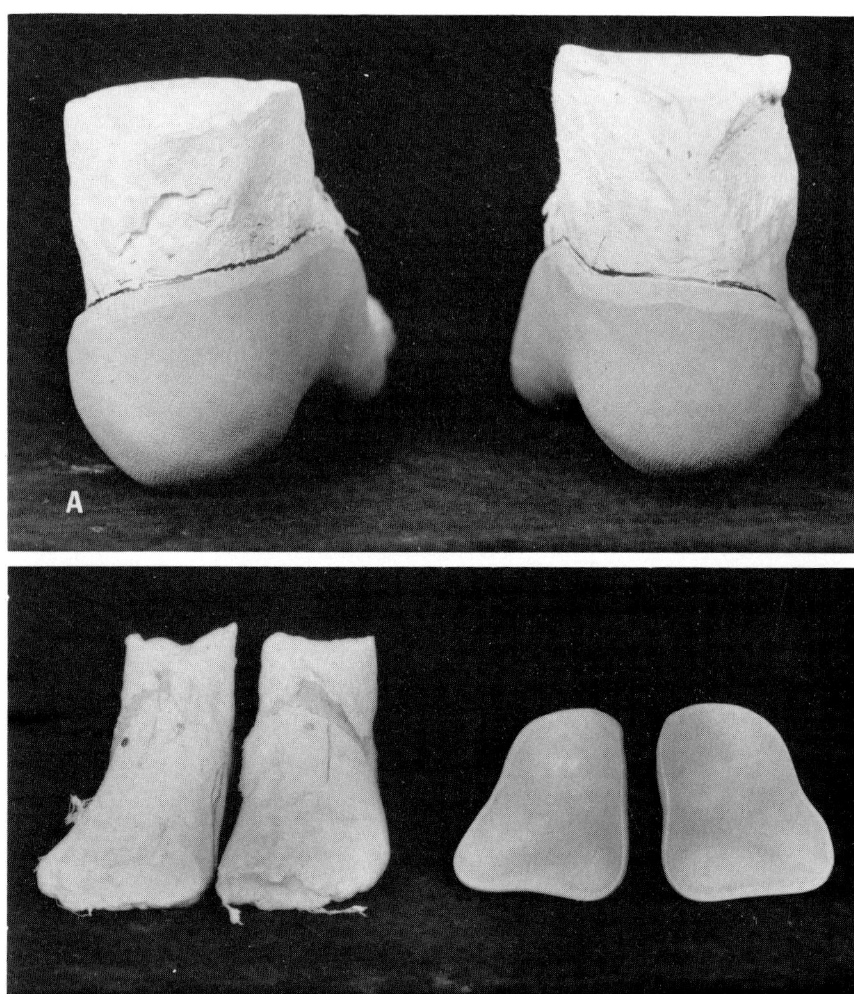

Fig. 9-21 Hind view of: (A) Heel molds built on a corrected plaster positive of the patient's foot. (B) Front view of the corrected plaster positive and of the finished heel molds.

tween chair and bed. Trunk control and at least one good upper limb are required for this activity.

Hoffer and associates (1973), reviewing 56 patients who were mostly in their teens and who were followed for over 5 years, have found that none of the ones with thoracic levels of deficit have ultimately become functional ambulators and that the children with sacral levels achieved functional ambulation. Our experience is identical.

At the lumbar neurological levels, surprisingly, they found no significant difference between higher and lower levels regarding ambulation. In their series of 40 patients with lumbar levels, 14 were community ambulators, 5 household ambulators, 2 exercise ambulators, and 19 wheelchair bound. It is at these levels that circumstances other than the level of motor deficit are important in defining the ultimate ambulatory status. The presence of brain damage, spasticity, decreased upper limb function,

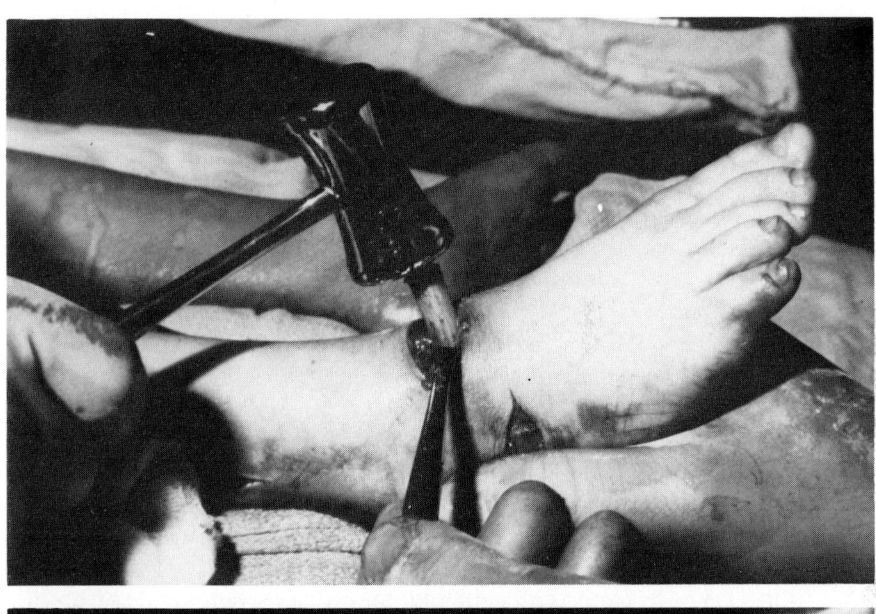

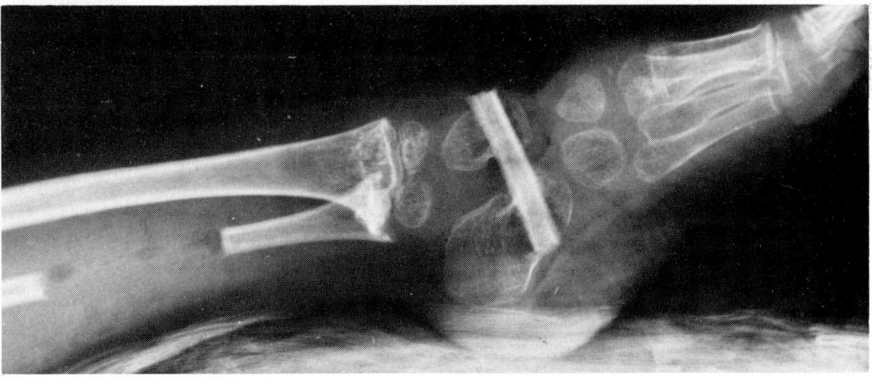

Fig. 9-22 Batchelor procedure. While the surgeon holds the patient's foot in the correct alignment, the assistant drives a segment of fibular shaft through the talus and the oscalis. A lateral radiograph of the foot after completion of the procedure shows the defect in the fibula and the segment of the fibular shaft locking talus and calcaneus in the desired position.

scoliosis requiring extensive spinal fusion, fractures, hydrocephalus, and lower limb contractures were a hindrance to ambulation. The level of motivation (perhaps related to intelligence), over-protection and other factors also may play a major role.

In Hoffer's experience, a few young children made the upward transition in ambulatory status mainly with age and a concomitant neuromuscular development. Upward transition occurred in our experience only as surgical procedures were performed to gain control of a distal joint, as in the case of hip control achieved after a Sharrard procedure. All of those who achieved community ambulatory status did so by 9 years of age in Hoffer's series and well before school age in our experience.

The exercise and the household ambulators are almost always transient groups. While the majority of exercise ambulators become wheelchair ambulators in their teens, about half of the household ambulators become community ambulators and the other half end up as wheelchair ambulators in adolescence.

This transition to a wheelchair takes place at about 13 years of age for several reasons (S. E. Stauffer, personal communication, 1972). The main reason is that the energy expended in walking becomes prohibitive because of the increase in weight and height. As the height increases, the vertical distance through which the body has to be lifted also increases. With each step, the patient expends the effort equivalent to a push-up. On the other hand, the child is increasingly unable to keep up with the pace of his peers, and also by this time the wheelchair is esthetically more acceptable than the pattern of gait to which he was accustomed.

There is considerable disagreement about the early management of the exercise ambulators. Some are of the opinion that it is best to train them for the sitting existence from the beginning, since they eventually end up in a wheelchair in their early teens. They argue that this saves the funds invested in their braces, saves the time and effort of the therapist, and avoids the sense of frustration and failure when the child realizes that he is not going to walk after all.

It is our opinion, shared by others (B. H. Curtis; S. E. Stauffer, and G. E. Sharpless, personal communications, 1972), that exercise ambulators should stand and ambulate for as long as possible. Even eventual wheelchair ambulators should be stood up while supported by braces for as long as feasible.

From a physical standpoint, standing is important not only because the major joints of the lower limbs have to adopt the functional position during stance, but, according to the experience gained by NASA with the Space Programs, about 4 hours of standing a day will prevent disuse osteoporosis of the weight-bearing skeleton. Thus, with standing alone, we are able to prevent postural deformities as well as pathological fractures. In addition, there is an improvement in cardiorespiratory functions and urinary drainage, bowel function, and reflex vascular function of the limbs.

Perhaps as important as the physical benefits of standing are the psychological benefits. The goal of treating these children, according to Sharples (personal communication, 1972), is the "maximalization of normalcy." The physical appearance of any person in society has associated expectations. The physically handicapped person thus is surrounded by negative expectations even with regard to skills not associated with the nature of the disability. For instance, anyone in need of directions and having the choice will more readily ask the man *standing* at the street corner than another one in a wheelchair. The implication is clear: the person in the wheelchair is not expected to know his way around as well as the one who has full use of his legs. Conversely, a wheelchair-bound person who is stood up for even part of the time will be expected to do, to learn, and to know more. He will have a better access to his environment, particularly if his hands are freed from the process of standing and ambulation. He will be challenged more because he is regarded as being less disabled. He will have had a more human experience.

Proper timing is important: a normal experience has to be learned at a normal age. To learn to walk at the age of 3 or 4 is abnormal. Therefore, the skills of standing and ambulation should be taught at an age (neurodevelopmental age) when children normally learn these skills. Even though standing and ambulation may be utilized for only a few years, the exposure to the environment and the feeling of normalcy make the invested effort well worthwhile (B. H. Curtis, G. E. Sharpless, personal communications, 1972). However, the *exercise ambulators never should be pushed towards functional ambulation.* Parents and sometimes the child should understand that we do not expect him to walk functionally. As the age of 13 or 14 approaches, he begins to fall back in his ambulatory skills.

ORTHOTIC DEVICES

Orthotic devices (orthos-straight, erect) are external aids to assist the child with meningomyelocele to sit, to stand, and to ambulate. They include not only braces, but wheelchairs, crutches, and motorized assisting devices.

More specifically, some serve as external "stiffeners," replacing paralyzed muscles, fighting the deforming forces of posture, gravity, and unopposed active muscles, and keeping the joints in the functional position; other orthotic devices help the patient to move about. In general, orthotic devices should make the patient less dependent on other people and on his environment.

The devices are made of different materials, such as lightweight metal alloys, occasionally steel, leather, laminated plastics, etc. The design of the devices and the materials used in their fabrication have to be considered in relation to their availability, ease of assembly, lightness, cosmesis, durability, ease of application and removal, adjustibility, ease of cleansing, expense, simple maintenance, and good tolerance. The devices can be classified as attendant operated or patient operated.

THE UMBROLLER

This device (Fig. 9-23) is attendant-operated and is excellent for the transport of the paraplegic child between the car, the clinic, the school, or the home. It consists of an aluminum frame and vinyl or canvas backing and it rolls on eight wheels. It is foldable and can be carried on the arm as an umbrella. It weighs less than 6 lbs. It was developed in England under the name of "Baby Baggy" and may be obtained at many department stores. There is a larger size for teenagers called "Baggy Major." This weighs 8 lbs. and has to be ordered from England.

WHEELCARTS

These are toys which can be used as prewalking devices. They are operated manually by the patient and help the child to explore his home environment. "Crawligator" carts (Fig. 9-24) or "Crazy Wheels" are very popular. The "Prone Scooter" is efficient on carpeted floor and can even manage small changes of level (single steps). The use of shoes will prevent the development of friction sores on the toes.

THE WHEELCHAIR

This is a most important orthotic device for many patients. Some depend on it for ambulation for the rest of their lives. The size should be adequate for

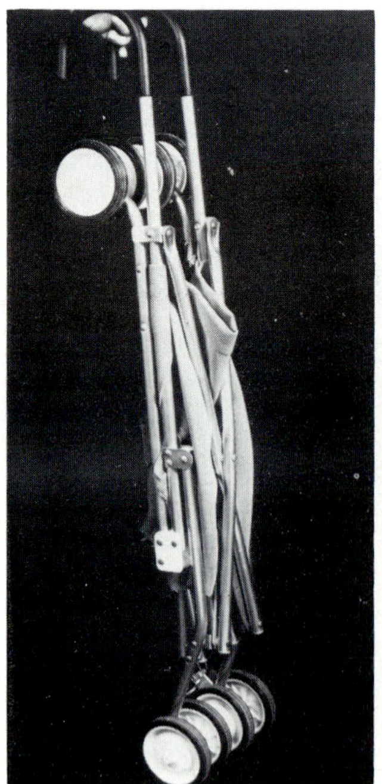

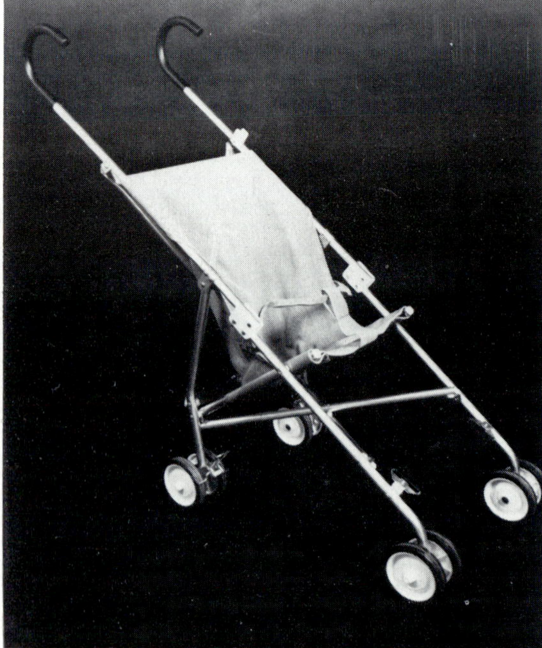

Fig. 9-23 The Umbroller, closed and open.

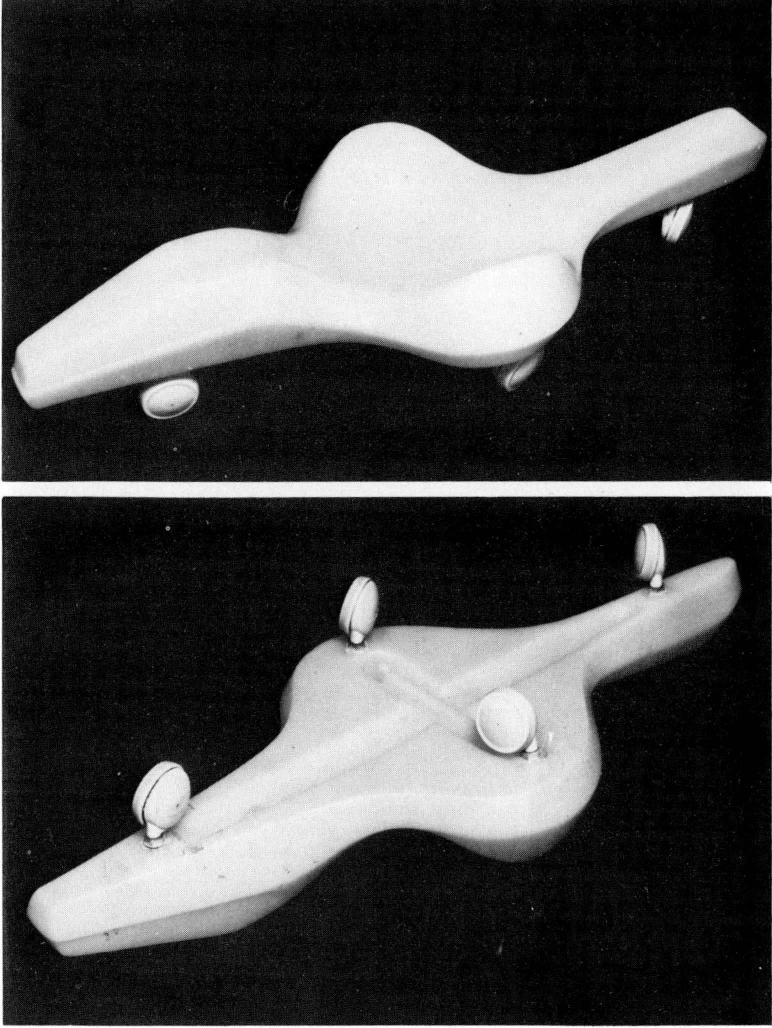

Fig. 9-24 Top and bottom view of the Crawligator.

the age of the patient. It serves not only as a means of locomotion, but as a positioning device. Unfortunately, the hips are flexed while the child is sitting in it, but the knees should be kept extended in the small child. The feet should be placed against the foot rests, with the ankles at right angles. The patients with additional disability of one upper limb can be provided with one-arm-driven wheelchairs.

SIEBENS' BRACE

This device (Fig. 9-9) is a back brace attached to the back of a wheel chair (Siebens et al., 1972). The brace supports the patient by his lower rib cage and relieves his buttocks from weight bearing. It allows free respiratory expansion of the upper chest. It is ideal for the thoracic or thoracolumbar lesion where ischiococcigeal pressure coexists with a paralytic scoliosis. In addition, it relieves the effect of gravity on the spine, thus slowing the progression of paralytic curves.

LAMINATED PLASTIC BACK BRACE OR CORSET

These may be used to prevent gross progression of paralytic scoliosis and thereby to give the spine time to grow before fusion is performed.

PARAPODIUM

This is an external standing device worn over clothes (Fig. 9-25). It is used in cases of complete paralysis of the lower limbs and also controls pelvic obliquity and scoliosis. It allows sitting, standing, and limited walking with a swing-through gait. Developed by Motloch (1971) at the Ontario Crippled Children's Centre, it has multiple advantages. For example, it has standard parts which are easily exchangeable, allowing for growth; its application and removal are easy and probably faster than those of other similar devices; and it is not cosmetically fashioned to the patient's body, giving the impression of being more a piece of therapeutic equipment than a brace in the classic sense. It is not suitable for the development of a pattern of reciprocating gait.

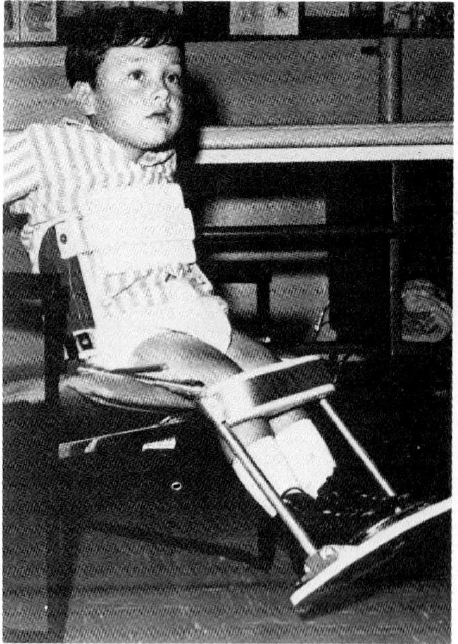

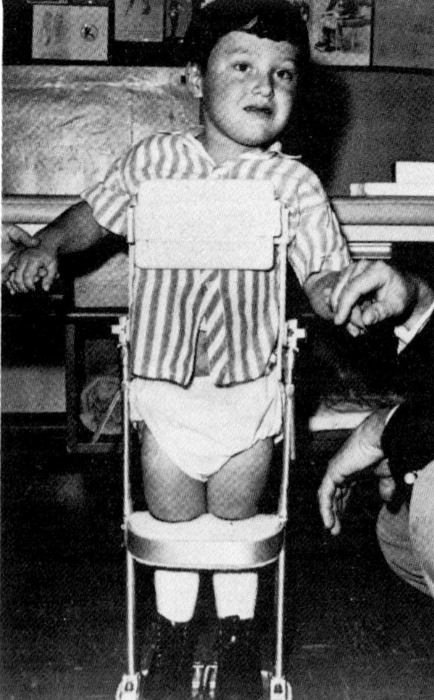

Fig. 9-25 The Parapodium, developed at the Ontario Crippled Children's Centre by Motloch. Published by kind permission of the author and of Artificial Limbs.

NEWINGTON BRACE

This device (Fig. 9-26) is made of "vitrothene," a laminated plastic material, and was developed at the Newington Children's Hospital. It is an inexpensive posterior splint applied to the back and lower limbs in which the

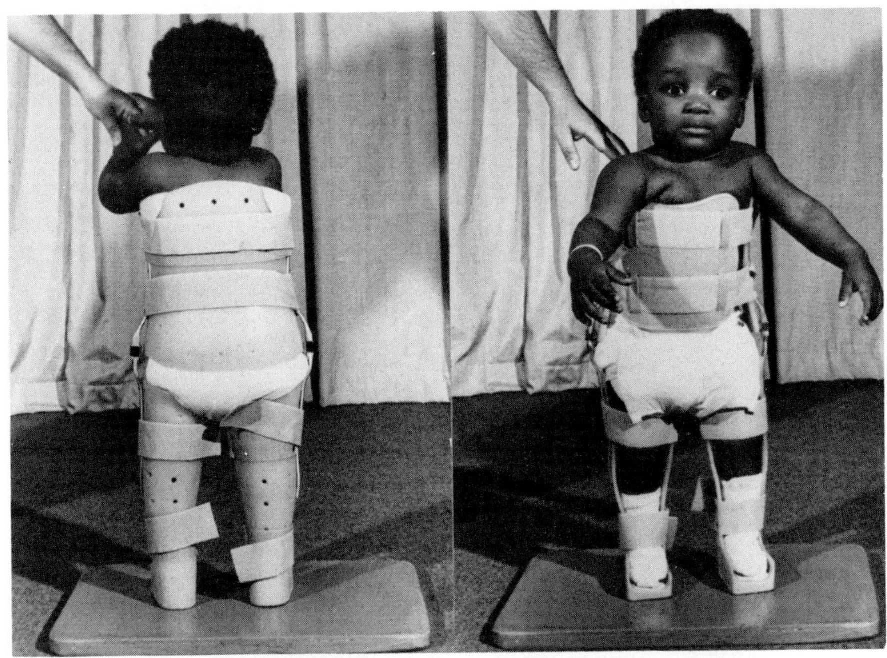

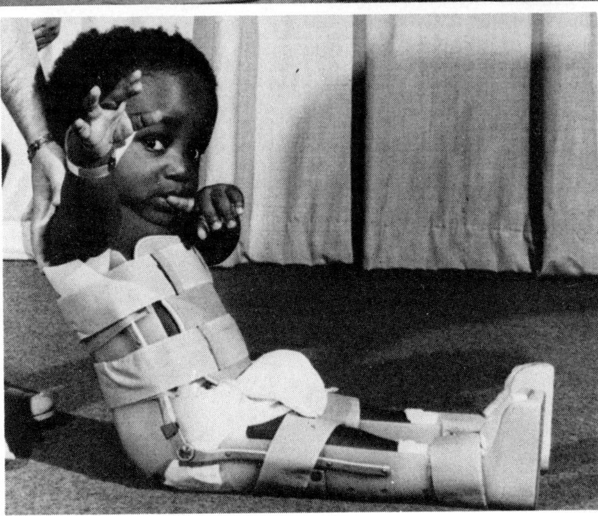

Fig. 9-26 The Newington Brace developed at the Newington Children's Hospital (Courtesy of Dr. Burr H. Curtis).

patient can stand passively supported. Hip hinges may be added later to allow sitting. Early gait training is started in this brace at Newington. It is a preliminary step toward the long leg braces with pelvic band.

BILATERAL LONG LEG BRACES WITH THE PELVIC BAND

These are the standard braces of the paraplegic who does not have hip, knee, or foot control. The pelvic band provides hip control, the long leg part provides knee control, and the short leg part, ankle and foot control. Double uprights held to the limbs by appropriate cuffs join a padded pelvic band and attach to shoes by split stirrups. Hip and knee joints with drop-locks allow for flexion-extension. The pelvic band has to be modified often to avoid friction over the stoma of the ileostomy. A full back brace instead of the pelvic band can be attached to the long leg braces if the patient transiently needs additional pelvic control. Permanent lack of pelvic control is an indication for the wheelchair. We tend to use the long leg braces with the pelvic band to begin ambulation even in those children who have fair hip control. This provides them with additional stability in the beginning, and the pelvic band can be removed at a later time.

This brace with a back extension and the feet attached to skis (Fig. 9-27) may be used as a standing brace. A removable anterior ankle lock is added. The few degrees of ankle motion given permit the patient to swing his trunk back and forth a few degrees while standing, which helps the development of standing balance and encourages the action of antigravity muscles. The back extension can be entirely removable and the brace used later for full gait training. With minor changes, it allows for about 2.5 to 3 years of growth. While it is more versatile and probably somewhat more expensive than other braces, its cost is only the equivalent of 3 to 4 hospital days.

We place children in this standing brace for several hours a day starting at about the age of 10 to 12 months if they have head and upper trunk control. As the ability of the child to ambulate increases, and if he gains hip control either by his normal development or secondary to surgery, the pelvic band is first unlocked, then removed.

LONG LEG BRACES

Few patients remain in long leg braces permanently. These provide knee control and are indicated in case of either quadriceps or hamstring weakness. A less frequent indication is the need for control of rotary displacement of the knee, with the tibia being externally rotated to the femur.

SHORT LEG BRACE

This is the most frequently indicated brace in our clinic. It controls the position of the ankle and foot, and with special provisions of construction it also may control the knee from buckling into flexion or from going out into recurvatum. As a rule, we have used the Phelps' brace (Fig. 9-28). This is a single lateral (or medial) upright bar attaching to high-top shoes by a built-

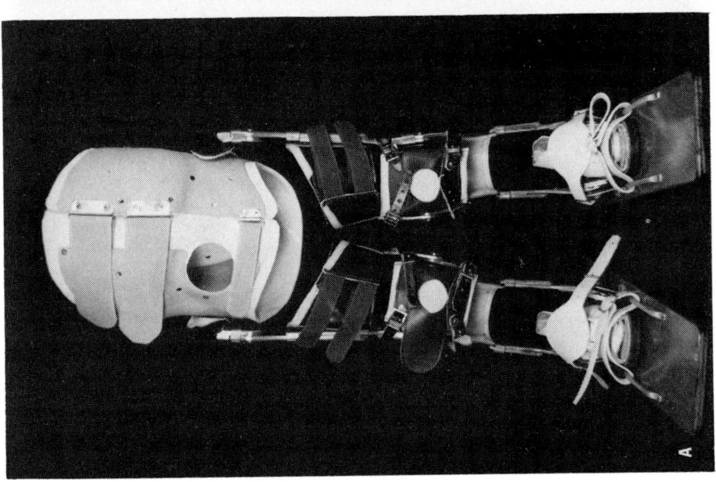

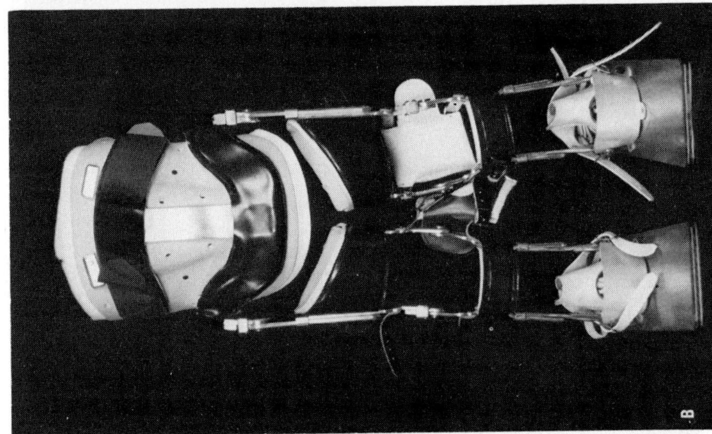

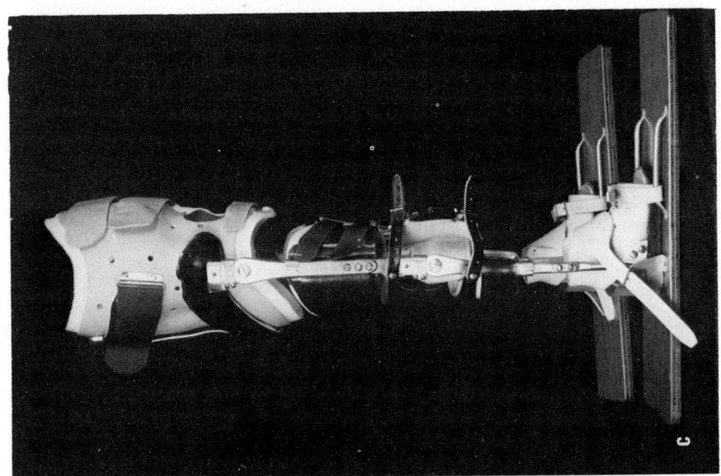

Fig. 9-27 (A) Front, (B) back, and (C) right side view of the brace used at our Birth Defects Center. It serves as a passive standing brace when mounted on skis. It is useful for training in all modalities of gait. The laminated plastic corset may be detached and worn separately while the patent sits for several hours a day (Courtesy of Mr. Robert Denison).

in foot plate and to the calf by a cuff and a Velcro strap. This is a static brace of great versatility. For limitation of dorsiflexion or plantarflexion, an anterior or a posterior ankle stop is added, respectively. Lateral control of the foot is achieved by the right-angle bend of the upright bar as it joins the foot plate and by the addition of a "T" strap. Such a strap is based on the inside of the shoe and is strapped around the lateral upright for correction of the supple valgus deformity and opposite to that for correction of varus deformity.

By fixing the ankle joint of the brace and raising or lowering the heel, one can control the knee. This is the principle on which the Saltiel brace was built (Saltiel, 1969). The Saltiel brace (Fig. 9-29) is a low-weight, one-piece, laminated plastic brace with a fixed, prepositioned ankle. It is primarily indicated to lock the knee in extension, replacing or complementing the action of a weak quadriceps. Its great merits are that it obviates the need for a long leg brace and does away with the heavy metal construction.

An excellent brace for a dropfoot deformity is the one-piece, laminated plastic, posterior splint designed by Yates (1968). Although it has no ankle

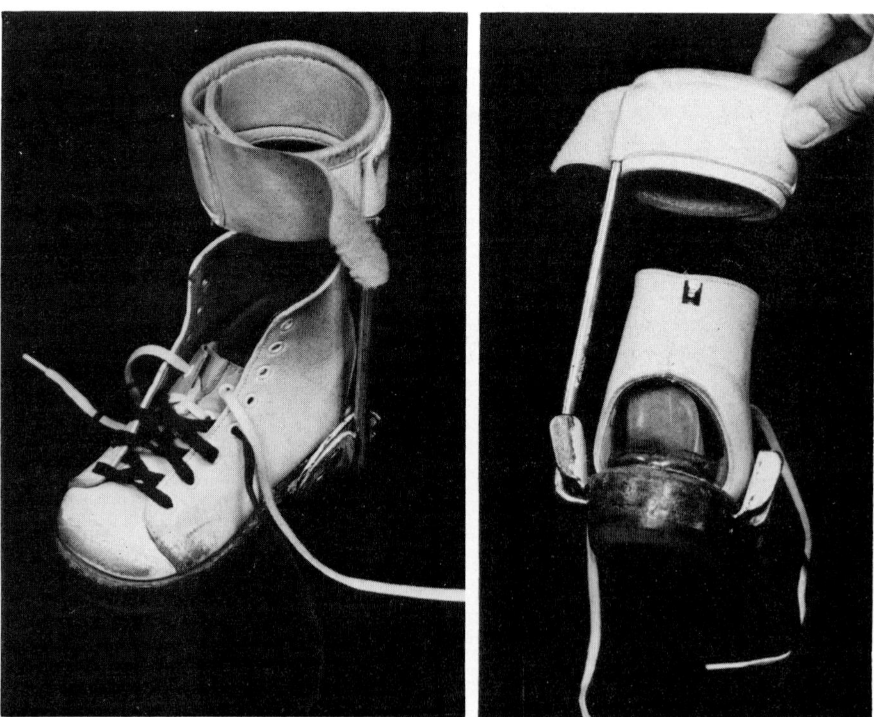

Fig. 9-28 Phelps' short leg brace. The lateral upright is attached to the high-top shoe by a footplate and to the leg by a Velcro strap. The ankle motion can be limited as seems desirable by anterior or posterior stops. The clear plastic heel window is useful to check the position of the patient's heel in the shoe.

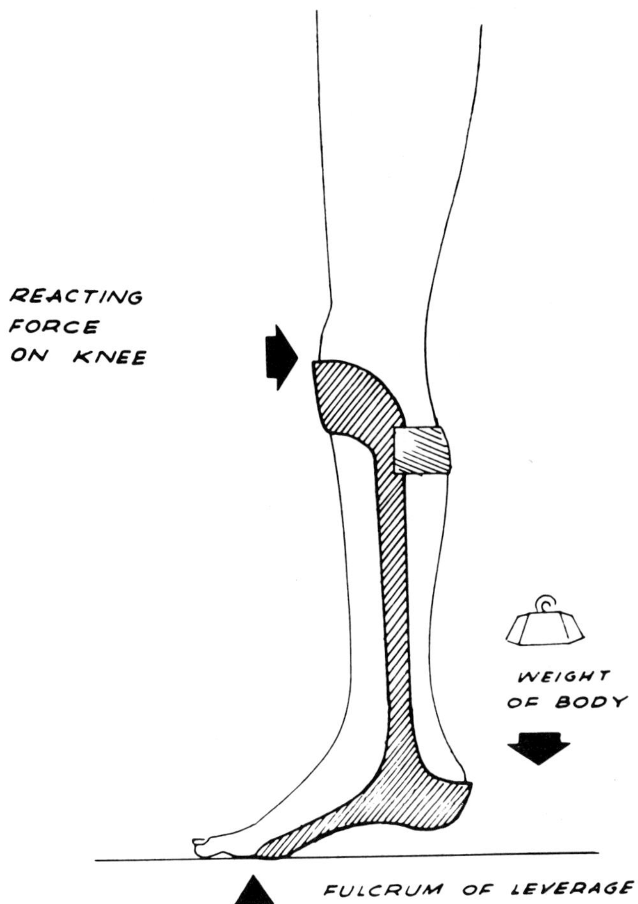

Fig. 9-29 The Saltiel brace (Courtesy of Mr. J. Saltiel, published with permission of Orthotics-Prosthetics).

joint, it permits some measure of dorsiflexion by the elasticity of the material and the type of design, but prevents plantarflexion beyond the right angle.

HEEL MOLDS

At the lowest level of motor involvement, ankle control is no longer a problem, but the subtalar joint may be unstable and the hindfoot displaced in valgus, overcome by the weight of the body because of the weakness of the posterior tibial tendon. Such supple valgus deformity of the heel may be corrected either surgically (Brown, 1968) or by plastic heel-cups (Yates, 1968) molded on a plaster model of the foot with the heel in the corrected position (Fig. 9-21). These may be inserted in low-cut laced Oxfords, and they effectively correct the displacement of the subtalar joint. We find that shoe wedges are ineffective.

SHOES

Worn by the patient with meningomyeloceles, shoes serve to protect the feet from friction sores and offer some measure of protection against foot deformities.

The shoes should be part of the patient rather than of the braces which may be attached to them, and high tops are preferable. Shoes should lace down to the toes, if possible, to prevent the big toe from flexing while the foot is slipped into the shoe. If the anesthetic toe remains flexed, it will develop a pressure sore on the tip.

PHYSICAL THERAPY

The purpose of physical therapy is to *teach* the patient and his family techniques which will make him more functional and independent. The emphasis is on teaching, for if the family and patient are able to carry out the physical therapy, they will be able to do it far more frequently than possible with visits to a physical therapist. The role of the physical therapist, then, is to continue supervision of therapy as carried out by the patient and his family.

The purpose of physical therapy is to circumvent absent function and to develop existing ability through the proper utilization of orthotic devices. The process starts with an assessment of the degree of functional loss and of the amount of remaining function. The principles and techniques described here are those used on patients of the Birth Defects Treatment Center by a team of physical therapists of the John F. Kennedy Institute under the direction of Susan Harriman, R.P.T.

In the paraplegic with meningomyeloceles, the functional goals are independent transfer and ambulation.

TRANSFER

Independent transfer between the wheelchair and the bed, from wheelchair to another chair, and from the wheelchair to the commode eases the nursing care and provides the child with a degree of independence. This independence is particularly important to those who will not become functional ambulators. Transfers should be taught early, between 1 and 2 years of age. A wheelchair of adequate size is a basic, yet often overlooked, requirement. All too often, children are mistakenly provided with an adult-sized wheelchair. The size of the wheelchair and its height may be of importance and should be tailored to the child and his disability. For children who are nonambulators, the chair should be higher to permit transfer to other pieces of furniture. For ambulators, the chair should be lower to permit the child's feet to reach the floor with him in a sitting position, thus enabling him to stand up. The length of the seat should not exceed the length of the child's thighs.

STANDING AND AMBULATION

We begin passive standing at about 1 year of age in long leg braces and a trunk brace extension attached to skis. We start with more bracing than will ultimately be needed, because it gives more support and security to the patient and permits him to start ambulation earlier and progress faster.

Gait training is started on parallel bars. Attempts are made by the therapist to unlock the hips as early as possible and to teach the child a four-point reciprocating gait. If this is not possible in the beginning, the hips are kept locked and a pivoting gait is taught. A swing-to swing-through gait may provide speed; however, it is less secure than a reciprocating gait. We prefer not to teach the swing-through gait until after the child has learned the elements of a four-point gait, since we find that children who have mastered the swing-through gait are less likely to use the four-point gait and more likely to remain dependent on crutches (Hoffer et al., 1973).

Training progresses from the parallel bars to quadcanes and finally to Lofstrand crutches (short arm crutches) (Fig. 9-30). The quadcanes give maximum stability while providing greater mobility than the parallel bars. Once the child has learned the four-point gait with Lofstrand crutches, a swinging gait with these crutches is the next step, although the patient may have to switch transiently to axillary crutches to learn this modality of gait.

Those children who have some hip control are forced to use it when utilizing quadcanes. If they are left to hang on axillary crutches, they will walk with a swinging gait and throw the limbs in front of them, not making use of the available hip muscles.

Whether or not the child becomes a functional ambulator depends on his ability to ambulate with the braces unlocked at the hips. Children are physically unable to unlock the hips themselves, and as soon as they have to depend on others to stand them up and lock their braces at the hip level, their gait will not be functional. Most children can manage the knee locks, unless they have hamstring tightness.

There is a growing debate as to the best course of management for children who are nonfunctional ambulators (exercise ambulators). One group feels that forcing a child to ambulate for exercise provides only frustration and accomplishes little. This group feels that the expense of braces and of physical therapy is not justified in these children who will not ambulate for function and who will ultimately end up in wheelchairs. A second group feels that the experience of standing and ambulation has multiple benefits. They feel that in addition to the benefit derived from standing, which prevents osteoporosis and fractures, the upright child is perceived as being more normal and thereby acts more normally. This second group feels that even exercise ambulation gives the child a feeling of accomplishment and provides the family with a more positive approach and outlook towards the child. They feel that as long as the parents and the children do not

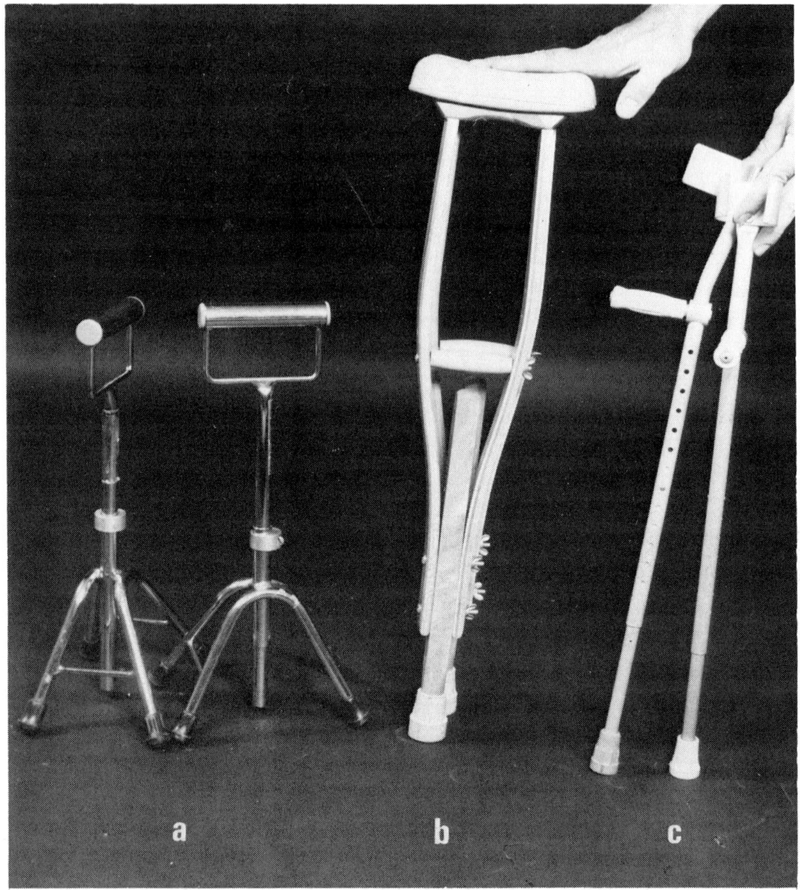

Fig. 9-30 (a) Quadcanes; (b) axillary crutches; (c) Lofstrand crutches.

acquire false hopes regarding ultimate ambulation, the benefits derived far outweigh the expense and trouble.

While we are inclined to agree with the second group and to encourage standing and ambulation, we feel that the ultimate decision must be modified depending on the child, his intellectual capacity, and the family constellation. We feel that ambulation, even for exercise, and standing as much as possible should be encouraged but not forced. We realize, however, that children who are unable to ambulate functionally will not continue to ambulate for exercise except under duress and will revert to a wheelchair. The attitude of the parents towards ambulation of their child is critical in determining his degree of ambulation.

FALLING

Parents should abstain from conveying the fear of falling to the child. This fear does not exist in the child at first, but is instilled in him by his parents and other persons in his immediate environment. The child should be provided with a helmet at the beginning of gait training, and falling should not be discussed. The parents should not respond to crying or screaming; instead such behavior on the part of the child should be ignored, and only positive attitudes should be reinforced. Sessions of standing with the canes should be brief and not last over 2 minutes at the start. Parents should hold onto the canes rather than onto the child, since this creates less dependency on the part of the child. It is easier to remove one's hands from the canes than from the child. The child, in turn, holds onto the canes with much more vigor.

The parents should encourage the child's ambulation to fit into the movements of the rest of the family. Ambulation should not be encouraged only at fixed times. For instance, instead of walking from 10:00 to 11:00 every morning, the child should be encouraged to get up from the dining table with the rest of the family and walk away. This encourages the concept that ambulation is not an exercise, but a useful, natural phenomenon.

Most parents can be taught to give physical therapy to their children at home and to return to the therapist periodically for supervision of old skills and the learning of new ones. Children are admitted for intensive in-patient therapy only if the above measures are unsuccessful or under unusual circumstances. Often, however, an admission of several weeks for gait training may permit far more rapid progress than that which could be achieved at home.

Therapy should be a game, and games can be incorporated into much of therapy. For instance, falling may be taught as part of a game that several children play together on the mat. Standing up is easier with the quadcanes because the cane is stable on the floor and the child is able to get back up again, working his way up from the base of the cane.

As soon as the child is able to step up enough, he is started on 2-inch curbs and on the ramp. The child can be started on stairs if one knee can be unlocked. If the knee cannot be unlocked, the child will have to wait until his arms grow long enough so that he can raise himself on the 2- to 3-inch curbs by elbow extension. The children use quadcanes and later Lofstrand crutches to walk the stairs. They should not be walking stairs if they need axillary crutches.

In summary, physical therapy should be used to teach the child and the family the techniques which will enable him to use his existing musculature and proper orthotic devices to achieve maximal function. The maximal function which can be obtained can be determined readily from assessing the joints which are under the patient's control. The use of these joints may be modified by factors such as intelligence, motivation, and dependency. The goal of the orthopedist is to determine what function is present and what procedures can be utilized to maximize that function. He also must utilize the minimal amount of surgery and the minimal amount of orthotic help to achieve maximal function. Careful and conscientious use of these techniques and devices will maximize function and minimize disability.

Acknowledgment. The author wishes to acknowledge the help with the manuscript received from T. Ravalli, the art work done by B. Robbins and L. Schlossberg, and the photography work by Suhair Karem.

REFERENCES

Brown, A. 1968. A simple method of fusion of the subtalar joint in children. J. Bone Joint Surg. 50-B:369.

Crenshaw, A. H. (ed.). 1971. Campbell's Operative Orthopedics. Fifth Ed. The C. V. Mosby Co., St. Louis, Mo.

Curtis, B. H. 1969. Congenital hypertension with anterior subluxation of the knee. J. Bone Joint Surg. 51-A:255.

Drennan, C. 1970. The role of the lumbar muscles in the development of human lumbar kyphosis. Develop. Med. Child Neurol. (Suppl.) 22:33.

Freehafer, A. A., J. C. Vessely, and R. P. Mack. 1972. Iliopsoas muscle transfer in the treatment of meningomyelocele patients with paralytic hip deformities. J. Bone Joint Surg. 54-A:1715.

Grice, D. S. 1952. An extra-articular arthrodesis of the subastragalar joint for correction of paralytic flat feet in children. J. Bone Joint Surg. 34-A:927.

Hoffer, M. M., D. Feiwell, R. Perry, T. Perry, and C. Bonnett. 1973. Functional ambulation in patients with myelomeningocele. J. Bone Joint Surg. 55-A:137.

Hoppenfeld, S. 1967. Kyphosis in myelomeningocele. J. Bone Joint Surg. 49-B:276.

Japas, L. M. 1968. Surgical treatment of pes cavus by tarsal V-osteotomy. J. Bone Joint Surg. 50-A:927.

Kopits, J., and I. Kopits. 1942. Orthopaedia Tankonyve [Textbook of Orthopaedics], p. 123. Magyar Orvosi Konyvkiado Tarsulat, Budapest.

McKibbin, B. 1973. The use of splintage in the management of paralytic dislocation of the hip in spina bifida cystica. J. Bone Joint Surg. 55-B:163.

Motloch, W. 1971. The parapodium: An orthotic device for neuromuscular disorders. Artificial Limbs 15:36.

Ogston, A. 1902. A new principle of curing club-foot in severe cases in children a few years old. Brit. Med. J. 1:1524.

Peabody, C. W. 1949. Tendon transposition in the paralytic foot. Am. Acad. Orth. Surg. Instr. Course Lect. 6:178.

Saltiel, J. 1969. A one-piece laminated knee locking short leg brace [Abstr.]. Orthotics Prosthetics 23:68.

Sharrard, W. J. W. 1959. Congenital paralytic dislocation of the hip in children with myelomeningocele. J. Bone Joint Surg. 41-B:622.

Sharrard, W. J. W. 1964. Posterior iliopsoas transplantation in the treatment of paralytic dislocation of the hip. J. Bone Joint Surg. 46-B:426.

Sharrard, W. J. W. 1968. Spinal osteotomy for congenital kyphosis in myelomeningocele. J. Bone Joint Surg. 50-B:466.

Sharrard, W. J. W. 1969. Newer aspects of myelomeningocele. *In* A. W. Wilkinson (ed.), Recent advances in pediatric surgery, p. 171. J. & A. Churchill, Ltd., London.

Sharrard, W. J. W. 1971. Pediatric orthopaedics and fractures. Blackwell Scientific Publishers, Oxford & Edinburgh.

Shiram, K., W. P. Bobechko, and J. E. Hall. 1972. Surgical management of spinal deformities in spina bifida. J. Bone Joint Surg. 54-B:666.

Siebens, A. A., J. P. Hohf, W. E. Engel, and N. Scribner. 1972. Suspension of certain patients from their ribs. Hopkins Med. J. 130:26.

Steindler, A. 1920. Stripping of the os calcis. J. Orthoped. Surg. 2:8.

Turco, V. J. 1971. Surgical correction of the resistant club foot. J. Bone Joint Surg. 53-A:477.

Winter, R. B., J. H. Moe, and V. E. Eilers. 1968. Congenital scoliosis: A study of 234 patients treated and untreated. J. Bone Joint Surg. 50-A:1.

Yates, G. 1968. A method for the provision of lightweight aesthetic orthopedic appliances. Orthopaedics (Oxford, 1968) 1:153.

10

The Genitourinary Tract in Patients with Meningomyeloceles

Rainer M. E. Engel, M.D.

Since the advent of early closure of the spinal defect and treatment of the hydrocephalus, the major cause of death in patients with meningomyeloceles has shifted to the urinary tract. Hydronephrosis and pyelonephrosis gradually lead to renal decompensation, hypertension, and slow death from chronic renal disease.

To prevent this slow renal death, one must understand normal bladder function as a prerequisite to understanding the abnormal physiology of neurogenic dysfunction and the pathophysiology of renal decompensation in children with meningomyeloceles.

NEUROANATOMY OF THE BLADDER

The urinary bladder serves as a reservoir for urine, which can then be evacuated voluntarily. In a healthy bladder, this evacuation leads to complete emptying with only an insignificant amount of residual urine left. In addition, reflux to the upper urinary tracts is prevented. Voluntary emptying of the bladder is a "learned," or acquired, ability, bladder distension serving as a stimulant for micturition. The phylogenetically lower control centers, located in the sacral area of the spine, are retained and have been studied intensely; anatomical and histological studies have been augmented by numerous experimental animal models. Still, a large number of the facilitating pathways involved in micturition escape our knowledge, despite the fact that we have found numerous areas in cortex, basal ganglia, midbrain, medulla, and cerebellum which obviously play a role in the act of micturition.

Muscles which facilitate micturition include the detrusor muscle of the bladder and those muscles of the abdominal wall and diaphragm which increase intra-abdominal pressure and, therefore, aid in expulsion of the urine. Micturition is inhibited by the sphincteric mechanism of the urethra as well as by the muscle entity of the pelvic floor. Any or all of these muscles may be involved in the neurological deficit of a patient with a meningomyelocele. Our prime consideration, however, is the involvement of the bladder itself.

The nerve supply to the bladder and sphincter is depicted in Fig. 10-1. The parasympathetic motor supply originates in the cord segments of S_2 to S_4. These motor fibers leave the cord through the anterior root and form the medial branch of the pudendal plexus. The branches to bladder, prostate, and seminal vesicles approach these organs from their posteriolateral aspects and terminate, in the case of the bladder, in the vesical plexus or in the wall of the bladder itself. The short postganglionic neuron then ends in the bladder muscle.

The sympathetic motor supply of the bladder takes its origin at T_{11} to L_2, leaving the spinal cord through the anterior root and coursing through the ganglionic chain to form the presacral nerve, terminating in the pararectal hypogastric ganglia. The postganglionic neuron starts from here and ends in the smooth muscle of the trigone, ureteral orifices, and vesical neck.

The pelvic floor derives its motor innervation from the sacral segments of S_2 to S_4. The nerve fibers originate in the anterior horn and leave the cord through the anterior root, whence they form the lateral branch of the pudendal plexus leading into the pudendal nerve. The internal pudendal

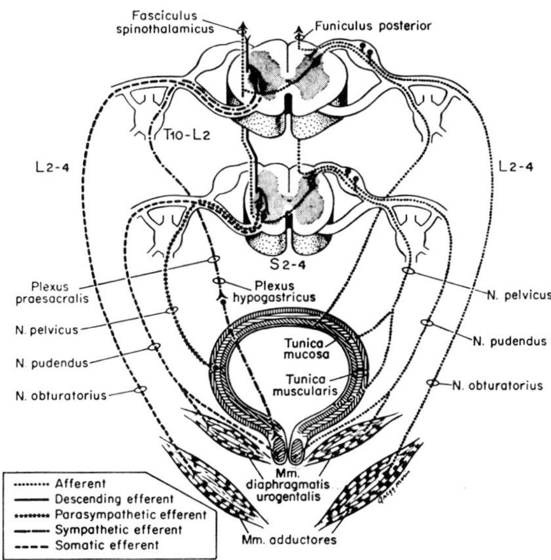

Fig. 10-1 Schematic diagram of the autonomic and somatic pathways which mediate potential reflexes between smooth and striated muscles of bladder, pelvic floor, and lower extremity. (Courtesy of Bors and Porter, Urol. Int. 25:114, 1970.)

nerve courses through Alcock's canal and, after sending off motor fibers to the striated muscle of the pelvic floor, trifurcates into middle, anterior, and posterior branches. The middle branch supplies the external urinary sphincter, whereas the posterior branch supplies the anal sphincter.

Sensory impulses from the bladder are divided into exteroception, for pain and temperature, and proprioception, for contraction and distention, and course along both autonomic and somatic nerves.

Proprioceptive and exteroceptive impulses pass through the posterior root into the posterior horn where, through short interneurons, they form a reflex arch to the anterior horn. Upper and lower cord segments are interconnected through fasciculi proprii. These pathways then mediate the potential reflexes between vesical mucosa, smooth and striated muscle of the bladder, and pelvic floor musculature.

Vesicocutaneous reflexes and visceral reflexes, such as vesicoureteral or rectovesical, are of clinical importance for the urologist who is faced with the problem of determining further care of the patient with a meningomyelocele and a neurological bladder dysfunction. It is important to remember that supraspinal pathways, including the brainstem, hypothalamus, and basal ganglia, also play a significant role in both facilitation and inhibition of the act of micturition.

The cerebral cortex becomes involved during bladder training and allows man to override volemic bladder stimulation with inhibitory impulses, or, on the other hand, to achieve voluntary voiding in the absence of such a stimulus.

CLASSIFICATION OF NEUROLOGICAL BLADDER DYSFUNCTION

Clinicians and researchers have tried to classify neurological dysfunction of the bladder. Much of our knowledge in this field has been gained by observation of patients with traumatic cord lesions. In these patients, it is relatively easy to correlate the anatomical defect with the physiological disturbance. Various classifications have only added to the confusion in this field, but most urologists classify these bladders into the following groups:

1. Spinal cord lesions
   a) Motor
   b) Sensory
   c) Sensory-motor neuron lesions
2. Lower motor neuron lesions (peripheral nerve)
3. Mixed lesions (upper and lower motor neuron)

It is the *mixed* lesions that are found most commonly in the patient with a meningomyelocele. The subclassification in this group depends essentially on the location of this lesion—whether it is above the conus medullaris, which contains the primary reflex center for bladder function, or whether it is at or below the conus. With an intact conus medullaris, the micturitional

Table 10-1 Classifications of Neurogenic Bladders (Adapted from Bors and Comarr, 1971)

I. SPINAL CORD LESION (UPPER MOTOR NEURON)	
A. *Motor neuron lesion* Sensation: NL Detrusor function: ↓ Residual urine: ↑ Capacity: NL to ↑ Bulbocavernosus reflex: NL	Causes: Parkinsonism, amyotrophic lateral sclerosis, poliomyelitis
B. *Sensory neuron lesion* Sensation: ↓ Detrusor function: NL to ↓ Residual urine: ↑ Capacity: NL to ↑ Bulbocavernosus reflex: NL	Causes: diabetes, tabes, chordotomy
C. *Sensory-motor neuron lesion*	
Complete Sensation: ↓ Detrusor function: ↓ or ↑* Bulbocavernosus reflex: ↓ to ↑* Residual urine: ↑ Capacity: ↑ to ↓	Causes: complete cord transsection secondary to trauma, vascular accident, myelitis
Incomplete Sensation: NL to ↑ Detrusor function: ↑ Bulbocavernosus reflex: ↓ to ↑* Residual urine: ↑ Capacity: ↑ to ↓	Causes: partial cord transsection (trauma, vascular accident, neoplasm, infectious or demyelinating process), hemiplegia
II. LOWER MOTOR NEURON LESION	
Complete Sensation: ↓ Detrusor function: ↓ Bulbocavernosus reflex: absent Residual urine: ↑ Capacity: ↑	Causes: cord trauma at conus medullaris or cauda equina
Incomplete Sensation: ↓ Detrusor function: ↓ Bulbocavernosus reflex: ↓ Residual urine: ↑ Capacity: ↑	Causes: cord trauma at conus medullaris or cauda equina
III. MIXED LESIONS—UPPER AND LOWER MOTOR NEURON	
Combinations of upper and lower somato-motor and upper or lower visceromotor lesions are seen	Causes: myelodysplasia (partial or total), sacral agenesis, spina bifida, meningomyelocele, conus medullaris and cauda equina trauma, lipoma of cord

*Depending on stage of recovery.

reflex arc will also be intact. This reflex pattern is transmitted via the pelvic and internal pudendal nerves.

The bulbocavernosis reflex is mediated through the same reflex arc as the micturitional reflex. This reflex is tested by squeezing or pricking the dorsum of the glans penis (or clitoris), and is assessed by contraction of the external anal sphincter. This reflex utilizes the third and fourth sacral nerves and the conus medullaris. Since this is the same reflex arc utilized for involuntary micturition, the bulbocavernosis reflex may be utilized to separate upper and lower motor neuron lesions of the bladder. If present, it indicates that the neurogenic dysfunction is above the level of the conus, and is therefore an upper neuron lesion. If the defect is at a level where it involves the conus medullaris or the peripheral nerves, then this reflex arc will be interrupted, and the dysfunction will be a *lower motor* neuron lesion.

Again, the neurological bladder deficit found in patients with meningomyeloceles usually represents a *mixed* lesion. A schematic classification of neurogenic bladders in general, as adapted from Bors and Comarr (1971), is given in Table 10-1.

HISTORY AND PHYSICAL EXAMINATION

As has been pointed out, the history and physical examination of the child with a meningomyelocele are of utmost importance. The examination includes a number of tests designed to help specifically in the differential diagnosis of the bladder lesion.

Most mothers will be able to give a fairly accurate description of the child's voiding pattern. They will notice whether the child continuously dribbles and leaks urine when crying or straining, or whether the child is able to produce a full stream and dribbles some urine between voidings, or is dry between voidings. The force and size of the urinary stream can also be described; the stream may be full and forceful, thin and weak, or intermittent. Abdominal straining to initiate the stream may be necessary. Crying during the act of micturition may signify urinary tract infection with pain on voiding. Pyuria, hematuria, or malodorous urine may be another expression of urinary tract infection. Pain can rarely be localized by these children because of both their age and their neurological deficit. They may be able to state some general suprapubic discomfort or backache. Tenderness in these areas cannot be demonstrated, but the discomfort may be increased by palpation of these areas. A history of fever or chills may indicate preceding upper urinary tract infection.

Urinary incontinence is classified by Bors and Comarr (1971) as follows:

> "1. *Incontinence of 'precipitate' micturition* characterizes the 'uninhibited neurogenic bladder' of incomplete upper motor neuron lesions.

"2. *Reflex incontinence* is present in complete upper motor neuron lesions.

"3. *Stress incontinence* may be due to either lower motor neuron lesions or to muscular damage of the pelvic floor. Loss or urine on laughing, lifting, walking up or down stairs, is a characteristic symptom. Uropathic obstruction must be excluded.

"4. *Overflow incontinence* occurs with imbalanced bladder function in patients with upper or lower motor neuron lesions or with sensory lesions. Obstructive uropathy must be excluded.

"5. *Incontinence of nonresistance* is manifested by continuous dribbling. This may be caused by a spastic detrusor and flaccid pelvic floor in some cases of myelodysplasia, or it may be surgically induced by resection of the external and internal sphincters in patients with upper or lower motor neuron lesions.

"6. *Psychologic incontinence* occurs either on an emotional basis (fear, agression) or following leukotomy which impaired the judgment of the patient."

Close association between urinary and bowel training, between bowel continence and urinary continence, and between continuous fecal soiling and urinary incontinence has been alluded to. In our institution, the pediatric surgeon guides the mother in the bowel training of her child (see Chapter 11).

The urological examination centers on several basic questions:

1. Does the patient have significant urinary tract infection?
2. Does reflux of urine into ureters or kidneys occur?
3. Are the upper urinary tracts damaged by either infection or reflux or a combination of both?
4. How much voiding pressure can the bladder musculature generate?
5. How much resistance does the external sphincter exert?
6. How much residual urine does this bladder carry?
7. What reflex arcs are intact? Are we dealing with an upper or lower motor neuron lesion?

Children with meningomyeloceles face continuing life-threatening situations. One such situation is that of septicemia secondary to urinary tract infection fostered by a large quantity of residual urine in the bladder or poorly emptying upper tracts. Recurrent infection will also cause lowered renal clearance as an expression of progressive renal failure.

A broad range of mortality rates is found in patients with traumatic cord lesions who have bladders with neurogenic dysfunction. Between 30% and 75% of all deaths are due to renal causes, renal failure clearly related to repeated urinary tract infections being the leading cause of death. The renal mortality rate with adequate urological care is as low as 12.5%, whereas it can reach 78% with inadequate care (Damanski and Sutcliffe-Kerr, 1964). It is thus of paramount importance to prevent urinary tract infections, urinary stones, and reflux.

THE UROLOGIC EXAMINATION

The initial urological evaluation includes a detailed history, as well as a physical and neurological examination. Initial laboratory tests include urinalysis and quantitative urine culture, electrolytes, urea nitrogen, and creatinine clearance. A cystometrogram, with determination of the residual urine and urinary sphincter manometrics, is obtained. An intravenous pyelogram is followed by cystoscopy under general anesthesia. A voiding cystourethrogram is included in this work-up. This rather complete work-up is performed when the child is first seen, regardless of age, and forms the basis for urological prognostication and follow-up. In the newborn the work-up is performed during the first weeks of life, as soon as the back is healed. An occasional child with an L_5–S_1 lesion may have hydroureter and hydronephrosis at birth and require evaluation and drainage even earlier.

Re-evaluation is performed at four- to six-month intervals. The re-evaluation includes an interval history, physical examination, electrolytes, serum urea nitrogen, quantitative urine culture, and an intravenous pyelogram. A cystometrogram, a voiding cystourethrogram, and a cystoscopy are done if any of the parameters shows changes when compared with preceding examinations.

The value of the excretory urogram or intravenous pyelogram is self-explanatory; it should not be interpreted as an expression of renal functions but, rather, as a means to delineate the anatomic outlines of the urinary tract. It affords us an excellent means of following a patient in whom reflux and infections with calyceal distortion, dilation, and hydroureteronephrosis are a constant threat. The number of films should be kept to a minimum to minimize the amount of radiation.

The voiding cystourethrogram with spot films on a filmstrip or a videotape offers an excellent way to document reflux and to study ureteral peristalsis. Poorly peristalsing ureters obstruct the urinary flow just as effectively as would an anatomic obstruction. It is well to remember that reflux is not a disease but a symptom, and that its underlying cause must be sought and treated.

Cystometry can give us a number of informative clues about bladder function. The residual urine can be measured, as well as the total bladder capacity; a possible impairment of sensation can be assessed, and the contractile force of the detrusor can be measured; also, the increase in pressure exerted with Valsalva's maneuvers, such as straining, can be recorded. Thus cystometry may aid us in establishing whether the patient has an upper or lower motor neuron lesion. It is the feeling of most urologists concerned with the care of children with meningomyeloceles that such a classification is of little prognostic value (Ridlon, 1971). The resistance exerted by the relaxed external sphincter is measured by running sterile saline across the external sphincter into the bladder and recording its resistance at the moment that fluid passes freely into the bladder lumen.

Cystoscopy not only will permit us to rule out anatomic obstruction at or below the bladder neck, such as prostatic valves, but will allow us to see the absence or presence of bladder trabeculation. Most important, however, we can judge the configuration and location of ureteral orifices in children with reflux; these orifices are important in determining the prognosis of this symptom. It has been shown that the degree of lateral displacement, and also the degree of malconfiguration of the ureteral orifice, have a significant bearing on the need for future reimplantation (Lyons, Marshall, and Tanagho, 1970).

After the initial evaluation, the patient is presented to the members of the team, and immediate care and long-term plans are decided upon. If the patient does well in general, and particularly as far as his urological status is concerned, no urological surgery is contemplated. Credé maneuvers have helped in emptying the large hypotonic bladder; a reflex bladder can be triggered by stimulating a reflex area, such as the inner thigh or the scrotum, or by tapping the suprapubic area. Catheter drainage via an indwelling bladder catheter or "bladder training" through repeat catheterization in these children is not recommended. In contrast to the case of traumatic cord lesion, improvement of bladder function cannot be expected.

UROLOGIC PROCEDURES

All urologic procedures for children with meningomyeloceles are designed to achieve the same goals: 1) to prevent urinary tract infection and to preserve renal tissue, and 2) to allow the child to be dry and attend school. Three different approaches have been utilized: catheter drainage, condom drainage, and urologic diversion.

CATHETER DRAINAGE

Catheter drainage of the neurogenic bladder would seem to be, at least on the surface, a workable solution. It should permit adequate drainage of the bladder thereby preventing reflux and infections, and provide continence. It is of interest that several institutions both in this country and abroad use this method with fair results in patients with acquired cord lesion. Unfortunately, there are a number of drawbacks to catheter drainage.

Intermittent catheter drainage requires a large, well trained "catheter team." Intermittent catheterization requires multiple instrumentations with the inherent risk of introducing infection via this route. As this procedure has to be done under aseptic precautions, it is a type of care that would *not* be feasible for home care. Continuous catheter drainage carries with it, also, the risk of infection, which occurs in approximately 70% of all patients on such drainage regardless of precautions, even with the most meticulous care. In patients who have an acquired lesion, one can hope for some degree of bladder recovery, but this is not to be expected in the child with meningomyelocele. In addition, a catheter may predispose to other problems, namely, that of calculus formation due to chronic irritation of the bladder, increased shedding of mucosal debris—which then forms a nidus for calculus formation; also, stricture formation of the urethra is a very true risk. Furthermore, breakdown of the urethral mucosa, particularly at the penoscrotal junction, is seen not infrequently in paraplegic patients. This breakdown, then, rapidly will lead to a urethrocutaneous fistula.

Temporary catheter drainage may be necessary at times (for example, when a child is undergoing orthopedic surgery, long period of immobilization is expected, and urinary diversion has not been performed as yet). The catheters used should be of small caliber so as to avoid urethral irritation. The material should be medically as inert as possible. A high fluid intake should be maintained to dilute the urine. This will achieve two goals, namely, (1) the urinary hypotonicity presumably can interfere with bacterial reduplication, and, (2) the concentration of urinary solutes will be low, thus decreasing the possibility of sedimentation and stone formation. In addition, we like to add systemic acidification. For this, we use ascorbic acid, by mouth. The dosage is titrated by determining the urinary pH. Bacterial growth in acid urine is usually retarded. Also, precipitation of urinary solutes usually occurs in alkaline rather than acid urine.

Local measures in the care of catheters are extremely important: The meatus should be cleansed twice daily with a bactericidal solution, for which Betadine is an excellent choice as it will coat the area of the meatus *and* the catheter with a bactericidal film. Should the catheter need irrigation, this again should be done under stringent sterile precautions.

Catheters, when used, should be changed only when they fail their purpose, namely, adequate drainage of the urinary tract.

CONDOM DRAINAGE

A second approach which has been used is to render the patient incontinent with a large wide V plasty of the bladder neck, and to collect the draining urine in external catheters. In particular, this has been used by some centers with males because of the ease in fitting external catheters. These external condom catheters, commonly called Texas catheters, consist of a large draining tube which is fitted about the penis with a snugly adhering rubber condom. The disadvantage of this catheter, and that of other incontinence devices, is that part of the skin is constantly bathed in urine, leading to severe maceration and cellulitis, even with the best of skin care.

The external catheter may be adequate on a temporary basis, but as a permanent appliance we have found it to be extremely unsatisfactory.

UROLOGICAL SURGERY AND DIVERSIONS

Many research projects are directed toward improving urinary drainage through an intact urinary tract. Devices such as an implantable bladder pump (Hughes and Scott, unpublished data) or electrical stimulation (Boyce, Latham, and Hunt, 1964) of the detrusor and external sphincter are examples. But at present all urological surgical procedures are mutilating and require external collecting devices as the price for maintenance of renal function.

A number of operations designed to reduce outflow resistance have been employed in the past. These include Y-V plasty of the bladder neck (Emmett and Simon, 1956), transurethral resection of the bladder neck (Emmett and Simon, 1956), sphincterotomy (Ross, Gibbon, and Damanski, 1963), sacral rhizotomy (Hutch, 1957), and pudendal neurectomy (Ross and Damanski, 1953; Tasker, 1961). Attempts to increase the voiding pressure by reducing bladder capacity and simultaneously leaving the total muscle mass undiminished have not been very successful. Operations on the bladder neck as well as sphincterotomy have been reported to decrease outlet obstruction, but the results seem to be only temporary in many instances.

Pudendal neurectomy may be worthwhile in a small, select number of patients, in whom the manometric examinations show that the detrusor force cannot overcome the external urethral sphincter contraction. Such a patient would show marked straining to void, with hesitance and intermittency. Overflow incontinence, a large quantity of residual urine, bladder walls which are thick and trabeculated, and a hypertrophic bladder neck may be seen. Preoperative evaluation of such a patient must include a temporary pudendal nerve block. If the results indicate a significant improvement of the patient's voiding pattern, then we will proceed with a pudendal neurectomy. The pudendal nerve can be reached through a parasacral approach; we prefer to reach its branches at Alcock's canal where the median branch is identified. This is then resected, thus sparing sexual function and retaining control of the external anal sphincter. A transurethral resection of the hypertrophic bladder neck is sometimes performed (Emmett and Simon, 1956). In addition to significantly improving the patient's voiding pattern, a unilateral pudendal neurectomy should improve overflow incontinence by decreasing residual urine. Presacral and hypogastric neurotomy, pelvic neurotomy, and posterior sacral rhizotomy have been recommended but are not done at our institution (Engel and Schirmer, 1973).

Catheter diversion is only occasionally used. Catheters placed transurethrally, suprapubically, or through a nephrostomy have in common the complications of a foreign body in the urinary tract, including foreign body irritation of the mucosa, increasing risk of urinary tract infection, and the precipitation of supersaturated urinary solutes leading to encrustation and stone formation. Catheter diversion via the transurethral route also adds the risks of urethrocutaneous fistula formation (predominantly at the penoscrotal junction), urethritis, epididymitis, and prostatovesiculitis.

The tubeless cystostomy (Fig. 10-2) has the advantage of not utilizing

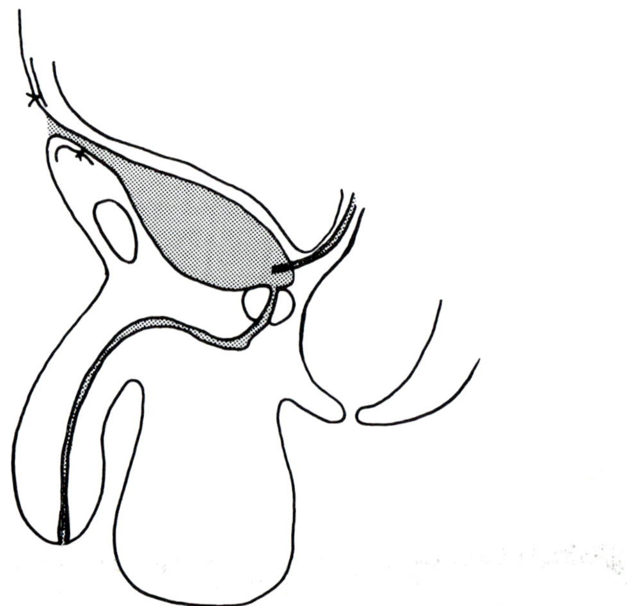

Fig. 10-2 Diagram of cutaneous vesicostomy. Urinary tract shaded.

a foreign body (Lapides, Koyanagi, and Diokno, 1971), but it is difficult to fit the patient with a tightly sealing appliance. The residual urine with this diversion can be considerable. We agree with Brady et al. (1971) in not recommending this procedure.

Ureterostomies can be done as a temporary diversion procedure or on a permanent basis. A temporary ureterostomy (loop cutaneous ureterostomy, Fig. 10-3) is useful only when there is reasonable assurance that the lower urinary tract will regain function. Thus its application in patients with meningomyeloceles is limited (Flinn et al., 1971; Eckstein, 1963). Temporary diversion, or loop cutaneous ureterostomy, is accomplished by bringing a loop of the dilated ureter to the skin, much as one would do in a double-barrel colostomy. The upper segment should be as short and as straight as possible to keep "urinary deadspace" to a minimum. We find *permanent* ureterostomy useful only in children with a dilated upper ureter and a non-functioning contralateral kidney. In our experience, normal-sized ureters have a tendency to scar-down at the cutaneous stoma; and in these patients, interposing an intestinal segment or an ileal loop is recommended.

ILEAL LOOP

The ileal loop is the preferred method of diversion in this clinic. It is a permanent procedure, provides an adequate stoma for fitting a faceplate, and can be done before there is gross enlargement of the ureters. The prime reasons for an ileal loop are preservation of the tract function and prevention of reflux and infection. However, the ileal loop is also performed to provide continence so that the child will be socially acceptable for entering school.

TECHNICAL ASPECTS

The ileal conduit was proposed by Bricker in 1950 and is shown in Fig. 10-4 (a, b, and c). A detailed description of the operation would be beyond the scope of this discussion, but a few important points of this diversion need emphasis. The ileal segment should be as short as possible, since its function is to be that of a conduit, not a reservoir. An intestinal reservoir of urine will lead to hyperchloremic acidosis. The site of the cutaneous stoma should be selected with care, preferably in conjunction with the orthopedic surgeon, because many patients will require various types of orthopedic braces with pelvic bands which may interfere with stoma function. In addition, a child who will be sitting and leaning forward may need a higher stoma than a more ambulatory patient. Thus the lower quadrant is not necessarily the best location.

The faceplate of the external appliance has to be measured with care and adjusted to the patient's individual stoma so as to expose only a minimum of the skin surrounding the stoma to the continuous urinary bathing, since this predisposes to acanthosis and keratosis, which frequently lead to stenosis of the cutaneous stoma.

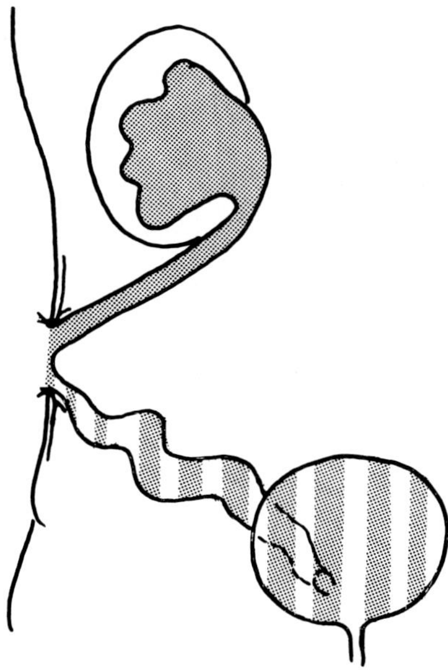

Fig. 10-3 Diagram of cutaneous loop ureterostomy. Urinary tract shaded; striped segment temporarily excluded from flow.

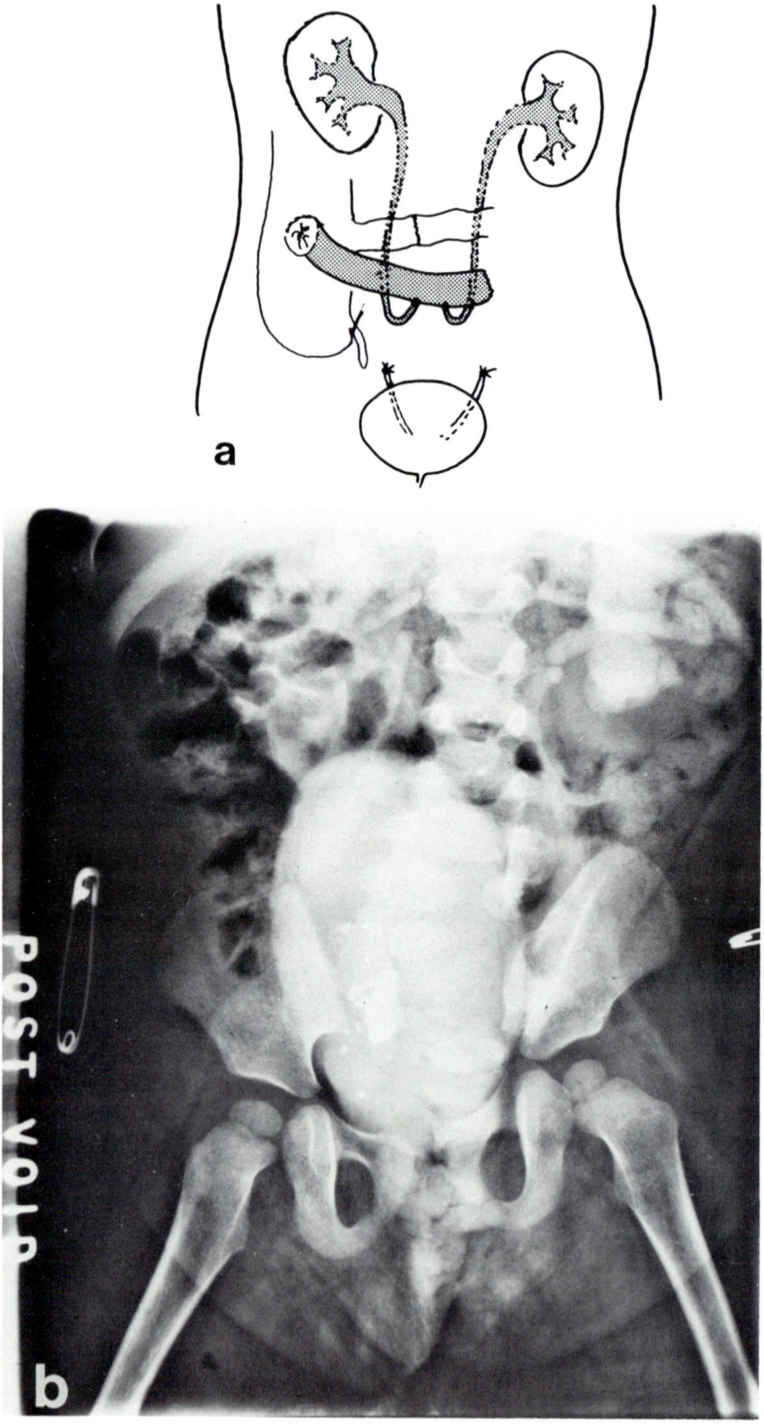

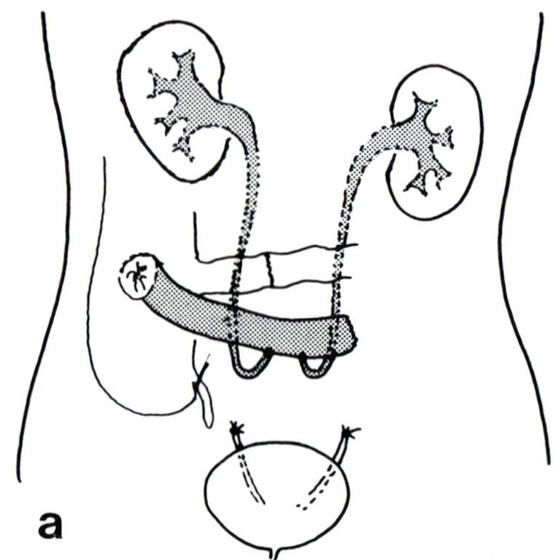
a

POST VOID
b

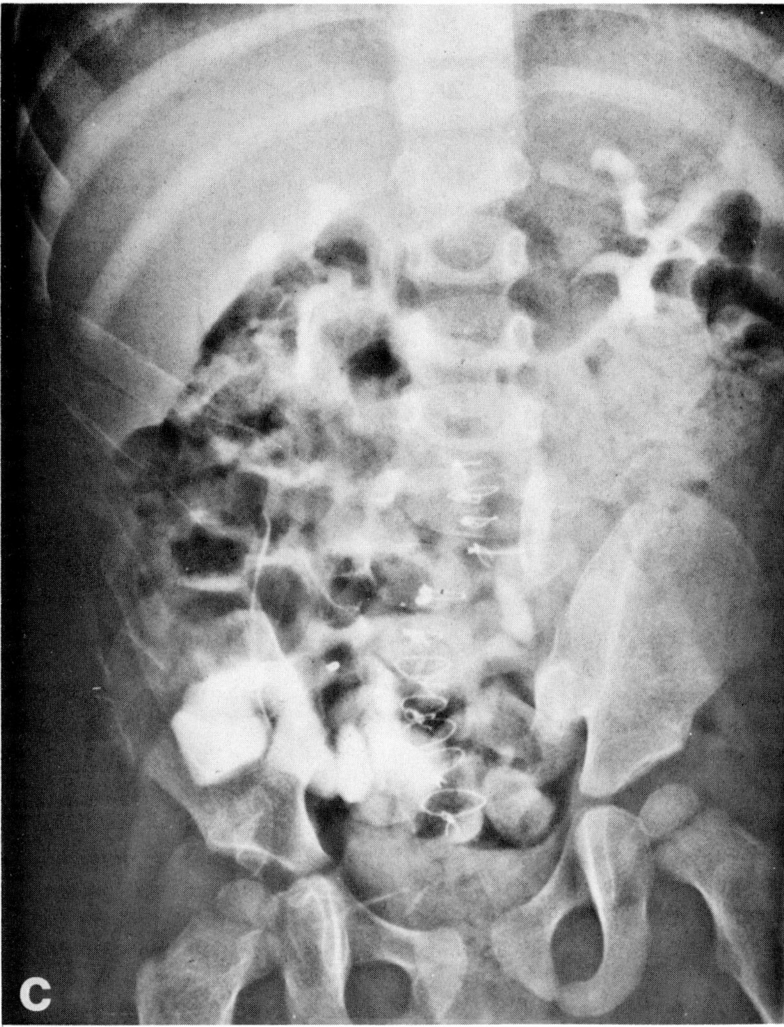

Fig. 10-4 (a) Diagram of bilateral uretero-ileo-cutaneous urinary diversion (ileal loop). Urinary tract shaded. Lower urinary tract defunctionalized or removed. (b) Eighteen-month-old patient with a meningomyelocele. Post-void film of double-dose IVP. Note bilateral hydroureteronephrosis. (c) Postoperative IVP of same patient two months after uretero-ileal urinary diversion. Note marked improvement in radiographic appearance of upper tracts.

We place special emphasis on proper bowel preparation prior to surgery. Patients with meningomyeloceles often suffer from atony of the bowel, which leads to a large amount of fecal residuum within the colon and, not infrequently, also to stagnation in the small bowel. Preparation should include administration of a nonabsorbable sulfonamide and clear liquids for two days, followed by repeat enemas on the day prior to surgery until the return is clear.

INDICATIONS FOR AN ILEAL LOOP

The decision to perform an ileal conduit is arrived at by the team during the follow-up sessions on our patients. The indications for such extensive surgery must be weighed with care:

1. Urinary incontinence not only leads to social ostracism but in many states prevents these unfortunate children from entering the public school system. External collecting devices for the female are nonexistent and for the male, by and large, unsatisfactory.

2. An increase in residual urine with repeated urinary tract infections, reflux, and/or radiological deterioration of lower or upper urinary tract are among the prime indications to divert the urine. Azotemia is a rare occurrence in such patients, since we tend to divert their urine prior to such large loss of renal parenchyma. It should be stressed that the decision to perform an ileal loop is made only after consideration of each patient on an individual basis by the entire team.

AGE

The loop can be performed at any age, but is ideally performed between two and four years so that the child can adjust to the appliance before he begins school (see Chapter 11).

COMPLICATIONS

In reviewing our own experience (Engel, 1969) with over 200 patients, of whom more than 50 were children, we find that a total of 28.6% had postoperative complications. These complications included empyema of the bladder, calculus formation, stomal stenosis, peristomal herniation, and uretero-ilial stenosis. Calculus formation was found in 8.2% of our patient group and occurred only in patients who, preoperatively, either had significant urinary tract infection with colony counts of more than 100,000/cc and/or radiographic evidence of upper tract deterioration. The incidence of bladder empyema, 21.5% in our total patient group, was significantly higher (40%) in patients with urinary tract infections and who preoperatively had undergone multiple catheterizations and instrumentation of the lower tract. We therefore adopt a more aggressive policy and suggest diversion before the upper tracts deteriorate or repeated urinary tract infections become a threat.

Progressive hydronephrosis and renal attrition, however, *can* be seen following a supravesical urinary diversion. This is more frequent in patients who have markedly dilated ureters prior to diversion. Patients with badly diseased ureters do poorly with conventional uretero-ileo-cutaneous anastomosis (King and Scott, 1964). Patients with markedly dilated ureters fare better when the "deadspace" of the dilated ureter is excluded from the diversion and the ileal segment is anastomosed directly to the renal pelves, as shown in Fig. 10-5 (Holland et al., 1967). Hydronephrosis and renal attrition may also be attributed to reflux of urine through the widely open ureteral anatomoses.

Logan, Scott, and Laskowski (1965) report no deterioration of renal function and no deterioration of electrolyte balance in 26 children, and worsening of the excretory urogram in only one kidney, following diversion. Smith (1964) reports, in 16 patients, one child with radiographic worsening of the upper tracts and evidence of pyelonephritic scarring. Glenn, Small, and Boyarski (1968), in 30 children, report a 19% deterioration of renal units following diversion. Eckstein (1965), in 68 children, cites one child with pyelonephritis and one with subsequent hydronephrosis following diversion. The results of others (Bowles and Tall, 1967; Cordonnier, 1968; Grossman, Winchester, and Colston, 1968; Retik, Perlmutter, and Gross, 1967) are similar. The consensus is that such complications are less likely if diversion is performed prior to deterioration of the urinary tract. In the past, urologists have followed children over the first two years of life in the hope that myelination of the pyramidal tract would improve the neurological status of the bladder. Unfortunately, such waiting has frequently led to progressive deterioration of the renal status in these unfortunate children and thus worsened their prognosis. Evidence for improvement in function with myelination is lacking.

Recently, the ileotrigonal diversion, whereby the intact trigone is implanted into the ileal conduit (Fig. 10-6a through d) has been utilized in this institution (Pond and Texter, 1970). The reasoning is that prevention of reflux with an intact ureterovesical junction might prevent some of the renal

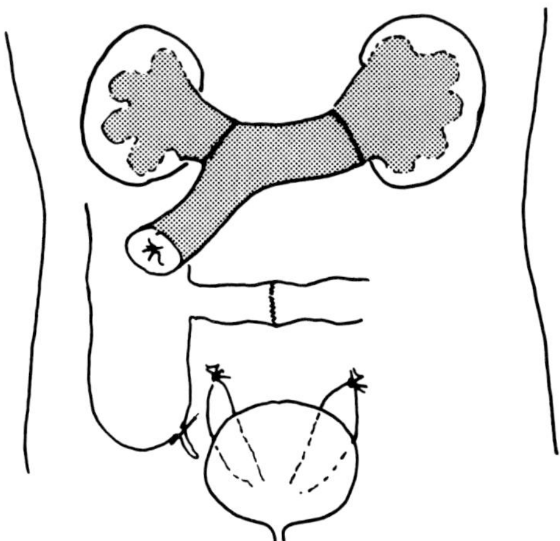

Fig. 10-5 Diagram of bilateral pyelo-ileo-cutaneous urinary diversion (high loop). Urinary tract shaded. Lower urinary tract defunctionalized or removed.

deterioration seen after urinary diversion with an ileal conduit. Though we are enthusiastic about our results, it is yet too early to draw any statistically significant conclusions. Following urinary diversion, and with the assurance of adequate urinary drainage, specific antibiotic therapy is administered to eradicate any urinary tract infection. This is followed by suppressive therapy and acidification of urine in children who are not azotemic.

Bishop, Smith, and Graley (1971) have shown that the stoma and the lumen of the conduit can be contaminated with growth of up to 10^3 organisms/ml. Heavy pyuria, where pus cells are clearly distinguished from epithelial cells, is felt to be a more reliable indicator of urinary tract infection in a urinary tract that is diverted by an ileal loop. We feel strongly that urinary tract infection and alkaline urine are among the factors that predispose to stomal stenosis. Jeter and Bloom (1971) were able to show that acidification of the urine in their patients with an ileal diversion reduced the need for surgical revision of stomal stenoses, from 31% in those with alkaline urine to 10% for those who were maintained on systemic acidification. Stomal stenosis, which has occurred in 22% of our children, is the most common postoperative complication; and we do forewarn the patient's parents that future surgery might be necessary.

After their urinary diversions, patients are re-evaluated at three- to six-month intervals for the first year, and thereafter on a yearly basis. Follow-up is more closely scheduled if the clinical condition warrants. These follow-up evaluations include, again, a quantitative urine culture, creatinine clearance, electrolytes, an excretory urogram, and a loop injection. At the

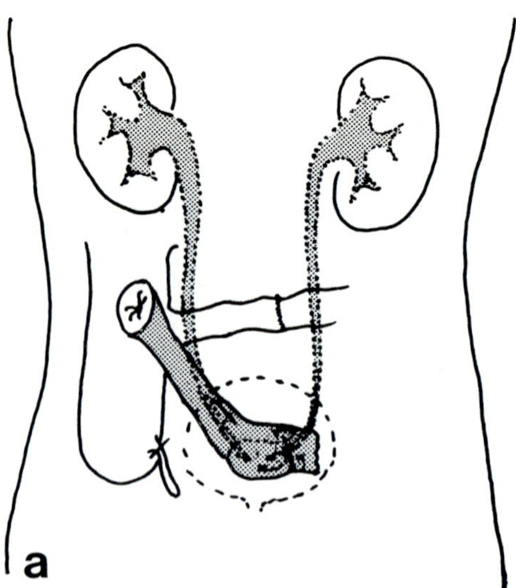

Fig. 10-6a Diagram of ileo-cutaneous urinary diversion. Bladder removed. Urinary tract shaded.

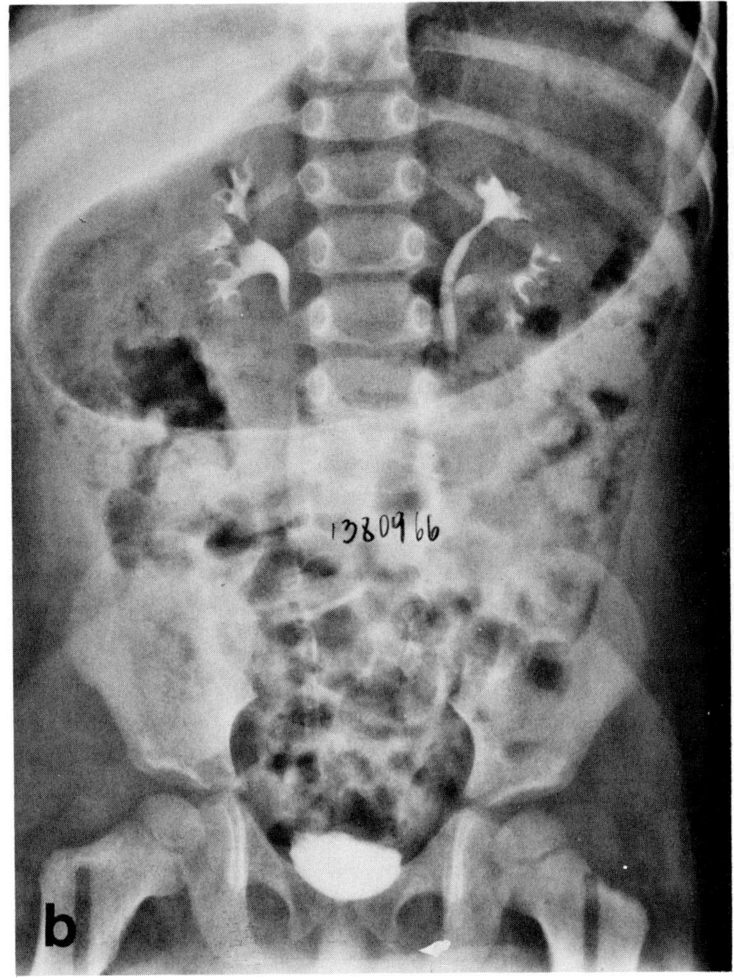

Fig. 10-6b Preoperative intravenous pyelogram (IVP) of two-year-old patient with a meningomyelocele. Partial reduplication of left upper tract.

same time the ileocutaneous stoma is calibrated and the loop checked for residual urine.

Sexual "adequacy" in patients with meningomyeloceles and neurogenic bladder lesions has not been studied sufficiently. A number of investigators (Comarr, 1965, 1971; Comarr, in press; Bors and Comarr, 1960; Zeitlin, Cottrell, and Lloyd, 1957) have dealt with the subject in patients with traumatic cord lesions, and it seems that patients with upper motor neuron lesion have reflexogenic erections but cannot ejaculate. Patients with incomplete upper motor neuron lesions may show ability to ejaculate (29%). Lower motor neuron lesion allows only psychogenic erections. Ejaculation

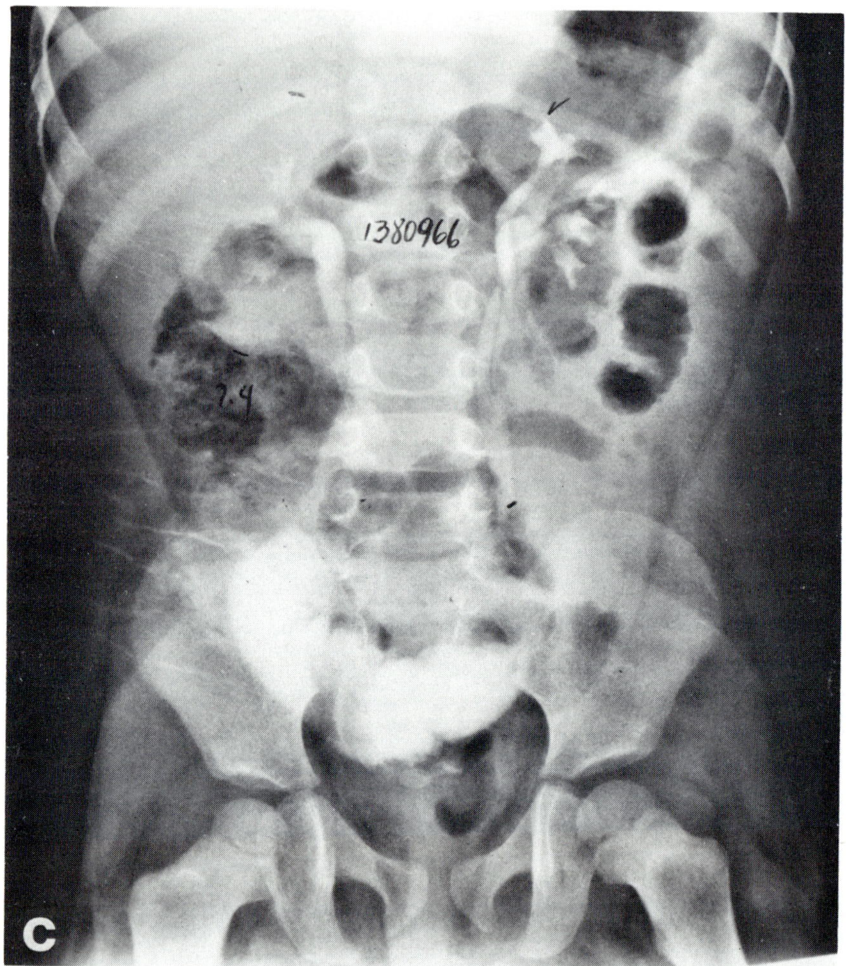

Fig. 10-6c IVP six months after ileo-trigonal urinary diversion.

is possible for 17% of patients with complete lower motor neuron lesions and in 60% of those with incomplete lesions (Comarr, 1971).

The main sexual problem encountered in the male child with a meningomyelocele is that of a virtual absence of sexual experience or training. In addition, the few patients that we have been able to follow past puberty failed to show any sperm in their thin and mucoid ejaculate.

Female patients have shown the ability to conceive and carry a pregnancy to full term without any urinary tract complications. Much investigation of the various aspects of these sexual problems, and guidance for patients, is needed.

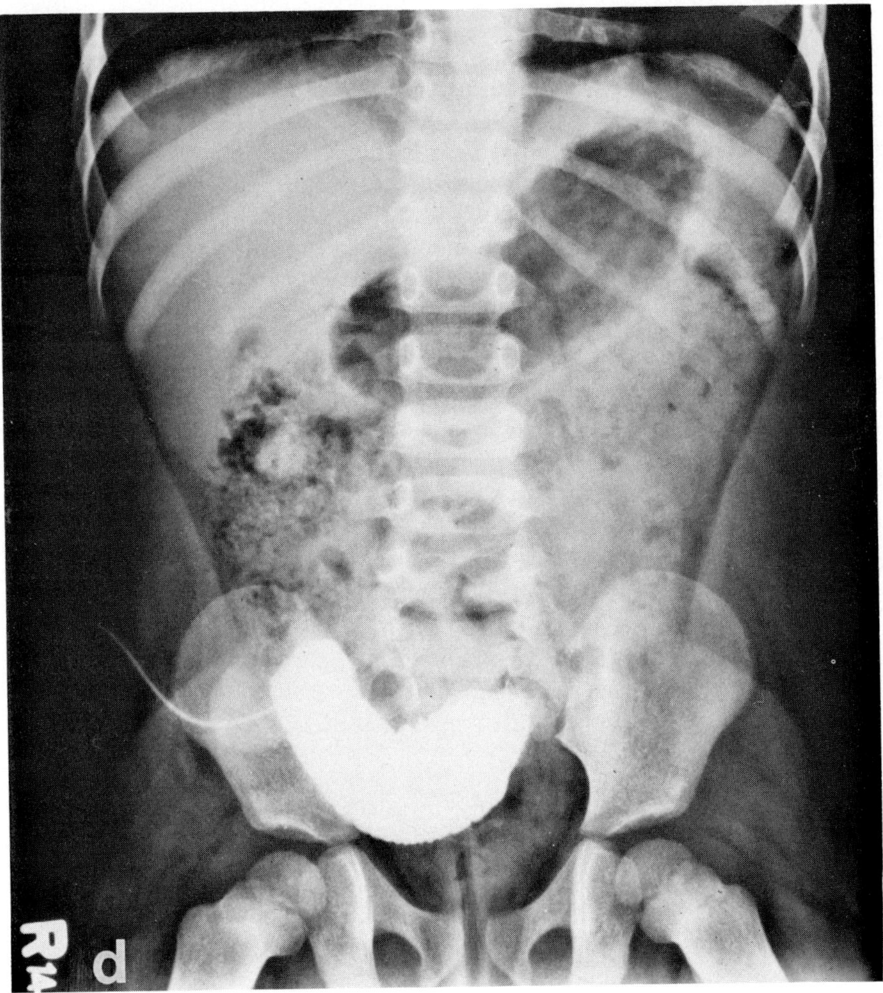

Fig. 10-6d Loop injection of same patient. Note absence of reflux.

SUMMARY

Children with meningomyeloceles have a complexity of problems, of which not the least is the threat of progressive deterioration of the upper urinary tract with ensuing azotemia and renal death. Close follow-up of these children from birth on, in a multi-specialty setting, is the optimal way of ensuring good care. The decision to perform a urinary diversion should be made by the entire team after consideration of the long-term outlook for the individual patient. Close follow-up is necessary to prevent and treat complications. Urinary diversion should be performed before the upper tracts deteriorate.

Since the initial writing of this chapter, several interesting publications have appeared in the literature. These deal with intermittent catheterization of the bladder in patients with neurogenic bladders. Patients who carry significant residuals are taught to catheterize their own bladders three to four times daily. Rabinovitch[1] reported his experience in a number of children with neurogenic bladder dysfunction, and Lapides[2] had similar results with intermittent catheterization in his patients. Sterile technique was *not* required, but rather what he describes as a "clean technique." This involves washing of the hands and the genitalia; no gloves are required; the catheter is cleansed by boiling but manipulated with nonsterile instruments and inserted after sufficient lubrication. The results in children with meningomyeloceles, in children with neurogenic bladder dysfunction, are promising: Fifty percent had excellent results, 35% were markedly improved, and in only 15% were the results discouraging (those were patients with small or spastic bladders). Of the entire patient group, half were free of urinary tract infection. However, longterm results and followup are needed to assess the survival and function of the upper tracts before we can definitely state whether intermittent nonsterile self-catheterization is superior to permanent supravesical urinary diversion.

(We have recently begun to train a few of our patients in this technique and are encouraged to continue. However, longterm results, as stated, are needed to assure us that renal function is at least as well maintained as in those patients who undergo urinary diversion.)

REFERENCES

Bishop, R. F., E. D. Smith, and M. Graley. 1971. Bacterial flora of urine from ileal conduit. J. Urol. 105:452.

Bors, E., and A. E. Comarr. 1960. Neurological disturbances of sexual function with special reference to 529 patients with spinal cord injury. Urol. Survey 10:191.

Bors, E., and A. E. Comarr. 1971. Neurological urology. University Park Press, Baltimore.

Bors, E., and R. W. Porter. 1970. Neurosurgical considerations in bladder dysfunction. Urol. Int. 25:114.

Bowles, W. T., and B. A. Tall. 1967. Urinary diversion in children. J. Urol. 98:597.

Boyce, W. H., J. E. Latham, and L. D. Hunt. 1964. Research related to the development of an artificial electrical stimulator for the paralysed human bladder. J. Urol. 91:41.

Brady, T. W., W. K. Mebust, W. L. Valk, J. D. Foret, and T. B. Sloss. 1971. Cutaneous vesicostomy reappraised. J. Urol. 105:81.

Comarr, A. E. 1965. Management of the traumatic cord bladder today. Urol. Int. 20:1.

---

[1]Rabinovitch, H.: Intermittent bladder catheterization in children with meningomyelocele. (In press, 1973).

[2]Lapides, J.: Self catheterization for urinary dysfunction. *Medical World News 14* (20), 1973.

Comarr, A. E. 1971. Sexual concepts in traumatic cord and cauda equina lesions. J. Urol. 106:375.

Comarr, A. E. In press. Sexual function among patients with spinal cord injury. Urol. Int.

Cordonnier, J. J. 1968. Ileal conduit in children. Urol. Int. 23:82.

Damanski, M., and A. Sutcliffe-Kerr. 1964. Paraplegia of non-traumatic origin and disseminated (multiple) sclerosis: urinary complications, their nature and treatment. Acta Neurol. Psychiat. Belg. 64:495.

Eckstein, H. B. 1963. Cutaneous ureterostomy. Proc. Roy. Soc. Med. 56:749.

Eckstein, H. B. 1965. Urinary diversion in children. Develop. Med. Child Neurol. 7:167.

Emmett, J. L., and H. B. Simon. 1956. Transurethral resection in infants and children for congenital obstruction of the vesical neck and myelodysplasia. J. Urol. 76:595.

Engel, R. M. 1969. Complications of bilateral uretero-ileo cutaneous urinary diversion: review of 208 cases. J. Urol. 101:508.

Engel, R. M. E., and H. K. A. Schirmer. In press. Pudendal neurectomy in selected patients with neurogenic bladder dysfunction. J. Urol.

Flinn, R. A., L. R. King, J. H. McDonald, and S. S. Clark. 1971. Cutaneous ureterostomy: alternative urinary diversion. J. Urol. 105:358.

Glenn, J. F., M. P. Small, and S. Boyarski. 1968. Complications of ileal segment urinary diversion in children. Urol. Int. 23:97.

Grossman, H., P. H. Winchester, and W. C. Colston. 1968. Neurogenic bladder in childhood. Radiol. Clin. No. Amer. 6(2):155.

Holland, J. M., L. R. King, H. K. A. Schirmer, and W. W. Scott. 1967. High urinary diversion with an ileal conduit in children. Pediatrics 40(5):816.

Hutch, J. A. 1957. Treatment of hydronephrosis by sacral rhizotomy in paraplegics. J. Urol. 77:123.

Jeter, K., and S. Bloom. 1971. Management of stomal complications following ileal or colonic operations in children. J. Urol. 106:425.

King, L. R., and W. W. Scott. 1964. Pyeloileocutaneous anastomosis. Surg. Gynec. Obstet. 119:281.

Lapides, J., T. Koyanagi, and A. Diokno. 1971. Cutaneous vesicostomy: 10-year survey. J. Urol. 105:76.

Logan, C. W., R. Scott, Jr., and T. Z. Laskowski. 1965. Ileal loop diversion: evaluation of late results in children. J. Urol. 94:544.

Lyons, R. P., S. Marshall, and E. A. Tanagho. 1970. The ureteral orifice: its configuration and competency. J. Urol. 102:504.

Pond, H. S., and J. H. Texter. 1970. Trigonal-ileal anastomasis: experimental studies. J. Urol. 103:746.

Retik, A. B., A. D. Perlmutter, and R. E. Gross. 1967. Cutaneous uretero-ileostomy in children. New Eng. J. Med. 277:217.

Ridlon, H. C. 1971. Urological management of child with meningomyelocele. Unpublished paper presented at Section on Urology, American Academy of Pediatrics, Oct. 16-21, Chicago.

Ross, J. C., and M. Damanski. 1953. Pudendal neurectomy in the treatment of the bladder in spinal injury. Brit. J. Urol. 25:45.

Ross, J. C., N. O. K. Gibbon, and M. Damanski. 1963. Further experiences with division of the external urethral sphincter in the paraplegic. J. Urol. 89:692.

Smith, E. D. 1964. Ileo-cutaneous ureterostomy in children. Austral. New Zeal. J. Surg. 33:169.

Tasker, J. H. 1961. Pudendal neurectomy. Brit. J. Urol. 33:397.

Zeitlin, A. B., T. L. Cottrell, and F. A. Lloyd. 1957. Sexology of the paraplegic male. Fertil. Steril. 8:337.

11

Care of the Child with an Ileal Loop

Charlotte Blackmon, E.T.
Johanna R. Bengel, E.T.
Marvin M. Schuster, M.D.

CARE OF THE CHILD AND FAMILY

The majority of children with meningomyeloceles require urinary diversion to prevent renal deterioration as well as to provide continence so that the child can attend school and function in society. The loop is usually created between the ages of two and four years so that the child and the family can become adjusted to its care prior to school.

The time of loop surgery is a period of emotional crisis for the family, and at times for the child as well. While the child has usually already had a number of operations, these have all been corrective surgery. Surgery to repair the back, relieve the hydrocephalus, and correct orthopedic deformity are all performed to make the child "more normal." The loop represents the first major surgery in which the child is made less normal. It reawakens the realization that the child will never be like other children. Thus creation of the ileal loop represents a major crisis which the parents often face with considerable reluctance.

A child's adjustment to any urinary diversion depends on the understanding and attitude of the family. The family's attitude in turn depends on that of the health team, who must share the responsibility of caring for and dealing with problems that develop. Members of the family should be given an opportunity to express their feelings and concerns and to reveal their misconceptions, and should be given correct, factual information.

Whenever possible, they should receive reassurance and advice. Above all, the parents must be prepared psychologically to make adjustments, enabling them to relate to the child without feelings of guilt or anxiety.

Initial instructions should be kept as simple and straightforward as possible. Frequent repetition is necessary, since both the patient and the family are often upset and preoccupied, with the result that their attention span is diminished. Many questions concerning daily routines such as bathing, playing, and school activities are to be anticipated, but often behind these routine questions there is an urgent plea for reassurance. It is advisable during the early sessions to provide parent and child with literature that will bring further understanding and raise additional questions that can be handled in subsequent visits.

It cannot be too strongly emphasized that each child is an individual with specific attitudes and sometimes with physical, emotional, or mental limitations that must be fully understood and carefully managed. In all instances, problems are much more easily prevented than corrected.

CARE OF THE LOOP

SKIN AND STOMAL CARE

Placement and physical characteristics of the stoma. The selection of the appropriate site for the stoma is crucial to good postoperative management. The stoma should be placed in an area that is free of scars, depressions, creases, and bony protuberances. Since the body contour changes in different positions, measurements must be made in three cardinal positions: recumbent, sitting, and standing. If the child wears braces, the braces should remain on while measurements are taken.

A protruding stoma (Fig. 11-1) is always preferable to one which is flush or retracted into the abdominal wall, since leakage can be more easily prevented when the stoma protrudes slightly into the faceplate of the appliance. Some patients find that they derive some degree of reassurance, as well as helpful hints about placement, if they wear an appliance filled one-third full of water (simulating urine) for several days prior to surgery. This also permits them to adjust to the feel of the appliance on their body.

It is advisable routinely to test an area of skin distant from the stoma with the adhesive that will be used for the applicance. This is especially important when there is a history of allergy. If skin breakdown does occur as a result of allergy, a different form of adhesive can be selected without having risked the difficulty of applying the faceplate over excoriated skin in the peristomal area.

MECHANICS OF THE APPLIANCE

The temporary appliance—postoperative pouch. Immediately after the operation a transparent pouch with a karaya-gum seal is applied to the stomal site. The transplant material readily allows inspection of the stoma

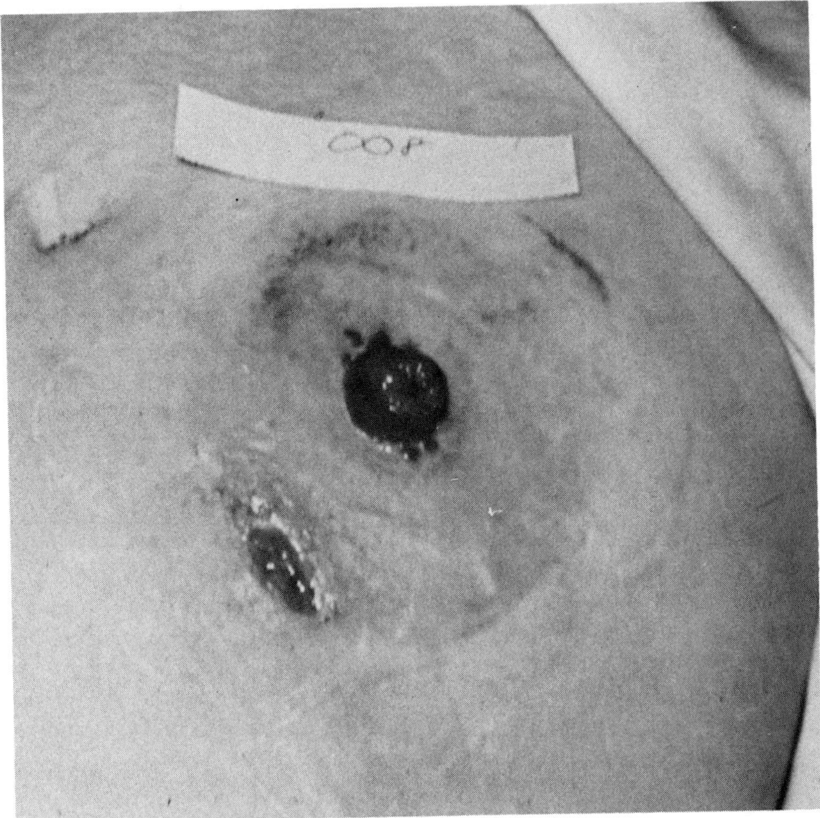

Fig. 11-1 Stoma and ulcer secondary to belt pressure. Stoma is properly fashioned and protrudes appropriately. Skin ulcer (upper margin of faceplate outline) resulted from belt pressure.

by the surgeon. Since the patient will be on bedrest immediately after surgery, this pouch should be placed transversely on his body to allow free drainage without twisting of the appliance. This bag is connected to a straight drainage bag, and the output is measured at frequent intervals.

Replacement of this temporary appliance is necessary as soon as leakage occurs.

The hematuria observed during the first few postoperative days is transient and should not cause any concern.

The permanent appliance. By approximately seven to ten days after surgery, the stoma will have attained a fairly stable size and the patient can be measured for a permanent appliance.

HOW TO MEASURE: The opening in the faceplate (mounting ring) should measure no more than 1/16 of an inch larger than the stoma. Accurate measurement can best be accomplished by using a stoma measuring gauge with openings in graduated sizes. This will ensure a good fit and will decrease leakage and skin breakdown.

SELECTION OF A FACEPLATE: The selection of the proper size of faceplate is of the utmost importance in order for the child to be comfortable and dry. The "infant flat" faceplate is designed especially for babies and small-framed children, and the "pediatric all soft flexible" faceplate for the older child or teenager. The soft faceplate conforms to the contour of the body and allows for a wide range of movement and activity.

EQUIPMENT SHOULD CONSIST OF:

Two faceplates (one on the body and one as a spare—the collection pouch attaches to the faceplate)

Clear plastic urinary pouches (infant and pediatric sizes)

O-Ring seals (to hold pouch onto faceplate)

Adhesive tape discs (double faced—for making faceplate adhere to body)

Stoma guide strips (for centering and guiding faceplate over stoma)

Drainage fittings (screw-type valve in bottom of pouch for emptying)

Night drain kit (used at bedtime in conjunction with the pouch for the child who sleeps through the night)

Solvent (for removing adhesive and for cleaning peristomal skin and the faceplate)

Child's size belts

One-inch Micropore 3M tape (used in strips around the faceplate for a more waterproof seal)

HOW TO APPLY TO BODY:

1. Lay assembled appliance (consisting of faceplate, pouch, and drainage fitting) on flat surface with faceplate side up.

2. Remove backing from one side of the adhesive tape disc and center over opening in faceplate. If cement is used, it must be applied in thin coats and allowed to dry for three to four minutes.

3. Remove backing from remaining side of tape disc.

4. Roll a stoma guide strip on finger and place in opening of faceplate (Fig. 11-2a and b).

5. Clean peristomal skin with solvent or soap and water. Rinse skin with plain water and pat skin dry.

6. Take applicance in both hands on edges of faceplate by the belt hooks, and direct the guide strip over the stoma. Push faceplate against body and press around outer edges. It is essential to apply the faceplate well centered over the stoma to avoid skin irritation or trauma to the stoma. The strip will dissolve in the pouch.

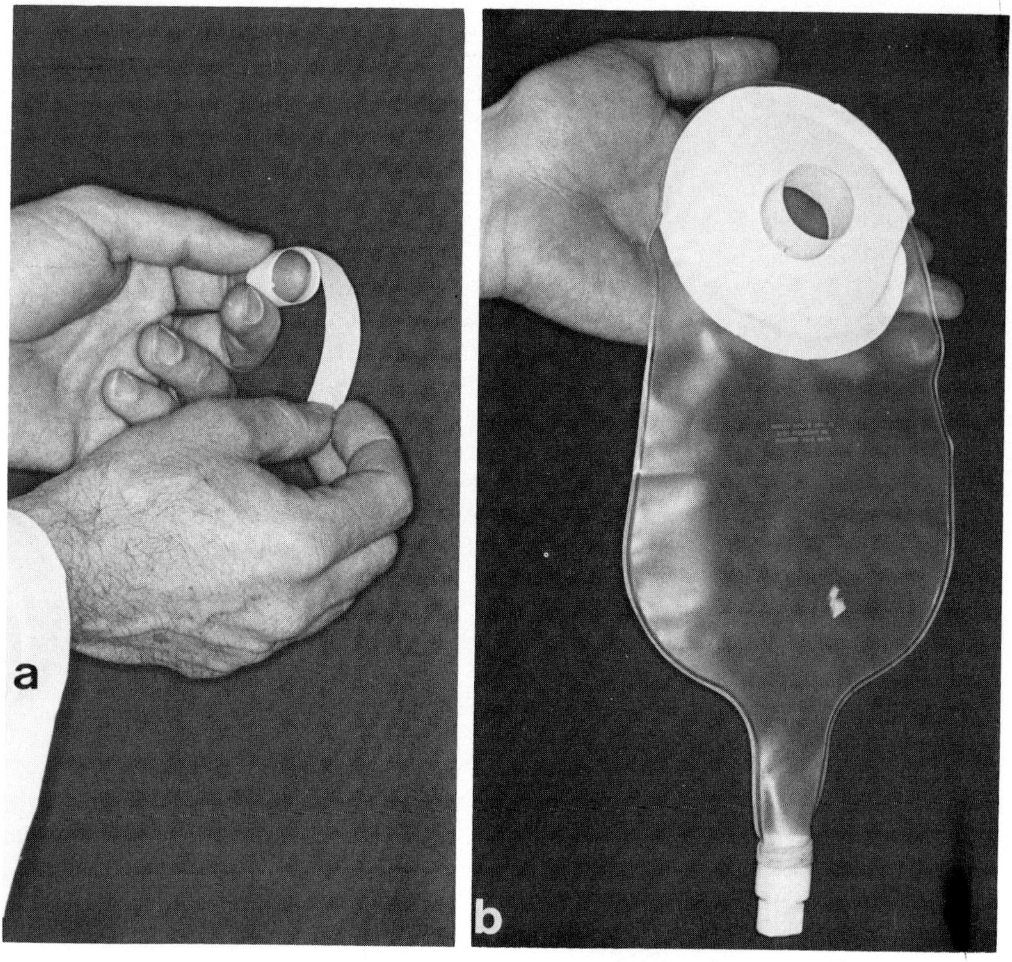

Fig. 11-2 Use a stoma guide strip to center faceplate over stoma (see text). (a) Roll a stoma guide strip on finger. (b) Place in opening of faceplate.

7. Attach belt and reinforce by placing strips of the one-inch Micropore tape around the faceplate.

GENERAL GUIDELINES: A bath or shower is permissible with or without the appliance on. The belt can be removed during this time—reinforce the faceplate with the Micropore tape. Rubber belts, used for swimming and bathing, are available from most companies that handle ostomy supplies.

The appliance may be left on for a week unless leakage occurs, and then it should be changed to prevent skin breakdown. For the patient who changes on a regular basis, the best time is first thing in the morning, before much liquid is ingested and while the urine output is slow.

For overnight care attach a night drainage kit. The urine then empties into the larger container and the pouch does not fill up and cause leakage. During the day, it is wise to empty the pouch every three to four hours depending on the amount of intake and the output of the individual. The pouch should never be allowed to get more than half full.

REMOVING THE APPLIANCE: Before removing the appliance it is best to have the spare one assembled and prepared; this will make for a faster change.

It is best to use solvent to remove the appliance in order to prevent peeling or injury to the underlying skin. The easiest method is to have a medicine dropper filled with solvent and allow it to drip between the skin and the adhesive backing of the pouch while gently pulling off in a downward direction. Cotton balls soaked in solvent can be used instead of the medicine dropper to drop the solvent. Wash the peristomal area with soap and water, rinse with plain water, and pat the skin dry.

CLEANING THE APPLIANCE: Good cleaning of the appliance is essential to dispel odor. The appliance should be cleaned after each change. Soak the appliance for 15 minutes in a basin or sink to which detergent (Lux, Vel, Ivory) has been added. Rinse with clear water and hang to dry. Should salt crystals form on the inside of the faceplate and pouch, soak in full-strength vinegar and scrub with a baby-bottle brush. The night drainage kit should be cleaned in the same manner.

NOTES: A fresh pouch should be put on the faceplate approximately every 14 days so that salt crystals do not accumulate inside the pouch and rub against the stoma, producing a sandpaper effect, and cause the stoma to bleed. Appearance of a few drops of blood is not unusual during the cleansing process, particularly if the patient has used dry material, such as Kleenex or gauze, which sticks to the stomal mucosa. To avoid bleeding, only moistened material should be used.

SKIN AND STOMAL PROBLEMS

Stomal stenosis and acanthosis. Stomal stenosis and acanthosis are caused in part by too large an opening in the faceplate, so that urine "sloshes" against the exposed skin. Crystals may be deposited if the urine is alkaline. Bleeding may occur. Infected urine may then cause skin irritation, inflammation, and granulation with resultant scarring. The involved skin develops a grayish, cobblestone appearance. This irregular surface leads to poor fitting of the faceplate and leakage, which compounds the problem. Not infrequently, surgical revision is necessary. In milder cases, conservative management may suffice (Jeter and Bloom, 1971).

TREATMENT:

1. Remeasure stoma and fit with proper size opening (1/16 inch larger than the stoma). When the faceplate is applied to the body with the new opening, the patient may complain of some tenderness, which will subside in a couple of hours. Change the appliance at normal intervals.

2. Acidification of urinary tract: administer 0.5–1 gm of ascorbic acid four times daily; titrate urinary pH for proper dose.
3. Force fluids to make urine more dilute.
4. Into the appliance:
   a. Add acetic acid, one part white vinegar to eight parts of water, prior to bedtime.
   b. One 5-grain aspirin tablet ground up and added through the bottom spout will lower the urinary pH for two hours and eliminate the strong odor that accompanies alkaline urine.
5. Treat urinary tract infection if necessary.

Small ulcers or cuts around stomal site. These often result from belt pressure due to wearing the belt too tight. This pressure causes friction under the faceplate, which results in skin cuts or ulcers (Fig. 11-1). It may also cause the faceplate to slip and cut into the stoma. Since the belt tends to make the appliance ride up under the stoma, the lacerations on the undersurface of the stoma may go unnoticed for some time.

TREATMENT: Place a small bit of gauze on the cut or ulcer and apply the permanent appliance in the usual manner. Change in 24 hours. Shower or bathe and pat the skin dry, then reapply the gauze and the appliance. Change in 48 hours. Repeat this procedure, increasing the wearing time of the appliance by one day each time until the cut or ulcer heals.

If the ulcer is large enough, it may require cauterization and the application of a Bandaid. A temporary (postoperative) pouch may be worn until the cut or ulcer heals. If the stoma itself is cut, discontinue use of the permanent appliance and substitute the temporary pouch until the ulcer heals. Belts should never be worn tightly enough to leave an impression on the skin.

Red "spotty" rash around stomal area: Such a rash is usually due to leakage of urine with resultant skin irritation, and often with secondary fungal overgrowth. The best prophylaxis is a properly fitted appliance over an appropriately constructed stoma. The opening in the faceplate must be the correct size.

TREATMENT:

1. Take a shower or bath with the appliance off; pat the skin dry. Do *not* rub the skin.
2. Spray the skin with Kenalog spray (corticosteroid) lightly and wipe off any excess.
3. Dust the skin lightly with Mycostatin topical powder (antifungal antibiotic) and wipe off any excess.
4. Apply the permanent appliance in the usual manner. The Kenalog spray and Mycostatin powder are not greasy and will not interfere with the adherence of the appliance to the body. Change in 24 hours and repeat the above regime. As the skin heals, leave the appliance on one day longer each time it is changed. Shower or bathe after each change.

Solid red ring around stoma where faceplate contacts skin: This often represents an allergic reaction to the preparation used to make the appliance adhere, such as cement, tincture of benzoin compound, or, in rare instances, adhesive tape discs. Secondary fungal overgrowth is not uncommon. Allergy can be documented by patch testing at a distant site with suspected material. A positive test will manifest itself within 24 hours. The adhesive tape discs by Marlen Manufacturing Company and Relia Seal by Davol, Inc., appear to be the least irritating to the skin and the most effective as adhesives.

TREATMENT: Use Kenalog spray and Mycostatin topical powder as previously described. Place a large karaya-gum washer (unless there is an indication of sensitivity to the karaya) around the stoma, and then place the permanent appliance over this without any adhesive on the faceplate. Change in 24 hours. Shower or bathe and pat the skin dry. Repeat this regime until the skin has healed sufficiently for the appliance to be attached in the usual manner.

Stomal allergy to pouch material: If the stoma bleeds and is reddened and no other cause is apparent, test for allergy to the pouch material.

TREATMENT: Remove the pouch and apply a temporary pouch. Wait 24 hours. If bleeding stops, then allergy to the pouch material is indicated. Change to a pouch of a different material (e.g., from vinyl to rubber, or vice versa).

FOLLOW-UP CARE

Good follow-up care is essential for the child with an ileal loop. Since alterations in the size of the stoma may continue over prolonged periods, the stoma should be remeasured six weeks after surgery, three months after, and yearly thereafter. Any change in the color, size, or shape of the stoma should be reported to the surgeon, for these signs may indicate problems that require surgical correction.

GENERAL REMARKS

Some children with an ileal loop can attend regular public schools without undue difficulty, whereas others need special education because of their mental or orthopedic handicap. In either case it is usually desirable for the parents of a child with an ileal loop to explain to the school officials the nature of the child's condition and the necessity for frequent use of bathroom facilities to prevent overfilling of the pouch and consequent leakage.

The child should be encouraged to do whatever he is physically capable of doing. With the exception of bodily contact sports, the ileal loop itself is not a hindrance to play or sport activities. Emptying the pouch prior to strenuous activities may help ensure safe adherence of the pouch.

As long as the clothes are not so tight that they interfere with drainage of urine into the pouch, any style of clothing is acceptable. The appliance may be made less noticeable if the bottom of the pouch is turned up and tucked into snug underpants. Teenage girls may wear girdles so long as they are made of stretch material such as Spandex or Lycra.

To permit the smaller child to wear short pants in the summer without the spout of the pouch showing below the edge of the pants, many mothers make pockets on the inside of the pants and then tuck the pouch into the pocket. This procedure also works well with a bathing suit. It also prevents the pouch from lying directly on the leg, causing the child to sweat and develop heat rash.

A plastic bottle carried in the car will help prevent the need for frequent stops to empty the pouch. It is also wise for the child to carry extra supplies when traveling, since the type of equipment needed may not be available in some areas.

It is most helpful to have a list of "Ostomy Associations" (which are worldwide) available in case of lost supplies or need for a physician familiar with ileal loop patients. This list may be obtained from a local ostomy group.

CONCLUSION

The most perfectly constructed stoma is still vulnerable if not appropriately managed. Proper management includes:

1. Psychological preparation of the patient and family.
2. Accurate measurement and fitting of the appliance.
3. Instruction in the use of the appliance.
4. Continued follow-up care by the health team.

With this comprehensive approach, most stomal, skin, and adjustment problems can be avoided. Gibney (1970) provides an excellent guide for the parents of children who will be having conduit surgery.

REFERENCES

Gibney, H. 1970. Your child and ileal conduit surgery; a guidebook for parents. Charles C Thomas, Springfield, Ill.

Jeter, K., and S. Bloom. 1971. Management of stomal complications following ileal or colonic conduit operations in children. J. Urol. 106:425.

12

The Management of Neurological Fecal Incontinence*

John J. White, M.D.
Issam Shaker, M.D.†

Fecal incontinence is a frequent manifestation of the neurological deficit that may accompany a meningomyelocele. During the child's early years emphasis is placed on the management of the neurosurgical problems, corrective orthopedic procedures, and urological care. Fecal incontinence usually is not of overwhelming medical consequence, and manifests itself mainly as a social problem. All too frequently, fecal incontinence is tolerated or ignored until it becomes a pressing social problem at or just prior to entering school. Then, without adequate time for a trial and assessment of a training regimen, a permanent colostomy is frequently elected as the "last" and only resort to achieve social respectability.

Presented with the opportunity to follow many children with neurological fecal incontinence from early infancy in the multidiscipline Birth Defects Center at The Johns Hopkins Hospital, we have studied the pathophysiology of their incontinence, and have established a physiological approach for the provision of acceptable bowel control. With this approach, we have been able to avoid colostomy and help our patients achieve satisfactory bowel continence.

Ano-rectal manometry, a technique which assesses the state of physiological reactivity of the anal sphincters to rectal distension, coupled with

---

*Supported by the Surgery Graduate Research Training Program, Vanderbilt University School of Medicine, NIH, 5 to 1 GM 01742-05.

†Supported in part by Clinical Research Unit Grant 5-M01-RR-00052.

the clinical presentation and radiological findings, has provided a dynamic understanding of the neurological fecal incontinence in these children. Data from the children with neurogenic incontinence and from a concomitant study of normal children and children with constipation of a functional nature or due to Hirschsprung's Disease has increased our knowledge of normal defecation and continence, and of the role of the ano-rectal sphincters. With this improved understanding, we have satisfactorily utilized a daily clean-out regimen for children with neurological incontinence, one which takes advantage of their residual functioning sphincter mechanism and permits virtually complete continence.

ANATOMY OF THE ANO-RECTUM AND SPHINCTERS

Despite its ready accessibility and the frequency of operations on the ano-rectum, the anatomical relationships of this area are still matters of controversy.

The ano-rectum is the terminal part of the intestinal canal, extending proximally about 6 cm from the anal verge in the adult. This area can be considered as a unit insofar as it is the region of the ano-rectal sphincters and has been called the "surgical anal canal." The lining of the upper third of the ano-rectum is intestinal mucosa typical of the rectum; it ends at the pectinate (dentate) line. The lining of the distal two-thirds is ano-derm, or modified squamous epithelium; this terminal 4 cm comprises the "anatomical anal canal."

The measurements cited, however, must be modified for infants and children. Shapiro (1948) has recognized three periods of developmental anatomy. In the newborn (first three months of life), the ano-rectum is about 3.5 cm in length; in infancy (three months to three years of life), it is about 4.5 cm; thereafter, from childhood to adult life the growth rate is relatively slow, reaching an average of 6 cm. In the newborn, the ano-rectum is mostly below the coccyx; growth and development produce the pelvic and abdominal location in the adult.

The circular smooth-muscle coat of the rectum continues distally in the wall of the ano-rectum to about 1 cm from the anal verge (Fig. 12-1). Its ending is a palpable but not usually visible landmark, and comprises Hilton's line (Stonesifer, Murphy, and Lombardo, 1960). This groove represents the intersphincteric line between the internal sphincter and the superficial, corrugator bands of the external sphincter. The *internal ano-rectal sphincter* is the most terminal portion of the circular smooth muscle of the rectum and would probably be more suitably termed the "intrinsic" ano-rectal sphincter. It varies from 2 to 3 cm in length, is composed of circularly and obliquely oriented bundles of smooth muscle, and is about 1 mm thicker than the circular muscle layer of the rectum proximally (Stonesifer et al., 1960). There is an apparent reduction in the number of ganglion cells in this area, the level of the last ganglion cells varying from 6 mm to 25 mm proximal to the terminal portion of the internal sphincter (Leutenegger, 1969). This sphincter contracts in vitro to adrenergic agents (Friedmann, 1968; Bass, Ustach, and Schuster, 1970).

The longitudinal smooth-muscle coat of the rectum parallels the circular coat, and terminates in multiple septa which divide the outermost portions of the external sphincter into a number of circular bundles of muscle fibers. Whether this longitudinal intermuscular septum is purely smooth muscle or connective tissue is debated. Some dissections have demonstrated only smooth-muscle fibers which attenuate at the skin and do not become continuous with the striated muscle of the external sphincter (Stonesifer et al., 1960). Courtney (1950) and Gorsch (1960), on the other hand, noted extensions from the levator ani muscles, and from the corrugator cutis ani muscle.

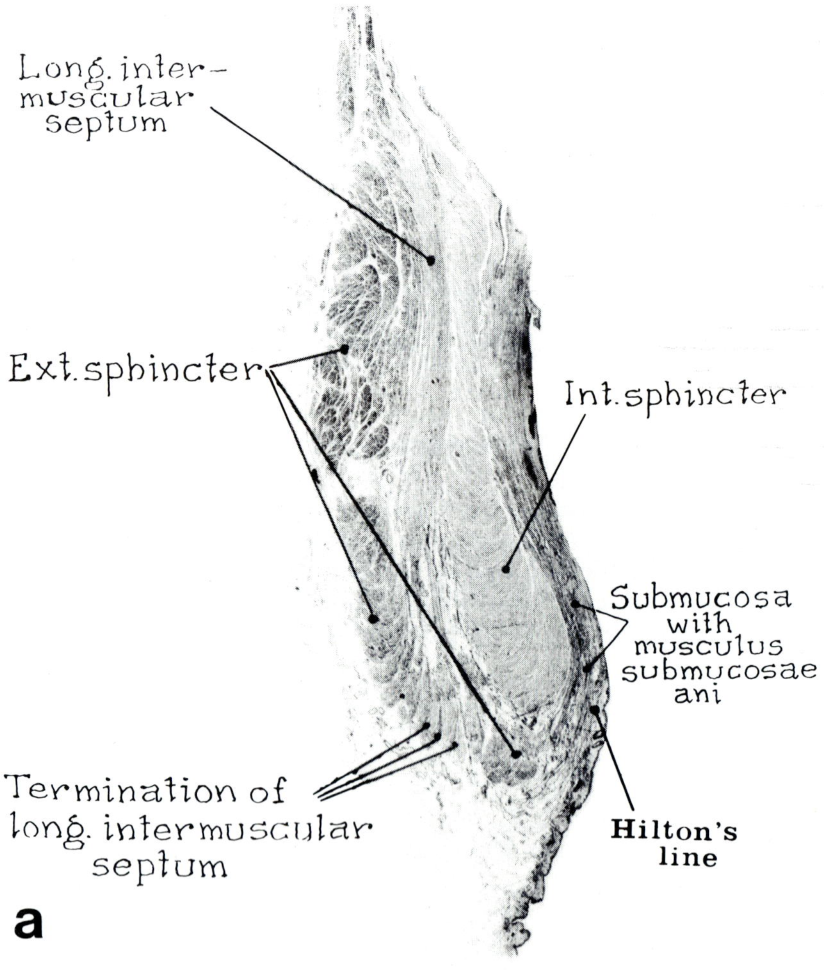

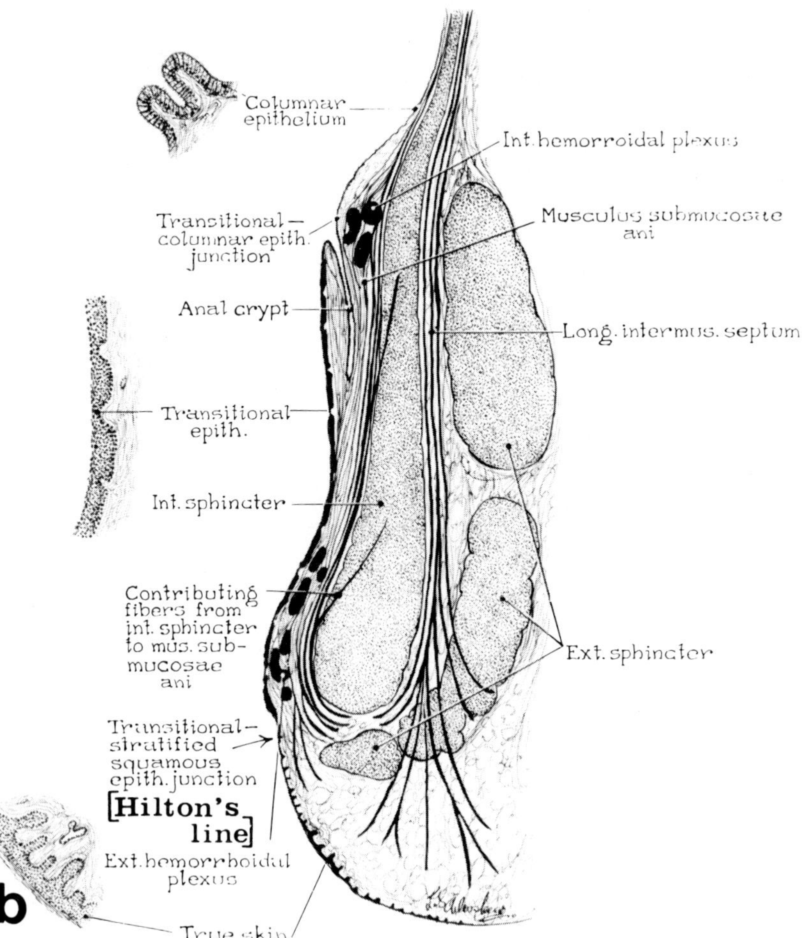

Fig. 12-1 Microscopic anatomy of the ano-rectal sphincters. (a) Photomicrograph of dissection specimen. (b) Artist's rendering of the same dissection. Note the distal termination of the smooth muscle internal sphincter at Hilton's line, about 1 cm from the anal verge. The longitudinal intermuscular septum separates the bowel from the striated-muscle deep external sphincters. The subcutaneous external sphincters lie within the septum. The outer bundles of the external sphincter encircle the ano-rectum and are constrictor in action. The deep bundles of the external sphincter are actually the puborectalis sling of the levator ani muscles, and exert a pinchcock action posteriorly. (From Stonesifer, Murphy, and Lombardo (1960) with permission.)

The *external ano-rectal sphincter* is composed of a conglomerate of striated, voluntary muscles of the pelvis, and would more suitably be considered as the extrinsic ano-rectal sphincter (Fig. 12-2). It has classically been divided into three separate portions: the subcutaneous or corrugator cutis ani muscle; the superficial portion which circles around the ano-

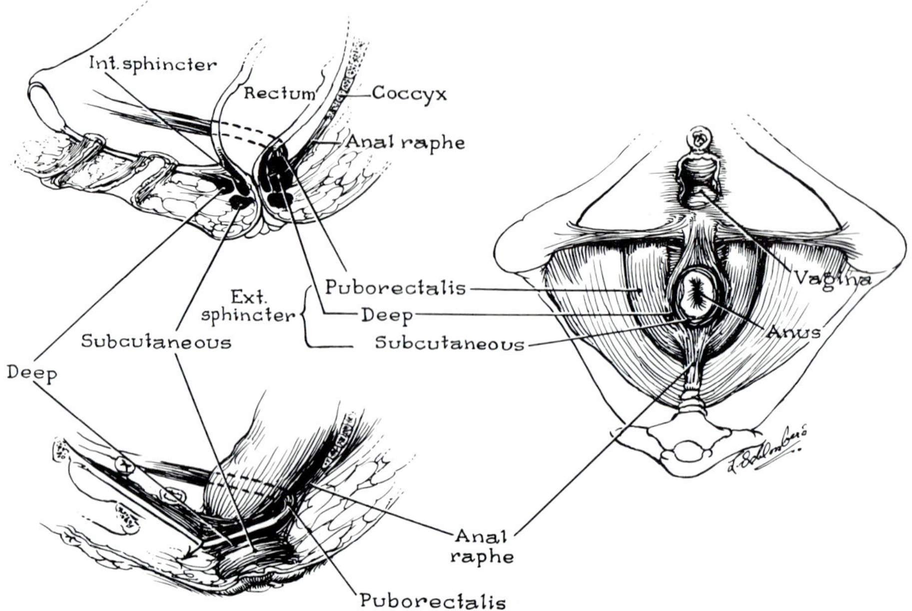

Fig. 12-2 Gross anatomy of the ano-rectal sphincters. The external or striated-muscle sphincters of the ano-rectum are separable into two distinct groups, the subcutaneous and the deep. The subcutaneous sphincter lies most superficially, within the longitudinal intermuscular septum, and surrounds the anus. It is attached to the perianal skin and subcutaneous tissues without lateral attachment, and has a corrugator or constrictor action around the anus. The deep external sphincter comprises the former "superficial" and "deep" bundles, an artificial distinction. It is derived from and actually constitutes the most caudal portions of the funnel-shaped levator ani muscles, namely the puborectalis muscle group. The deeper portions of the puborectalis loop about the ano-rectum posteriorly in its "sling" component; the more superficial portions have posterior attachment to the coccyx via the raphe of the levator ani muscles, and anterior stabilization via attachment in the perineum, especially to the transverse perinei muscles. While there may be some constrictor action from the more superficial fibers which encircle the ano-rectum, its main action appears to be pinchcock in nature via the puborectalis sling component, pulling the ano-rectum cephalad and anterior.

rectum somewhat deeper and more laterally, attaching to the coccyx behind and to perineal structures anteriorly; and the deep portion, an annular bundle about the upper third of the ano-rectum which blends with the puborectalis portion of the levator ani muscle (Milligan and Morgan, 1934; Gorsch, 1960). Others have noted difficulty in distinguishing these portions as separate (Hollinshead, 1961), and have suggested that division is an artificial one. Levy (1936) and Courtney (1950) have indicated that the muscle is divisible into only two portions, a subcutaneous and a deep. The deep part comprises both the superficial and deep portions previously described and originates from the inferior layers of the levator ani muscle, principally the puborectalis (Courtney, 1950). The deep portions of the external sphincter decussate and blend in anteriorly with the perineal structures and posteriorly with the coccyx, thus obtaining lateral attachment. The major part of the deep portion of the external sphincter, the puborectalis sling, is located posteriorly, with only minor fibers decussating anteriorly. The external ano-rectal sphincter can then be considered as having two anatomical functions: those muscles circling the ano-rectum (the subcutaneous sphincter and decussating fibers of the deep sphincter) may act as circular constrictors; the fibers looping around the ano-rectum (the puborectalis-sling part of the deep external sphincter) act as a pinchcock, drawing the ano-rectum forward and upward toward the pubis.

Summary. The ano-rectum is the termination of the intestine. It is guarded by two sets of sphincters. The internal sphincter is a terminal elaboration of the circular smooth muscle of the gut. It is involuntary muscle and under autonomic reflex control. The external sphincter is a conglomerate of pelvic striated muscles. It has a circular constricting action, primarily in its subcutaneous portion, and a pinchcock effect, primarily from the puborectalis-sling part of its deep portion. Like striated muscle elsewhere, it is under voluntary and reflex control.

ANO-RECTAL MANOMETRY

Ano-rectal manometry is used to assess physiologically the reactivity and function of the ano-rectal sphincters. Strictly speaking a kymography technique, it was developed by Schuster, Hendrix, and Mendeloff (1963). The apparatus consists of a double balloon device, with two separate components of a molded latex balloon tied around a hollow steel tube. Two holes in the side walls of this cylinder are connected to two separate pressure strain gauges and recording channels, one for each compartment. After rectal examination, the balloon system is placed in position inside the ano-rectal region and connected to the recording system. The balloons are distended with 1 to 3 ml of air, depending on the caliber of the ano-rectum and the age of the patient. A third balloon on a polyethylene tube is threaded through the hollow core of the tube and used briefly to distend the rectum with increasing volumes of air. The test is performed with the patient in the lateral position and under mild sedation if necessary.

The technique of ano-rectal manometry assesses three aspects of the physiological control of continence and defecation. Balloon inflation in the proximal rectum simulates the increase in pressure in a full rectal reservoir. The inner measuring balloon reflects the reflex pressure changes of the smooth-muscle internal sphincter. The outer measuring balloon responds to pressure alterations of the striated external sphincter. We have reported the accuracy and usefulness of ano-rectal manometry studies both for constipation problems (Schnaufer et al., 1967; Tobon et al., 1968) and incontinence problems (Schnaufer, Kumar, and White, 1970; White et al., 1972).

We have recently simplified the technique of ano-rectal manometry (El Shafie et al., 1972). This new system utilizes materials readily and economically accessible in office or hospital ward, but is otherwise similar to our previously described electronic technique. The balloon apparatus can be easily constructed from finger cots and available tubing, and a water manometer is used for measurements.

Children with constipation and incontinence problems were studied with this simplified system. At the same time, the usual electronic recordings were obtained. The simplified apparatus correctly reflected the graphic results and may provide an opportunity for more universal application of this technique in the physiological assessment of children with ano-rectal dysfunction.

Simple methods of investigation can fall into disrepute if they are not applied correctly. For this reason the following points are emphasized for accurate ano-rectal manometry:

1. The balloon must be positioned properly and remain there during the whole procedure. The best way of maintaining position is to use all three balloons in the system: the inner one for distending the rectum, the middle one for assessing internal sphincter reaction, and the external one for measuring the external sphincter reaction. The balloon for the external sphincter should be placed so that half of it lies within the anal canal and the other half is visible outside the anus all the time.

2. The length of the anal canal is different in various age groups, and one should not use a "standard" balloon system for all age groups. Different sizes of apparatus, suitable for infants and children, are presented in Table 12-1.

3. Digital rectal examination before the study is important to assess

Table 12-1 Recommended Measurements for Balloon Systems

	Infants (under 2 yr)	Children (over 2 yr)
Cylinder		
Total length	6.0 cm	10.0 cm
I.D.	0.4 cm	0.6 cm
O.D.	0.6 cm	0.8 cm
French size	20	24
Distance between side holes	1.3 cm	2.5 cm
Inner tubing		
O.D.	0.17 cm	0.28 cm
P.E. No.	190	260
Distance between rectal and sphincter balloons	2 cm	3 cm

the size of the rectum and judge the amount of distension that will be needed to stimulate the rectal wall in a given patient.

4. The balloon for rectal distension should be in the lower half of the rectum, which is the sensory receptor area. Insertion distances suitable for each age group are presented in Table 12-1.

Physiological assessment of ano-rectal function has been reported for a variety of techniques, most of which rely on open-tipped catheter recording (Duthie and Watts, 1965; Howard and Nixon, 1968; Collins et al., 1969; Scharli and Kiesewetter, 1970; Suzuki, Watanabe, and Kasai, 1970). Our method has utilized intra-anal balloons to measure the sphincteric responses. It is our impression that the balloon recording device more accurately assesses the combined responses of the anal sphincters than does the open-tipped catheter, which measures, in effect, local responses or forces in the area where it is located (Collins et al., 1969). Harris, Winans, and Pope (1966) have documented the difficulties attendant upon catheter measurements of the anal sphincters.

The two balloons, carefully positioned, accurately record the reflex reactions of the two sphincters. Concomitant electromyographic studies have demonstrated that the external balloon in our ano-rectal manometry method records the subcutaneous part of the external sphincter and those parts of the deep sphincter that circle anteriorly to insert in the perineal skin or perineal musculature and which provide the circular constricting action at the outermost level (Schnaufer et al., 1967; Alva, Mendeloff, and Schuster, 1967; Tobon et al., 1968).

Collins et al. (1969) have demonstrated that the puborectalis, or deep external sphincter, exerts positive pressure posteriorly and none anteriorly to provide the pinchcock action (Fig. 12-2). The inner recording balloon is thus not fully encircled by striated muscle and can truly register the reflex relaxation of the smooth-muscle internal sphincter; its reaction is not affected by any reflex reaction of the puborectalis or deep portion of the external sphincter, which exerts pressure only posteriorly.

Ano-rectal manometry has been used to assess the reflex responses of the internal and external ano-rectal sphincters in normal children and in those with incontinence or constipation problems. Coordinated with physiological and anatomical studies of others, a deeper understanding of normal and abnormal ano-rectal function can be provided.

NORMAL ANO-RECTAL PHYSIOLOGY

Defecation and continence appear to be dependent on proper rectal sensation and peristalsis, coupled with normal ano-rectal sphincter response. The rectum basically has a reservoir function (Scharli and Kiesewetter, 1970). The pressure in the closed anal canal, which abets fecal storage and prevents continuous defecation, is due mainly to the tone of the involuntary internal sphincter (Schuster et al., 1963; Bennett and Duthie, 1964). When the rectum is full, afferent nerves in the rectal wall (Brody, McCorriston, and Skoryna, 1960) and/or puborectalis muscle (Scharli and Kiesewetter, 1970) trigger a reflex relaxation of the internal sphincter that is independent of peristalsis (Schuster et al., 1963). The external anal sphincter is under both voluntary control and reflex influence from the distended rectum. It may contribute to the pressure within the anal canal only when a bolus is present (Duthie and Watts, 1965); or the external sphincter may be tonically contracted with a higher threshold than the internal sphincter, and with a capability for further, albeit temporary, contraction (Alva et al., 1967). The resting internal sphincter appears to maintain continence of liquid feces and flatus; its relaxation with rectal distension seems to prepare for defecation. The minimally contracted external sphincter reflexly tightens when the rectum is fully distended, facilitating continence; voluntary contraction can be superimposed in a sense as a "fine control," or to prevent accidents (Alva et al., 1967).

An illustration to summarize this natural sequence can be made in a case of diarrhea. A sense of rectal fullness usually appears first. This is followed by a feeling of urgency, as the internal sphincter reflexly relaxes, presenting a full bolus of liquid feces to the external anus. A reflex contraction of the constricting circular sphincter and pinchcocking deep external striated sphincter ensues, abetted by voluntary reinforcement such that continence is usually maintained until a "shelter" is reached.

Our data from ano-rectal manometry testing (Schnaufer et al., 1967, 1970; White et al., 1972) and data from others using this technique (Alva et al., 1967; Tobon et al., 1968) confirm these responses. With transient distension of the intrarectal balloon to simulate rectal fullness, we have observed slow relaxation of the internal sphincter and a contraction of the external sphincter of briefer duration that correlated with concomitant electromyographic tracing (Fig. 12-3).

Armed with this understanding of the normal physiology of defecation and continence, and supported by our observations from ano-rectal manometry, we have studied patients with abnormal ano-rectal function.

DISTURBED ANO-RECTAL FUNCTION

Abnormalities of ano-rectal function appear in two characteristic forms, constipation and incontinence. Thorough evaluation of patients with both conditions, coupled with ano-rectal manometry studies, have provided a deeper insight into normal function, and a better understanding of the disturbed physiology as a rational basis for therapy.

CONSTIPATION PROBLEMS

Constipation problems in children generally derive from two conditions, one organic and the other functional. The former, Hirschsprung's Disease,

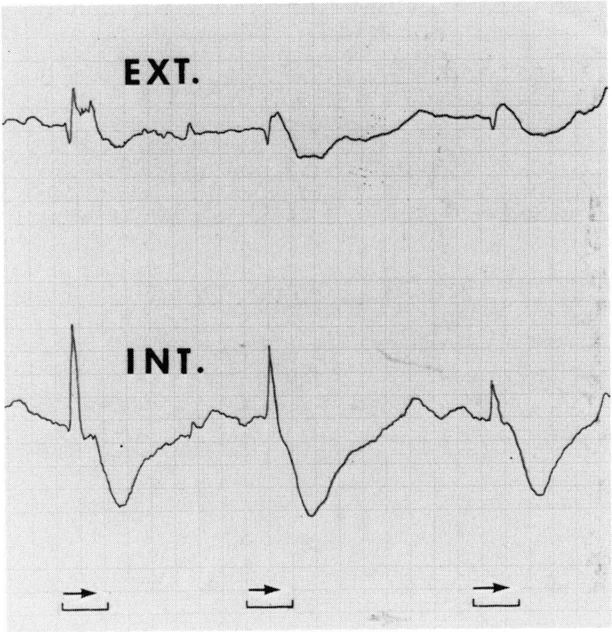

Fig. 12-3 Normal ano-rectal manometry response. In a patient with functional constipation, the tracing shows a reflex relaxation of the internal (smooth-muscle) sphincter and a contraction of the external (striated-muscle) sphincter to proximal rectal distension with an air-filled balloon. The underlined arrows indicate the time and duration of rectal balloon distension. The external sphincter responses represent actual contractions as determined by concomitant electromyography, and are not merely reflections of the rectal balloon distension (Schnaufer et al., 1967; Tobon et al., 1968).

is due to a congenital lack of ganglion cells in the ano-rectum and, perhaps, more proximal colon; the latter is due to an unconscious withholding of stool, and is properly termed functional constipation or functional megacolon. The term which has often been applied, "psychogenic," connotes mental illness and should be decried. Since this condition arises as a very natural defense mechanism of an infant or child to the pain from anal fissures, or to the psychic trauma of rigid toilet training, and is, therefore, truly functional, the term functional constipation would seem both descriptive and appropriate.

Differentiation between Hirschsprung's Disease and functional constipation can usually be made on clinical grounds (Schnaufer et al., 1970). Hirschsprung's Disease is congenital, and symptoms can usually be dated from birth; functional constipation is acquired later. Abdominal distension from a very dilated colon may occur in Hirschsprung's Disease, and the constipation is usually relieved only by enemas or the like. The abdomen is seldom distended in functional constipation, and the constipation is more periodic, with ultimate spontaneous evacuation. Encopresis, or overflow incontinence of liquid feces past impacted stool in the ano-rectum, is common in functional constipation and not present in Hirschsprung's Disease. The salient differentiating points are summarized in Table 12-2.

As might be expected, ano-rectal manometry responses in patients with functional constipation were perfectly normal in more than 100 such patients studied. With rectal distension, slow internal sphincter relaxation and rapid external sphincter contraction occur (Fig. 12-3). The constipation appears to result from voluntary, albeit unconscious, withholding of stool through the mechanism of contraction or nonrelaxation of the external striated-muscle sphincter. Sufficient tonus can be maintained to withhold stool over a somewhat protracted period of time. Not enough resistance can be maintained, however, to prevent encopresis, or periodic bulky bowel movements, or to produce a megacolon large enough to cause abdominal distension.

In Hirschsprung's Disease, which is basically a disorder of autonomic smooth-muscle innervation, the pathophysiology appears to reside mainly in the internal sphincter and the more proximally aganglionic colon. Due to lack of peristalsis or inertia in the distal colon and to an unrelaxing or actually contracting internal sphincter, constipation ensues. Rectal sensation appears to be intact. In more than 30 patients with Hirschsprung's Disease, ano-rectal manometry has demonstrated normal external sphincter contraction in response to transient distension of the rectal balloon. The autonomically innervated internal sphincter, that specialized termination of smooth muscle of the large bowel at the anus, either fails to relax or actually contracts (Fig. 12-4). Sufficient resistance is provided to obtain relentless constipation and normal distension of the bowel proximal to the aganglionosis. Aganglionosis limited to the internal sphincter alone,

Table 12-2 Differentiation of Constipation Problems

	Functional constipation	Hirschsprung's Disease
Onset	Infancy	Birth
History	Anal fissures, or coercive toilet training: colicky abdominal pain; periodic volume stools	No antecedent episode; no abdominal pain; assisted evacuation necessary
Encopresis	Present	Absent
Physical examination	Minimal abdominal distension Feces-packed rectum	Massive abdominal distension Empty rectum
Barium enema	Dilated rectum	Narrow segment
Biopsy	Ganglion cells	No ganglion cells

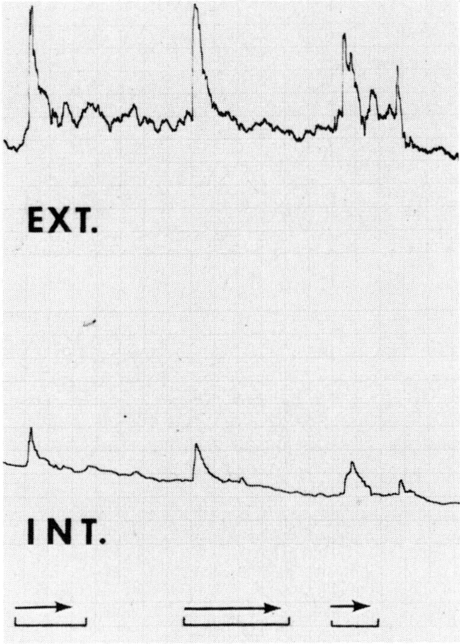

Fig. 12-4 Manometric response in Hirschsprung's Disease. The external (striated-muscle) sphincter contracts normally to the proximal rectal balloon distension. The internal (smooth-muscle) sphincter may remain unrelaxed or may actually contract.

the "form anale" of Hirschsprung's Disease, is associated with less severe constipation, which seems to respond to simple division of the internal sphincter. Internal sphincterotomy or sphincterectomy has been reported to be beneficial for such patients with low-segment Hirschsprung's Disease (Thomas, Bream, and DeConnick, 1970; Nissan and Bar-Maor, 1971; Backwinkle, Oakley, and Truffle, 1971).

These physiological studies of patients with constipation problems underscore our understanding of ano-rectal function. Disturbance of the smooth-muscle internal sphincter function such as occurs in Hirschsprung's Disease, with intact striated-muscle external sphincter function, manifests itself as constipation. Nonrelaxation of internal sphincter tonus does not allow the initiation of defecation, and constipation ensues. Faulty peristalsis and lack of relaxation in the aganglionic proximal colon certainly plays a role. Sphincterotomy alone, however, provides relaxed tonus and remedies constipation in many patients, emphasizing the role of the internal sphincter in this disease. It should be noted that incontinence is not a problem following internal sphincterotomy, a fact that emphasises the role of the external sphincters in maintaining continence. The capability of the striated-muscle external sphincters to prevent defecation is demonstrated by the functional constipation group. Nonrelaxation can be maintained for prolonged periods, thus preventing defecation, particularly of formed stool. Training regimens designed to overcome the unconscious withholding of stool have returned normal bowel habits without incontinence.

INCONTINENCE PROBLEMS

True incontinence problems, as opposed to encopresis or impaction with overflow, are almost always neurological in origin. Incontinence results from somatic denervation of the striated-muscle external sphincters. It is secondary to lower spinal cord injury, or to a congenital lesion such as a meningomyelocele.

Once the rectal reservoir is full, involuntary relaxation of the smooth-muscle internal sphincter occurs. Defecation cannot be avoided by voluntary sphincteric contraction since striated-muscle innervation is impaired, and "accidents" or fecal soiling occur. The external sphincter striated-muscle deficit is consistent with the other neurological skeletal muscle deficiencies that occur in these conditions.

More than 60 children with neurological incontinence have been studied with ano-rectal manometry. In the vast majority, particularly those with the most severe lesions, these patients had normally relaxing internal sphincters, as suggested by the earlier studies of Denny-Brown and Robertson (1935) and of Kuntz (1953). Thus the autonomic innervation of smooth muscle does not appear to be involved. On the other hand, reflex contraction of the striated-muscle external sphincter was generally absent or extremely weakened (Fig. 12-5). On examination these children were also found to have a patulous anus, with deficient anal closure.

Physiological studies of patients with neurogenic fecal incontinence underscore the importance of the external sphincter in maintaining normal continence. Consider again the previous analogy of the patient with diarrhea. With involuntary relaxation of the internal sphincter, the patient with neurogenic incontinence is unable to voluntarily contract his striated-muscle sphincters, and an "accident" ensues. The importance of the striated-muscle sphincters is stressed, as well, in the current concepts for repair of a high imperforate anus. No matter how much smooth-muscle internal sphincter residual has been left by nature, the best functional results have been obtained when the ano-rectum pullthrough segment has been accurately coated within the deep (puborectalis) and superficial (corrugator) striated muscle groups. The external ano-rectal sphincters, then, are responsible for continence, and their deficiency due to neurological embarrassment is the usual cause of true incontinence.

CHILDREN WITH NEUROLOGICAL INCONTINENCE

Neurological lesions of the lower spine accounted for all 59 cases in children with incontinence considered in this review. Thirty-eight of these cases have been reported previously.

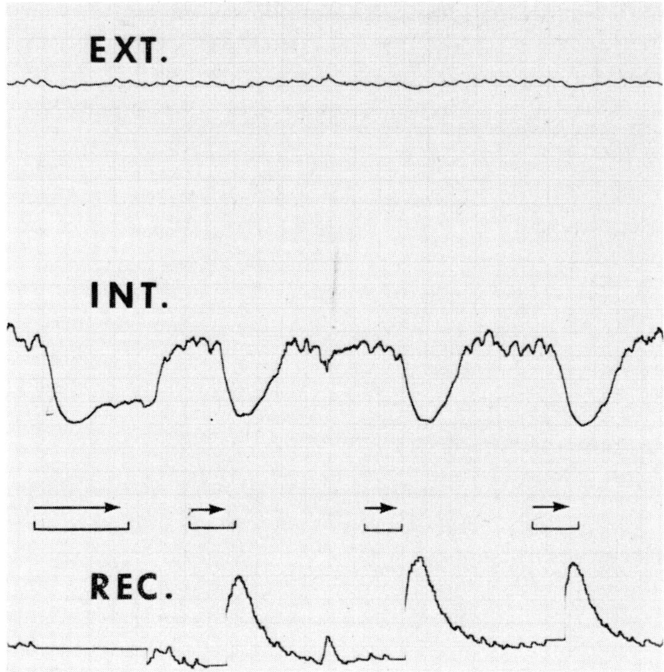

Fig. 12-5 Manometry response in neurological incontinence. In a typically severe spinal lesion (meningomyelocele), the internal (smooth-muscle) sphincter normally relaxes in response to proximal rectal distension. The usual external (striated-muscle) contraction is absent. The bracketed arrows indicate the time and duration of rectal balloon distension.

Most of the 59 children had severe incontinence problems; a few had apparent incontinence which proved to be encopresis associated with normal sphincteric function. Constant soiling with accidents (involuntary passage of bowel movements) was present in 20; another 12 patients had constant staining (fecal smearing always present on underwear or diapers); and 7 children had impaction usually with encopresis. There were 10 patients who exhibited only occasional staining (Table 12-3). There was usually a patulous anus with no external sphincter reaction to stimuli; only the relatively weak internal sphincter was present on rectal examination in the severe cases. An appropriate lumbo-sacral deficit was noted on neurological examination.

Ano-rectal manometry was performed in all cases (Table 12-4). With the exception of one patient who had serious damage from a spinal abcess, the internal sphincter relaxed normally. The external sphincter contractual response was absent in all patients with the more severe defects, including four children with sacral agenesis, in all those with meningomyeloceles, and in the patient with spinal abcess. In the less severe lesions (spina

Table 12-3 Neurological Incontinence—Bowel Function before Treatment

	Constant soiling with accidents	Frequent staining	Occasional staining	Impaction
Spinal cord malformations*†	0	1	0	0
Spina bifida occulta†	2	2	0	0
Sacral agenesis	3	0	0	1
Meningomyelocele‡	14	9	10	6
Spinal abscess	1	0	0	0
	20	12	10	7

*One case is too young to evaluate continence.

†Two cases had no symptoms.

‡Seven cases are too young to evaluate continence.

bifida occulta, cord malformation, etc.), the external sphincter reacted normally. This latter group generally exhibited soiling and encopresis rather than true incontinence.

With understanding of the physiopathology involved, suitable therapeutic regimens can be applied. In our series, those children with normal sphincteric reactions and minor neurological conditions, such as spina bifida occulta, were treated with training regimens similar to those used for functional constipation with encopresis (Schnaufer et al., 1970), namely, mineral oil, milk of magnesia, or an irrigation regimen. Sufficient mineral oil or milk of magnesia was given following cleansing enemas to produce one or two loose bowel movements daily. The medications were gradually discontinued following establishment of satisfactory bowel habits. Those with true neurological incontinence and deficient external sphincters were placed on a daily evacuation regimen. These regimens were designed to take advantage of the tonus of the only remaining sphincter, the autonomically innervated internal sphincter, to prevent soiling. With realization that internal sphincter relaxation occurs reflexly when the rectal reservoir attains a certain fullness, these regimes rely on regular evacuation before this fullness is reached to avoid inadvertent relaxation of the internal sphincter and "accidents."

THERAPEUTIC REGIMENS FOR NEUROGENIC INCONTINENCE

All the regimens consist basically of emptying the rectum electively and regularly before spontaneous defecation is reflexly initiated, the internal sphincter relaxes, and "accidents" occur. Initially, the colon should be evacuated completely by thorough enema cleansing. To take advantage of gastrocolic emptying reflexes, the colo-rectum is emptied at a time suitable for parents and child, generally after the evening meal. Most children respond promptly to a bisacodyl suppository (Ducolax); others benefit

Table 12-4 Neurological Incontinence—Ano-Rectal Manometry Results, and Bowel Function After Treatment

Diagnosis (No. of patients)	Results of manometry	Assisted evacuation necessary	Function			
			Occasional accidents	Frequent staining	Occasional staining	Clean
Spinal cord malformations						
1 vascular	Int. (↓)					
1 lipoma						
1 diastomyclomyelia	*Ext. (↑)	0/2	0	0	1	1
Spina bifida occulta	Int. (↓)					
(5 cases)	Ext. (↑)	4/5	0	2	1	2
Sacral agenesis	Int. (↓)					
(4 cases)	Ext. (↑)	1/1	0	1	0	0
	Int. (↓)					
	Ext. (O)	3/3	0	2	0	1
Meningomyelocele†	Int. (↓)					
(46 cases)	Ext. (O)	29/39	2	10	5	22
Spinal abscess	Int. (O)					
(1 case)	Ext. (O)	1/1	1	0	0	0
Total cases 59		38/51	3	15	7	26

*One case is too young to evaluate continence.

†Seven cases are too young to evaluate continence.

Legend: ↑ = Contraction; O = No reaction; ↓ = Relaxation

from an enema, either phosphate (Fleets), soap suds or saline, or by CO_2 evacuant suppositories (Ceo-Two).

In the bisacodyl suppository regimen, a half or whole adult-sized suppository, depending on the response of the child, is maintained in the anal canal by holding the buttocks together with the child in the lateral Sims position. It is allowed to dissolve; a reaction is obtained, usually within 30 minutes. The child is then placed on the toilet or potty chair for evacuation. The enemas are administered in similar fashion, holding the buttocks together to allow sufficient retention to accomplish full evacuation. The CO_2 evacuant suppositories are used in the same way as the bisacodyl suppositories. The Assisted Evacuation Regimen is summarized in Table 12-5.

The results of these regimens have been very gratifying in our series. A colostomy was not necessary in any case, with the exception of one child who continued to have accidents following a spinal abscess with morphological deficiencies of both sphincters.

The remaining children, all of whom had residual function of the internal sphincter which could be utilized and exploited, have been benefitted (Table 12-4). Accidents or impaction with encopresis no longer occur. About half (26 patients) are clean all the time; staining of the underwear occurs in 22 children and is considered only a minor inconvenience by both children and parents. Thirteen out of 51 children have learned regular bowel habits and no longer need any assistance; eight are still too young to evaluate. The remainder (38) require the daily emptying regimen; 13 of these children are always clean.

The ability to provide socially acceptable continence for these children has been enthusiastically received by patients and family alike. The necessity for the daily evacuation regimen is considered a small price to pay to avoid colostomy in these children, who are usually already encumbered with urinary conduit bags and orthopedic braces. We agree with Smith (1965) and Sieber (1969) that colostomy is seldom warranted for neurological

Table 12-5 Assisted Evacuation Regimen

1. Place child on side and give enema (soap suds or saline).
   Retain enema by holding buttocks together for 10 to 15 mins.
   Place child on toilet seat or potty chair, making sure that the feet are supported or are on floor. Repeat enemas as necessary until the rectum is clear of feces.
2. Thereafter, use a rectal suppository daily after supper (or breakfast, if perferred by mother and patient) if there has not been a spontaneous bowel movement. Allow suppository about 15 to 30 min to dissolve and take effect while the patient lies on his or her side. Then place the child on the toilet seat or potty chair with feet supported.
3. If no results are obtained within 60 min of the insertion of the suppository, give the child an enema (Fleet's, soap suds, or saline).
4. Do not allow the child to become impacted.

fecal incontinence, and with Forsythe and Kinley (1970) that bowel training regimens with regular evacuation are usually satisfactory.

Analysis of our series suggests that the sooner evacuation regimens are started, the more likely can spontaneous bowel habits be learned. The average age of those in our series who have developed adequate bowel habits and remain clean was 3.3 years at the initiation of the regimen; those who still require assistance averaged 6.6 years when started. Seventeen children of this latter group of 30 who need the daily regimen were over five years of age when first seen by us, and never had adequate evaluation or any training at an earlier age.

Fecal incontinence problems must not be "put aside," out of a concern for prior correction of urological and orthopedic problems, until the sudden realization that they may prevent the child from entering school. Early training can prevent this problem and markedly diminish, if not eradicate, the need for a permanent colostomy. We prefer to initiate the bowel training regimen in these children between one and two years of age, essentially when they are very capable of sitting on a potty chair.

The technique of ano-rectal manometry has provided us with a better understanding of the disturbed ano-rectal physiology of these children with neurological incontinence. Such testing is certainly not necessary for the routine management of children with clear-cut evidence of neurological embarrassment. When such a child is found on careful physical examination to have a gaping anus or an external sphincter that is easily distended and remains open, we have consistently noted an absent external sphincter and a normally relaxing internal sphincter on manometric testing. Indeed, the resting tone of the ano-rectum is maintained by the internal sphincter, which can be noted to close slowly following digital examination, a reaction similar to the slow return to normal tonus seen with manometry (Fig. 12-3). Such a child can be confidently managed with a daily evacuation regimen without further diagnostic testing. Ano-rectal manometry may be helpful in questionable or recalcitrant cases.

SUMMARY AND CONCLUSIONS

Neurological fecal incontinence is a frequent accompaniment to spinal malformations such as meningomyeloceles and appears to result from somatic denervation of the striated-muscle external sphincters. Anatomically and functionally, the external sphincters appear to have two components, a more superficial group which surrounds the anus and acts as a corrugator, and a deeper group, basically the puborectalis portion of the levator ani muscles, which acts as a pinchcock. The internal sphincter, a specialized continuation of the smooth muscle of the bowel, appears to provide the resting tone for the outlet of the rectal reservoir, but cannot prevent incontinence. In our cases of true neurological incontinence, the technique of ano-rectal manometry has demonstrated normal relaxation of the internal sphincter and absent or feeble external sphincter contraction in response to a rectal-distending stimulus.

From our Birth Defects Clinic, 59 children with neurological lesions of the lower spine were studied. Starting from a status of severe incontinence and constant soiling or staining, socially acceptable continence has been obtained by a careful training regimen. Regular assisted evacuation of the colo-rectum allows 50% of the children to remain clean; the others have minor staining of their underwear. Colostomy was not necessary and appears to be rarely indicated.

One-third of the group have learned regular bowel habits and no longer need assistance. The difference in age between those children not requiring assistance (3.3 years) and those who still need daily assisted evacuation (6.6 years) strongly suggests that bowel training regimens should be initiated early in children with neurological fecal incontinence.

REFERENCES

Alva, J., A. I. Mendeloff, and M. M. Schuster. 1967. Reflex and electromyographic abnormalities associated with fecal incontinence. Gastroenterology 53:101.

Backwinkle, K. D., D. W. Oakley, and G. A. Truffle, 1971. Rectal myectomy for short segment aganglionic megacolon. Surg. Gynec. Obstet. 132:109.

Bass, D. D., T. J. Ustach, and M. M. Schuster. 1970. In vitro pharmacologic differentiation of sphincteric and nonsphincteric muscle. Johns Hopkins Med. J. 127:185.

Bennett, R. C., and H. L. Duthie. 1964. Functional importance of internal and external sphincter. Brit. J. Surg. 51:355.

Brody, G. S., J. R. McCorriston, and S. C. Skoryna. 1960. Observation on fecal continence mechanisms. J. Am. Med. Assoc. 173:226.

Collins, C. D., B. H. Brown, G. E. Whittaker, and H. L. Duthie. 1969. New method of measuring forces in the anal canal. Gut 10:160.

Courtney, H. 1950. Anatomy of the pelvic diaphragm and ano-rectal musculature as related to sphincter preservation in ano-rectal surgery. Am. J. Surg. 79:155.

Denny-Brown, B., and E. G. Robertson. 1935. An investigation of the nervous control of defecation. Brain 58:256.

Duthie, H. L., and J. M. Watts. 1965. Contribution of the external anal sphincter to the pressure zone in the anal canal. Gut 6:64.

El Shafie, M., H. Suzuki, L. Schnaufer, and J. J. White. 1972. A simplified method of ano-rectal manometry for wider clinical application. J. Ped. Surg. 7:230.

Forsythe, W. I., and J. G. Kinley. 1970. Bowel control of children with spina bifida. Develop. Med. Child Neurol. 12:27.

Friedmann, C. A. 1968. Action of nicotine catecholamines on the human internal anal sphincter. Am. J. Digest. Dis. 13:428.

Gorsch, R. V. 1960. The sigmoid, rectum and anal canal. Relations, attachments, and pelvic spaces. CIBA Clin. Symp. 12:2.

Harris, L. D., C. S. Winans, and C. E. Pope. 1966. Determination of yield pressures: a method for measuring anal sphincter competence. Gastroenterology 50:754.

Hollinshead, W. H. 1961. Anatomy for surgeons, Vol. 2, p. 709. Hoeber-Harper, New York.

Howard, E. R., and H. H. Nixon. 1968. Internal anal sphincter. Observations on development and mechanism of inhibitory responses in premature infants and children with Hirschsprung's Disease. Arch. Dis. Childh. 43:569.

Kuntz, A. 1953. The autonomic nervous system, 4th ed. Lea and Febiger, Philadelphia. 238 pp.

Leutenegger, F. 1969. Untersuchungen des M. Sphincter Ani Internus Auf Ganglienzellen. Schweiz. Med. Wschr. 99:1431.

Levy, E. 1936. Anorectal musculature. Am. J. Surg. 34:141.

Milligan, T. E. C., and C. N. Morgan. 1934. Surgical anatomy of the anal canal. Lancet ii:1150.

Nissan, S., and J. A. Bar-Maor. 1971. Further experience in the diagnosis and surgical treatment of short-segment Hirschsprung's Disease and idiopathic megacolon. J. Ped. Surg. 6:738.

Scharli, A. F., and W. B. Kiesewetter. 1970. Defecation and continence: some new concepts. Dis. Colon and Rectum 13:81.

Schnaufer, L., A. P. Kumar, and J. J. White. 1970. Differentiation and management of incontinence and constipation problems in children. Surg. Clin. No. Amer. 50:895.

Schnaufer, L., J. L. Talbert, J. A. Haller, Jr., N. C. R. W. Reid, F. Tobon, M. M. Schuster. 1967. Differential sphincteric studies in the diagnosis of ano-rectal disorders of childhood. J. Ped. Surg. 2:538.

Schuster, M. M., T. R. Hendrix, and A. I. Mendeloff. 1963. Internal anal sphincter response: manometric studies on its normal physiology, neural pathways, and alteration in bowel disorders. J. Clin. Invest. 42:196.

Shapiro, S. 1948. Applied anatomy of infants and children. Rev. Gastroent. 15, 4 (April).

Sieber, W. K. 1969. Fecal incontinence of neurogenic origin. *In* C. D. Benson, W. T. Mustard, M. M. Ravitch, W. H. Snyder, and K. J. Welch [eds.], Pediatric surgery. Year Book Medical Publishers, Chicago.

Smith, E. D. 1965. Spina bifida and the total care of myelomeningocele. Charles C Thomas, Springfield, Ill.

Stonesifer, G. L., Jr., G. P. Murphy, and C. R. Lombardo. 1960. Anatomy of ano-rectum. Am. J. Surg. 100:666.

Suzuki, H., K. Watanabe, and M. Kasai. 1970. Manometric and cineradiographic studies on ano-rectal motility in Hirschsprung's Disease before and after surgical operation. Tohoku J. Exp. Med. 102:69.

Thomas, C. G., Jr., C. A. Bream, and P. DeConnick. 1970. Posterior sphincterotomy and rectal myotomy in the management of Hirschsprung's Disease. Ann. Surg. 171:796.

Tobon, F., N. C. R. W. Reid, J. L. Talbert, and M. M. Schuster. 1968. Nonsurgical test for the diagnosis of Hirschsprung's Disease. New Eng. J. Med. 278:188.

White, J. J., H. Suzuki, M. El Shafie, A. P. M. Kumar, J. A. Haller, Jr., and L. Schnaufer. 1972. A physiologic rationale for the management of neurologic rectal incontinence in children. Pediatrics 49:888.

13

Psychosocial Aspects of Meningomyeloceles

John M. Freeman, M.D.

The longest section of a book on meningomyeloceles should be devoted to the psychosocial problems related to this defect. Over the years it is these problems that are the most severe for the child, the parents, and the siblings. The fact that this is one of the shortest chapters, with fewer pages than are devoted to the care of the ileal loop, is an admission of the ignorance and perhaps arrogance of those of us who are dedicated to doing our best for these unfortunate children and their families.

Arrogance is perhaps a harsh word, but the medical profession has traditionally equated "doing our best" with technological advances in care rather than with psychosocial advances. We have looked at diseases and at patients and asked "What can we do?" rather than "What should we do?" We have looked at the child's back and found that it could be closed, and at the hydrocephalus and found that new shunting techniques could be devised. We have not, however, looked at the long-range effects of these procedures on the children, nor have we looked at the effects of the children on their families.

When we decide not to operate, or decide that we cannot operate, many of us turn our backs and leave the burden of the consequences of this decision on the family, or on the nurses and other personnel of the institution caring for the child. In these cases we have assessed our technical capacity, found it wanting, and turned away. In a sense we do the same thing when we decide to apply vigorous medical therapy. The specialists, even at a combined clinic, look at the sum of the involved organ systems. But the child is more than the sum of his organ systems, and the family more than just the child. All should be considered part of the total care of a child with a meningomyelocele. The use of a social worker–coordinator and a psychiatric consultant as part of the team is but a preliminary step toward total care.

It is significant that when questions about the efficacy of early closure of the back were raised, carefully controlled studies were performed to assess the medical benefits of early or late closure. Yet questions about the total effects of meningomyeloceles on children and families are just now being raised, ten years later. Indeed, Lorber's (1971) reassessment of the effects of treatment represents a courageous attempt to evaluate what we are doing with our vigorous treatment. His assessment is technological and founded on mortality, retardation, and motor handicap. What are we producing, even if we concentrate, as Lorber suggests, on those with "a better prognosis"? How good a life can we expect to provide even for these children with a lesser handicap?

Questions should be asked about the psychological adaptation of these children. What are their handicaps, not only in intellectual or motor terms, but in terms of adjustment and adaptation? Some have said that we have an anthropomorphic view of these handicapped children, meaning that we who are whole try, and fail, to empathize with children who are less than whole. We can imagine what life would be like if we suddenly became paraplegic, and indeed can inquire of those who have become paraplegic. But what does this tell us about the child who has never walked? Is loss of function equivalent to never having acquired it? What are our long-term goals for the newborn with a meningomyelocele? Is existence alone sufficient, regardless of participation in society? Do we demand that the child make some contribution to society? Or is it sufficient that the child merely be "happy" (whatever that is)? If our limited goal is "happiness" or "contentment," do we achieve that for these children? Some have said that the adolescent with motor impairment, a shunt, an ileal loop, and impaired performance will "only grow up to curse us." But do we know?

The answers to these questions may not only modify what we do, but should modify the type of care we give to children and families to produce the best results. We can divide the questions to be asked into two interrelated questions. First, what are the effects of a child with a meningomyelocele on the *family*, in social, emotional, and financial terms? What factors enable one family to cope and adapt, while another disintegrates? Second, what are the psychosocial effects of this disability on the affected *child* as he becomes an adolescent and adult, and are there things we do, or fail to do, which affect this outcome?

THE FAMILY

A limited number of excellent studies of the effects of chronic diseases on the family have been done. Such studies often concern progressive, fatal diseases, such as cystic fibrosis (McCollum and Gibson, 1970), which occur in a previously normal child, or an acute illness with chronic consequences, such as polio (Davis, 1963). Other studies deal with the grieving reaction to the diagnosis of a fatal disease such as leukemia. But the child with a meningomyelocele presents elements of all of these. The child with a meningomyelocele is unique in that the lesion is obvious from birth; thus the grieving for the normal child who had been expected is accompanied by grieving for the malformed child who is. The long-range motor effects of the lesion are in many ways similar to those of polio, but the child never has the chance to develop the relations of the polio victim. The "disease" is chronic, like cystic fibrosis, and requires frequent hospitalization and surgery, but it is usually not fatal.

Studies of the psychosocial effects of this malformation are just beginning to appear (Hare et al., 1966; Kolin et al., 1971; Freeston, 1971; Walker, Thomas, and Russell, 1971; Fye, Saunders, and Freeman, 1972). Some of these studies point up particular problems as perceived by the parents.

TELLING THE PARENTS

The initial recognition of the spina bifida and the initial information given to the parents may affect parental attitudes for the remainder of that child's life, for this early period is critical in the development of parental attitudes toward the defect and the child (Klaus et al., 1972). Who informs the parent, how this information is transmitted, and what is said may cause parental attitudes that can never be altered. Parents who have been told the child will die often avoid the psychological attachment required for mothering, and then keep waiting for the event to occur (Green and Solnit, 1964). Conversely, parents told that the lesion is insignificant tend not to trust physicians when they later learn the truth.

Frequently, the mother is aware that something is wrong at the time of delivery. The gasped "Oh, no!" by the nursing attendant, the muttered consultations by physicians in the delivery room, or the silence of those in attendance are all immediate indications of catastrophe (Walker et al., 1971; Fye et al., 1972). While it is difficult to know what, if anything, to tell the mother immediately, it is obvious that in these days of minimal sedation of the mother, delivery room personnel must be very circumspect about what they say.

Telling the parent or preferably parents the nature of the defect and its consequences requires the true art of medicine, as well as knowledge of the proper information to convey (Kennell and Rolnick, 1960). Yet, at this crucial time, we find parents being informed by nurses, relatives, or physicians who have little information about the implications of the defect. Information given ranges from "it's a small lump, easily covered by a skin graft" to "the baby will die within hours." *It is better for the physician to admit ignorance and tell the mother only that the lesion is serious and will require the help of a specialist, than for the physician to provide misinformation.* The correct information is there for people who have the experience to evaluate it.

Ideally, a physician associated with the team responsible for the long-term care of the child should be responsible for providing the initial information. Unfortunately, this is not usually practical. However, when the child is sent to a referral center, one physician and the coordinator should inform the father, who accompanies the baby, as fully as possible about the defect and its consequences. We usually ask the father to relay this information to the mother, and then follow up with a phone call to the mother the same day to repeat the explanation and answer questions. Follow-up studies (D'Arcy, 1968; Fye et al., 1972) indicate that parents want the truth explained in understandable terms and in a sympathetic way. They want an informed person to encourage them to ask questions and provide whatever answers are available. While parents may not remember exactly what was said, they all seem to recall the manner in which the matter was discussed.

SEPARATION OF PARENTS AND CHILD

Apart from the mechanism by which the critical information is delivered, the physical separation of mother from child may play a major role in determining parental attitudes. Klaus et al. (1972) have shown a major effect on mothering merely by allowing the mother of a normal infant to have 16 *extra* hours of contact during the first three days of life. What, then, must be the effect of total maternal deprivation during this time? What are the effects of separation over the first weeks of life on the maternal-child interaction? Perhaps we should do more to encourage maternal contact with the infant during the early hospital period.

Since these children have multiple hospitalizations over their first years of life, we must also consider the effects of separation on both child and mother. Indeed, it is possible that some of the mental impairment in these children is a consequence of repeated hospitalization.

EFFECTS ON THE FAMILY

The effects of a child with a meningomyelocele on a family are enormous. In one small sample (Kolin et al., 1971) almost half the parents were divorced, while in another study with a low divorce rate almost half the parents felt that the marital relationship had deteriorated (Walker et al., 1971). Two-thirds of the families were "discontinued" after the birth of an affected child (Timson, 1970). Three-quarters of the families found themselves isolated, subjectively by their anxiety about the child (Green and Solnit, 1964), or objectively by the inability to find babysitters who will cope with braces and ileal loops (Walker et al., 1971). Half of the mothers in this latter study were found to be depressed.

Fye et al. (1972) found a major tendency to infantilize the child. This was true in punishment, as well as in areas of self-care. This infantilization worked to the detriment of the child, as well as the parents, by inhibiting the development of independence.

While few in number and limited in scope, these studies indicate that the family with a child having a meningomyelocele needs far more extensive psychiatric help and social service work than is usually provided.

THE CHILD

Studies of the long-range effects of the defect on the affected children are virtually nonexistent, and are obviously badly needed. In one such study (Kolin et al., 1971), of 13 children, aged 7 to 11, who initially had mild to moderate neurological impairment, only four had good adaptation in terms of self-care skills, school performance, social interaction, and mental status. The adaptation of parents (or on occasion older siblings) to the defect seemed to be the major determining factor in the child's adaptation. The adaptation of the parents was determined less by the degree of physical impairment of the child than by the stability of the marriage. Parents who were married less than five years prior to the birth of the defective infant and who had no normal children had major difficulties adapting and providing an optimal environment for the affected child. Studies of these children during adolescence, of their ability to interact socially with peers, of their ability to be independent, and of their attitudes toward their handicap, are needed to give us a picture of the product of our vigorous treatment.

SUMMARY

In summary, we need considerable information about the effects of meningomyeloceles on the family and on the child. If we are to provide optimal care for children, this care must include major improvements in the psychiatric and social services available. These services are just as important, if not more so, than much of the medical care provided.

REFERENCES

D'Arcy, E. 1968. Congenital defects: mothers' reactions to first information. Brit. Med. J. 3:796.

Davis, F. 1963. Passage through crisis: a study of polio victims and their families. Bobbs, New York.

Freeston, B. M. 1971. An enquiry into the effect of a spina bifida child upon family life. Develop. Med. Child Neurol. 13:456.

Fye, B., Jr., B. Saunders, and J. M. Freeman. 1972. Psychosocial studies of the families of children with myelomeningocele. Unpubished manuscript.

Green, M., and A. J. Solnit. 1964. Reaction to the threatened loss of a child: a vulnerable child syndrome. Pediatrics 34:58.

Hare, E. H., K. M. Laurence, H. Payne, and K. Rawnsley. 1966. Spina bifida cystica and family stress. Brit. Med. J. 2:757.

Kennell, J. H., and A. R. Rolnick. 1960. Discussing problems in newborn babies with their parents. Pediatrics 26:832.

Klaus, M. H., R. Jerauld, N. C. Kreger, W. McAlpine, M. Steffa, and J. H. Kennell. 1972. Maternal attachment: importance of the first post-partum days. New Eng. J. Med. 286:460.

Kolin, I. S., A. L. Scherzer, B. New, and M. Garfield. 1971. Studies of the school age child with meningomyeloceles: social and emotional adaptation. J. Pediat. 78:1013.

Lorber, J. 1971. Results of treatment of myelomeningocele: an analysis of 524 unselected cases with special reference to possible selection for treatment. Develop. Med. Child Neurol. 13:279.

McCollum, A. T., and L. E. Gibson. 1970. Family adaptation to the child with cystic fibrosis. J. Pediat. 77:571.

Timson, J. 1970. Social factors in the incidence of spina bifida and anencephaly. J. Biol. Soc. Sci. 2:81.

Walker, J. H., M. Thomas, and I. T. Russell. 1971. Spina bifida and the parents. Develop. Med. Child Neurol. 13:462.

14

The Role of the Center Coordinator

Verna Klein

The arrival of an infant with a major birth defect has an immediate, overwhelming, emotional impact on parents. They are overwhelmed with grief at having an imperfect child, overwhelmed by the crucial and complex decisions thrust upon them by new and strange physicians, overwhelmed by the immediate necessity for operation on such a tiny infant, overwhelmed by the prospects for the future of the child, and overwhelmed at the child's probable effect on the family. In most major institutions, they are further overwhelmed by the number of physicians caring for the child and by the lack of any central, neutral figure to assist them in their confusion. Separation of the mother from the infant, who has usually been sent to another institution, and separation of mother from father, who accompanies the baby, adds to their anxiety.

At this crucial time the center coordinator can act as a stable, nonmedical figure to help the family comprehend the situation. The coordinator can help the family deal with feelings of guilt, frustration, and helplessness, the normal grief reactions surrounding such an event. From the first days, the coordinator remains the central figure in the clinic to parents and children. She becomes the guide to the medical and paramedical personnel, to the institutional bureaucracy, and to the financial agencies which assist in the child's care. In addition to this major role in making a long rocky road smoother, the coordinator has many other roles in the running of the clinic.

THE COORDINATOR AS AN ADMINISTRATOR

The clinic represents a multidisciplinary approach to the care of the whole child. This means that at a given clinic visit, each child is seen by full-time staff physicians from a number of specialties, each followed by his retinue of residents and students. One of the coordinator's jobs is to help bring order to this confusion. The scheduling of patients and collection of medical records and x-rays constitute one step in making the clinic work. Talking with patients and parents to uncover their problems and concerns, both medical and nonmedical, is essential. Parents are often afraid to ask questions of the physician, but will voice them to the coordinator. Every clinic session is followed by a conference in which each patient is discussed by the specialists (Fig. 14-1). It is here that an attempt is made to coordinate and integrate the child's care. It is here that the coordinator can most effectively act as the patient's advocate, making the physicians aware of particular family problems.

The coordinator then schedules admissions, laboratory tests, and x-rays, attempting to integrate them with clinic visits to save time and effort for the parents.

THE COORDINATOR AS A COUNSELOR

In addition to the initial feelings of guilt and grief, families of children with meningomyeloceles face continuous emotional problems as the child grows. They are isolated from friends, have difficulty finding sitters, are subjected to the child's repeated hospitalizations and surgery, and thus are often separated from the child. They overprotect the child, and continue to foster dependency when the child should be becoming independent. They are naturally ambivalent to the physicians and the clinic, and to the child as well. While an experienced psychiatrist is a part of the clinic staff, the bulk

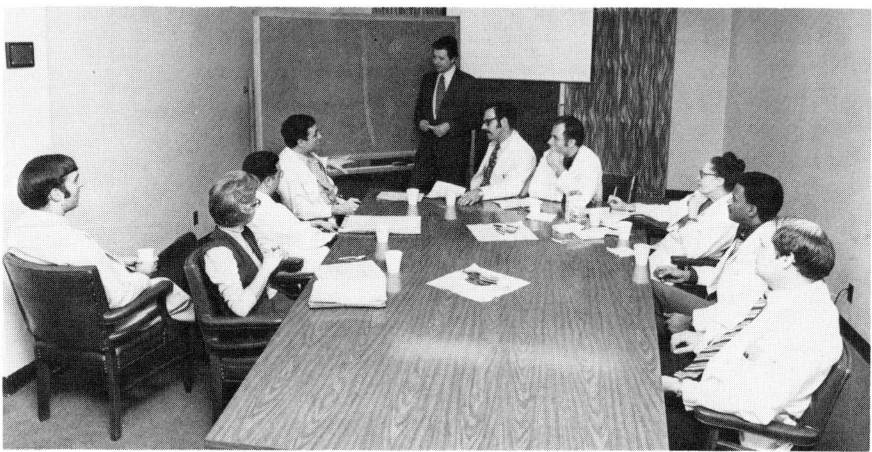

Fig. 14-1 Conference of Birth Defects Treatment Center staff following a clinic. Each patient is reviewed and the subspecialty care provided by the various staff members is integrated into a total program.

of the counseling and guidance falls to the coordinator. She acts as the psychiatrist's aide in helping parents to understand their feelings, and evaluates the parents' emotional resources. The coordinator attempts to strengthen these resources and to evaluate the parents' and child's ability to cope, using the psychiatrist as her consultant.

The value of such a mental health counselor may be seen from the case of one mother. After several years of her daughter's frequent admissions and regular attendance at the clinic, the mother firmly resisted a further necessary procedure on her six-year-old child. During a home visit, the mother sobbed to the coordinator: "She's so little, and she's already had so many operations, there won't be anything left of her. I don't want her hurt anymore." Indeed, the attractive, blue-eyed child had, in her short life, been admitted eight times: for spinal closure, for urinary diversion, for cystectomy, three times for orthopedic surgery, and twice for stomal revision.

The coordinator-counselor's problem was to understand and help the mother in order to help the patient. The young mother was physically and mentally exhausted after six years of anxiety and constant care for the child. She no longer had a husband to share the burden. A "breathing space" was arranged for her by enlisting a relative to take over the care of the patient for a few weeks. At the end of the "vacation," the mother readily agreed to the procedure and thanked us for insisting that her daughter be given another chance to walk. Fortunately, the operation was highly successful.

Today, at 10½ years of age, the daughter manipulates her crutches with skill and ease, does well in school, is a Camp Fire Girl, talks over the phone at every opportunity to her many friends, and plans to be a secretary to a doctor in, she says, "six years and six months."

THE COORDINATOR AS A FINANCIAL ADVISOR

Of the several nonmedical problems confronting the parents of a child with a meningomyelocele, the lack of adequate finances, though not the most heartbreaking one, can be the most persistent and corrosive.

A young couple may be prepared for the ordinary expenses of bringing a healthy baby into the world but quite unprepared for the greatly increased bills an infant with a meningomyelocele will create. Even parents who have insurance often find that the new child is not covered until after several weeks, and major surgery must be done the *first* day of life. Some insurance covers the baby only as long as he or she is in the hospital with the mother; accordingly, if the infant must be taken to another area or hospital immediately after birth, there is no coverage. Other insurance plans do not include care for a child with major birth defects at all. Further, most types of insurance pay only from 60% to 80% of the total hospital charges, and 60% of a $5000 bill leaves $2000 for the young family to assume.

If the original bill were the only one, the majority of families could eventually pay off the uncovered balance in small periodic payments, but the child may have to be readmitted to the hospital within a few weeks or months and will require frequent evaluation.

Medical institutions usually are unaware of the parents' financial plight, and do not try to get help for them. Bills may be allowed to accumulate to a total of $10,000 or $20,000. Finally, the father is presented with a demand for payment. Quite understandably, he is dazed, frustrated, and embittered, because he *can't* pay upon demand, and his child *still* needs treatment.

To avoid these situations, a financial evaluation of the family should be done as soon after the infant arrives in the hospital as possible. The state Crippled Children's Services is notified of the birth, the medical problem, and the family circumstances. Contact is established with public health personnel in the family's home county, who can be of continuous help to the family. Crippled Children's Agencies and other organizations are usually able to provide financial assistance to families not adequately covered by insurance, thus helping them avoid financial catastrophe.

In recent years when, for one reason or another, needy families were not eligible for agency help, funds have been requested and received from American Legion Posts, churches, lodges, appropriate foreign embassies, and the National Foundation–March of Dimes.

THE COORDINATOR AND EDUCATION

Children with meningomyeloceles usually have normal or low-normal intelligence; however, schooling presents particular problems. Psychological testing will document the child's intellectual capacity and may pick up evidence of specific learning disability, which is common in children with hydrocephalus. Parents and sibs, under guidance, can often help tutor the child with problems. However, even those patients with normal IQ's may have difficulties in school because of head size or shape, braces, canes, wheelchairs, and ileostomies. These children will appear different to most of the students in a regular school. Although many go to schools for the physically handicapped, a substantial number do attend regular schools. As the patient approaches school age, the team psychiatrist and the coordinator confer with the child and his parents in order to examine and fortify the patient's ability to cope with the new learning and social situation. The child is helped to realize that since he looks "different," "normal" students will be curious about him and will make comments that may hurt.

Not long ago we talked with a nine-year-old boy who was born with a meningomyelocele and developed hydrocephalus. Originally he adjusted to school very well but recently had become unhappy and reluctant to attend because some new students yelled "Mr. Big Head" every time they saw him. After minimizing the "insult" as much as was advisable, the suggestion was lightly made to him that perhaps the offenders' heads were a bit on the *small* side and maybe an appropriate name could be yelled back. Two weeks later, he asked to return. He came in grinning and immediately dismissed the whole problem by saying, "I called 'em peanut heads." He then went on to talk about whether he should become an accountant or a doctor when he grows up.

THE COORDINATOR AND COMMUNICATION

Patients come to the Birth Defects Center from 19 counties in Maryland and from seven other states. It is, therefore, important that reports of tests and surgery and copies of clinic notes be sent to those involved in the child's care: local pediatricians, family doctors, and public health services. Physical therapy may often be prescribed to be carried out in the home town schools. Referring doctors and schools, in turn, send us progress reports and requests for continuing prescriptions. In short, there is a steady flow of such information to and from the center.

The center also acts as a source for referral for a multitude of problems. Calls often come from the local March of Dimes office or from county chairmen describing a child who needs help. If the child is not an appropriate patient for our center, he is referred to the proper clinic or area. For example, a child with a congenital heart defect or cleft palate would be referred directly to specialty clinics equipped to handle those problems.

Occasionally, parents whose children are being treated by private physicians call us because they are in need of financial support. An effort is always made to evaluate the request and to give suggestions as to possible sources of funds. Follow-up telephone calls are usually made.

Calls come from organizations and schools that want doctors to speak to their members or students about "birth defects." Every effort is made by the clinic staff to assist in community education. Many teenagers call or write asking for brochures and information to use in school work; such requests are promptly honored.

Our youngest correspondent gave us great delight, and it pleases us to share her communication with you in its entirety:

> "Dear Center, I am nine (9) years
> old. Teacher said we have to write
> about anything and I guess it might
> as well be yours. Maybe it will do
> good. Goodbye
> Yours sincerely,
> PATTY"
> "P.S. send me everything"

SUMMARY

A Center Coordinator must be a secretary, administrator, integrator, psychiatrist, social worker, educator, patient advocate, and friend. It is she more than anyone else who translates the multidisciplinary medical effort exerted on behalf of a child into sympathetic care. It is the coordinator who plays a major role in transforming a medical, emotional, and financial catastrophe into a tolerable burden.

15

Perspectives in the Care of Children with Meningomyeloceles

John M. Freeman, M.D.

In the past 10 to 15 years enormous progress has been made in dealing with children born with meningomyeloceles. From neglect, the pendulum has swung to vigorous therapy. Centers for multidisciplinary treatment of these children have dramatically increased the number of survivors and improved the function of many of those survivors. With this dramatic increase in survival, however, has come a dramatic increase in the number of children with severe neurological handicaps, with or without mental retardation, and a dramatic increase in the nonmedical problems is to be anticipated. Most of the children treated have yet to reach the teenage period, a time of increasing need for independence, of need for jobs, and for marriage. It has been said that the infants we treat will grow up to curse us, that the adolescent who is ambulatory only in massive braces and crutches, or is in a wheelchair, with an ileal loop and an ever precarious shunt, when facing the difficulties of marriage and employment will hardly be thankful for the investment of time, effort, and money expended in bringing him or her to that state. Studies of the emotional aspects of such a chronic but nonfatal disease are only beginning to appear. These patients will indeed provide a fertile field for studies by psychiatrists and sociologists in an effort to improve our handling of their problems.

From a medical standpoint, much remains to be done in the care of children with meningomyeloceles. The management of hydrocephalus, while far better than 10 years ago, is still far from adequate. Better techniques must be devised so that the hydrocephalus can be managed with a single operative procedure or with only rare revisions, rather than the frequent revisions and unpredictable course now encountered. Until such a procedure or shunt is available, we must devise better methods of following and diagnosing shunt inadequacy and "occult" or "arrested" hydrocephalus. Such an advance will doubtless improve the mental function of our survivors.

The orthopedic management of these children is undergoing a change, and major changes are to be expected in the future. The cumbersome braces and crutches now utilized in children with high lumbar or thoracic lesions do not provide them with a functional gait. Indeed, many of these children have not been braced at all. Recent thinking indicates that these children should be braced early: from 9 months or a year onward. Bracing will allow the child to stand, improve circulation in the lower extremities, and prevent osteoporosis. Perhaps, even more important, it will allow the child to function in the normal upright position and alter the expectations of those who deal with him. As was indicated in the chapter on orthopedic management, most of these children can maintain some ambulation through childhood and up to the adolescent period. Then, because of the increase in weight and size, it is too difficult to lift the whole body for a swing through gait. However, assists can be developed. Hydraulic crutches which could lift the weight are in a development stage. Wheelchairs which come to a standing position may also assist these children during adolescent. Major efforts towards the development of orthotic devices are being undertaken. Indeed perhaps we can look to the day when the major determining factor for function will be less the degree of paralysis than the degree of mental impairment. A day when a bright motivated child with an L_1 lesion may have useful "ambulation" and be able to function as an independent adult.

Just as management of the bowel has evolved from the colostomy to nonsurgical management, so must management of the urinary dysfunction evolve. It should be possible to devise an electrical mechanism which will allow "voluntary" bladder contraction by stimulation and which will prevent incontinence by "tonic" sphincter contraction. Such repeated emptying should prevent reflux and kidney infection and eliminate the chronic urological problems and ileal loops of children with meningomyeloceles.

Children with meningomyeloceles will still be left with the neurological impairment, which cannot be corrected but only circumvented or prevented. Prenatal diagnosis of various genetic diseases is currently possible. Prenatal diagnosis of many types of structural disease is theoretically possible. Parents who have had a previous child with a meningomyelocele have a sufficiently high risk of recurrence (5 to 10%) to warrant prenatal examination. Amniocentesis with injection of a lipid-soluble radio-opaque dye such as Pantapaque or a water-soluble radio-opaque dye such as Hypaque should allow radiological delineation of meningomyeloceles in most affected fetuses. A mother carrying such an infant could then have her pregnancy terminated, if she so desired. Recent reports indicate that there may be elevated levels of alpha-fetoprotein in the amniotic fluid of women carrying a fetus with a meningomyelocele. Indeed, a small number of fetuses have been aborted on this indication. While amniocentesis would be limited to women having a high risk of an affected fetus, it is possible that this alpha-fetoprotein may be reflected in the maternal serum, thus permitting a suitable screening test to be developed. Thus many families who are fearful of having a second affected child, and who therefore avoid future pregnancies, would be able to have normal children. These techniques *would not* adequately distinguish meningoceles from meningomyeloceles and would bring about abortion of "mild" meningomyeloceles as well as severe ones.

Technological improvements in shunting procedures 15 years ago brought about major changes in the ethics and philosophy of management. From waiting until the child was 1 year to 18 months old, physicians began treating all children. This change in philosophy was the biggest factor in fostering further technological improvements and in improving the prognosis for the infant born with spina bifida.

The further evolution of ethics and the philosophy of management of these children over the next 15 years will be the major determing factors in meningocele management. This evolution may take the form of allowing or encouraging the death of children who do not have promise of becoming functional adults. It may take the form of the active, vigorous management of *all* children with meningomyeloceles, with society providing the necessary physical, emotional, and financial support. It is for physicians and society to decide which course we will take.

Index